SOURCEBOOK
for
MEDICAL
SPEECH PATHOLOGY

Second Edition

Clinical Competence Series

Series Editor
Robert T. Wertz, Ph.D.

SOURCEBOOK
for
MEDICAL
SPEECH PATHOLOGY

Second Edition

Lee Ann C. Golper, Ph.D.

Director, Department of Rehabilitation Therapy
and Communication Services
University of Arkansas for the Medical Sciences
Associate Professor, Audiology and Speech Pathology
Assistant Professor, Otolaryngology/Head and Neck Surgery

SINGULAR PUBLISHING GROUP, INC.
SAN DIEGO · LONDON

Singular Publishing Group, Inc.
401 West A Street, Suite 325
San Diego, California 92101-7904

Singular Publishing Ltd.
19 Compton Terrace
London N1 2UN, U.K.

e-mail: singpub@mail.cerfnet.com
Website: http://www.singpub.com

Typeset in 10½ /12 Times by So Cal Graphics
Printed in the United States of America by McNaughton & Gunn

Library of Congress Cataloging-in-Publication Data

Golper, Lee Ann C., 1948–
    Sourcebook for medical speech pathology / Lee Ann C. Golper. —
2nd ed.
       p.   cm. — (Clinical competence series)
    Includes bibliographical references and index.
    ISBN 1-56593-861-5
    1. Speech therapy. 2. Internal medicine. 3. Medicine—
— Terminology. 4. Speech therapists. I. Title. II. Series.
    [DNLM: 1. Speech-Language Pathology — handbooks. 2. Nomenclature—
handbooks. 3. Clinical Medicine—handbooks.   WL 39 G628s 1997]
RC423.G64 1997
616.85'5 — dc21
DNLM/DLC
for Library of Congress   97-24423
                                                  CIP

CONTENTS

FOREWORD

com•pe•tence (kom'pə təns)   n.   The state or quality
of being properly or well qualified; capable.

Clinicians crave competence. They pursue it through education and experience, through emulation and innovation. Some are more successful than others
in attaining what they seek. Much of being competent is being current. Lee Ann
Golper's *Sourcebook for Medical Speech Pathology* is a second edition. It
moves the Clinical Competence Series into its second generation, makes the
wealth of material in the first edition current, and provides a state-of-the-art
tool for speech-language pathologists who practice in medical settings. Here is
the information clinicians need to know about what their medical and allied
health colleagues do, the language they speak, and the avenues that lead to consultation and collaboration. Dr. Golper knows medical settings. The many hats
she wears—clinician, administrator, teacher, investigator—permit access to the
laboratory bench as well as the bedside, to medical cost recovery as well as
medical care. Her travels save us steps. Her careful presentation of facts and
figures save us time. If we are new to Speech-Language Pathology in a medical setting, Dr. Golper orients us to our environment. If we have accrued some
mileage in a medical setting, Dr. Golper provides us with what we always
wanted to know. Her book, I suspect, will become well-thumbed as a constant
reference. My first edition did. Most of all, a competent clinician has provided
the information that makes her that way. Our attention to what she provides
indicates our competence and our efforts to improve it, because competent clinicians seek competence as much for what it demands as for what it promises.

Robert T. Wertz, Ph.D.
Series Editor

PREFACE

The practice of Medical Speech Pathology includes evaluation and treatment of conditions that directly affect health and safety as well as communication. There has been a gradual acceptance of the speech-language pathologist's role in the assessment and treatment of patients with *dysphagia*, including infants, children, and adults, and a greater and earlier involvement with the cognitively impaired patient with *post traumatic head injury*. As technologies for the nonvocal patient have offered more options for improved communication, speech-language pathologists have had greater contact with the *nonvocal, tracheostomized*, and the *ventilator dependent patient*.

Occurring concurrently with the growth and development of speech-language pathology practices in hospitals, have been administrative efforts to trim the costs of health care by requiring shorter hospital stays in acute care facilities. Thus, hospitalized patients referred to speech-language pathologists are increasingly likely to be acutely, or seriously, ill.

Clinicians working outside of hospitals in rehabilitation, home health, and nursing home settings are also seeing patients much earlier after the onset of acute illness than they were previously. In both inpatient and outpatient settings, clinicians no longer have the luxury of saying, "Please re-consult when this patient is medically stable."

Clinicians who work in medical settings should have a basic understanding of the conditions that bring patients into the hospital and what is being done, medically or surgically, to manage them. Patients are not hospitalized because they have a communication problem; thus, we need to understand the relationship between illness and communication. We should be able to read medical terminology and interpret vital sign data to the extent that we gain a general understanding of the patient's status. Even if we are not entirely comfortable using words like "indurated" instead of "hard" or "erythematous" for "red" we still need to communicate, in notes, reports, and conferences, in a manner that conforms with the expectations of a medical facility. We should to be able to read and understand articles in medical journals written on topics related to speech, language, or swallowing. Unfortunately, exposure to the principles, procedures, practices, and vocabulary one encounters as a member of a health care team usually comes late in our clinical training. Speech-language pathologists learn how to work in a medical setting when they take their first job in a medical setting. This "on-the-job training" is also typical for other hospital staff such as psychologists, dietitians, physical therapists, occupational therapists, social workers, and even pharmacists who usually receive much of their professional preparation in a classroom.

In my own practice as a clinician and supervisor, I have observed and experienced the difficulties encountered when we attempt to translate what we are taught in academic training into the vernacular of a medical setting. I have puzzled over medical chart notes trying to decipher their abbreviations and terminology, and I have sat through conferences wondering, "What does that word mean?", "What does that finding reveal?" I once spent a considerable amount of time trying to define the diagnosis "G.O.K.," only to find out it stood for "God only knows."

I have read, and undoubtedly written, reports containing incorrect uses of medical terminology. I have written background summaries containing abstracted medical histories that listed two names for the same disease. But, worst of all, I have made recommendations regarding communication or swallowing management that were contraindicated by the patient's medical status. Through a great deal of trial and an embarrassing amount of error, I am gradually learning to communicate—to interpret and present information—in a credible manner in the hospital where I work. In addition, I have come to understand that if I choose to work in a hospital, I, like any other member of the medical staff, have to be prepared to play a role in health maintenance.

In my attempt to become more comfortable with a medically oriented practice, I have acquired a library of resource materials, including textbooks, manuals, dictionaries, hospital memos, charts and illustrations, conference handouts, and so on, which were consulted in the preparation of this *Sourcebook*. As a gauge for deciding what to include, I have drawn on comments and observations of my co-workers and from student clinicians, and included information that reflects their needs, problems, and confusions.

This text is intended to be a general resource book *about medical practices*. It is not about *how to practice* Medical Speech Pathology. Other texts in the Clinical Competence Series focus on particular clinical problems and populations. The information included here and the terminology reviewed cover topics and facts about illness and medical care that seem important to have readily available for clinicians who practice in a medically allied setting. Some of the information in this text is intended for reference only, some could be viewed as "nice to know," and some applies directly to Speech-Language Pathology. The definitions included come from an amalgam of resources available to me, including comments from individuals who were kind enough to review the manuscript. Additional or different abbreviations, definitions, or interpretations from those provided here can be found; and important terms, topics, or items probably have been inadvertently omitted or have received only a brief mention. Medical sciences are constantly changing, and new tests, technologies, and therapies introduce new vocabularies. Some items may not be found in this *Sourcebook* simply because I have not yet encountered them in the settings where I have worked.

This second edition has undergone revisions, elaborations, and clarifications of the text and terminology. Attempts were made to update and expand material, and new sections were added throughout the text. Now that clinicians increasingly are working in Neonatal Intensive Care Units, additional information about neonates is included.

Due to the broad scope of this text, definitions and descriptions are, by necessity, terse and superficial and may be vague and incomplete in places. Additional reference texts may need to be consulted for elaboration and clarification. The user is encouraged to augment this text with personal notes on the pages provided at the end of each chapter. Each chapter and appendix has been reviewed by at least one reader with expertise in that subject area, as well as the Series Editor and publication editors, and content questions were checked against multiple reference texts.

The information contained in this text is organized in the manner in which conditions are typically discussed by physicians. Concepts and terminology are introduced within the context of various medical conditions, rather than related to disciplines of medical practice. For example, we did not chose to address "geriatrics" or "pediatrics" specifically but discussed medical conditions throughout the life span, and the practices one encounters in a medical setting treating those conditions. To use this text as a reference, it is best to familiarize yourself with the chapters, both the content and the organization. All of the material is concise, and cross references are provided. Related terminology, abbreviations, tables, figures and explanations are organized to aid in understanding basic concepts. This second edition of the *Sourcebook for Medical Speech Pathology*, like the first edition, is intended for use by clinicians practicing in medical care facilities, rehabilitation programs, private practice, and home health agencies. It is aimed at clinicians who are new to practices in a medical setting, especially practicum students and Clinical Fellows.

ACKNOWLEDGMENTS

This text contains some previously published material and data used with permission from reference texts and journals. These sources are cited and are reproduced with gratitude. The reference texts that were used in preparing this *Sourcebook* are listed following each chapter and the general text and appendix references are listed at the end of the book.

This second edition has built upon the material contained in the first with new sections where needed and deletions, corrections, updates, expansions, and clarifications of the original text. I remain indebted to those people who helped with the expert reviews of the first edition of this *Sourcebook*: Marvin N. Golper, M.D.; Lillian O. Seligman, M.S., CCC-SLP; Suzanne Boone, R.D.; Nancy Owen, R.D.; Bernie McIntyre, R.D.; Lisa Green, R.D.; Janice Sargent, R.N., N.P.; Pamela Hagen, R.N.; Ann Teaford, O.T.R.; Jane Salat, P.T.; Kara Carr, M.D.; Todd Kirchoff, M.D.; and Dennis Briley, M.D. My husband, Thomas A. Golper, M.D. has been a patient teacher, kind critic, and partner in helping me with both editions of this book. I continue to have the highest regard for all of the great folks at Singular Publishing Group, Inc. Lastly, I want to express my gratitude to Robert T. Wertz, Ph.D., the series editor. Terry has sent me several wonderful career opportunities, including this text, and has truly been a mentor for me and for many others.

CHAPTER

1

Medical Speech Pathology

In medical settings, speech-language pathologists do essentially what they do in other professional work settings. They provide diagnostic consultation and rehabilitative treatment for communication, cognition, and specific motor and structural disorders affecting speech, language, and swallowing. Unlike practice in an outpatient clinic or school setting, however, medical speech-language pathologists work in an environment where *health* is the primary issue. For the most part, their clientele are patients who are acutely, critically, or chronically *ill*.

I. SPEECH-LANGUAGE PATHOLOGY PRACTICE IN MEDICAL SETTINGS

A. Concurrence, Cooperation, and Coordination

In most medical settings, speech-language pathologists see patients only by *referral*. They must work with the **concurrence**, and in most cases, upon the "order" of physicians, even though the physician may know less about speech-language pathology than the speech-language pathologist knows about medicine. Most of the diagnostic and treatment services provided by speech-language pathologists in medical settings, including home health services, require the written or

1

verbal approval of the patient's physician. For some procedures this approval is legally as well as ethically necessary; for other procedures, such as bedside screening of speech, it is a routine courtesy to inform the physician or the primary nurse of any activities involving patients under their care. Oftentimes payment for SLP services requires a "doctor's order." Nurses and physicians are the professionals with the greatest and most direct responsibility for a patient's health and, correspondingly, have the greatest authority in a health care setting.

In hospitals, physicians have the ultimate say about what transpires with their patients and carry the ultimate burden for any problems that may arise. Usually the patient's physician sees communication processes and swallowing abilities as important aspects of the health and well-being of the patient. For example, in cases where patients have had laryngectomies, a successful functional outcome depends on both successful surgical treatment *and* successful speech rehabilitation treatment.

Along with the need to have the physician's concurrence, medical speech-language pathologists often need to gain the cooperation of other health care professionals. The **cooperation** of nursing staff may be necessary to carry out recommendations regarding the best way to communicate with or feed a patient. The cooperation of the Dietetics Service may be necessary to have food trays prepared and presented in the manner the patient can manage best. The cooperation of Social Work Service may be necessary to ensure that the patient has access to continued speech-language rehabilitation after he or she leaves the hospital.

Finally, medical speech-language pathologists spend a considerable amount of time **coordinating** their activities with others. Scheduling assessments and speech-language therapies when the patient is least fatigued requires coordination and cooperation with the rehabilitation therapy services. Treatment with the ventilator dependent patient requires coordinating visits with the respiratory therapist. Diagnostic evaluations of dysphagic persons requires, at a minimum, coordinating the efforts of radiology staff, dietitians, nurses, and speech-language pathology staff.

B. Scope of Practice and Responsibilities

The following outline lists the problems typically referred to the speech-language pathologist and some additional responsibilities and concerns for clinicians working in medical facilities.

1. **Mental status assessment.** Bedside screening and formal assessments of *attention, memory, and orientation* are frequently required to determine the patient's mental status as it relates to communicative abilities and readiness for standardized testing, rehabilitation efforts, self-feeding, and independent living.

2. **Dysphagia evaluation and treatment.** Evaluation of dysphagia can include a clinical, or "bedside screening," *assessment of oral motor functions and swallowing status* to gain an appreciation of the patient's nutritional status and any medical concerns related to nutrition and hydration, and conducting or participating in studies of swallowing abilities. *Treatment of dysphagia* requires the ability to recognize indicators for a good or poor potential to regain functional swallowing and to understand the appropriate measures to improve swallowing or reduce the risks of aspiration. Treatment can include recommending dietary adjustments, special facilitative feeding procedures, or the use of adaptive equipment and positioning adjustments during meals. Treatment may also include training in safety procedures; behavioral therapies; oral, pharyngeal, laryngeal neuromotor stimulation therapies; and consideration of alternative, nonoral methods of nutrition and hydration support. Increasingly, medical speech-language pathologists are participating in *oral motor stimulation and feeding in Neonatal Intensive Care Units.*

3. **Neurogenic language disorders.** Diagnostic assessment of neurogenic language disorders involves both bedside screenings and *comprehensive standardized testing.* Neurogenic language disorders include aphasia, confusion, dementia, and the verbal characteristics associated with right hemisphere brain damage and traumatic brain injury. *Determining candidacy for treatment, selecting appropriate treatment avenues, implementing treatment services for neurogenic language disorders*, and *counseling* family members about communication disorders are clinical activities within the *practice domain* of a speech-language pathologist.

4. **Neurogenic speech disorders.** Like neurogenic language disorders, neurogenic speech disorders receive diagnostic evaluation and treatment by the speech-language pathology staff. The diagnostic assessment frequently requires the use of *special instruments to measure physiologic and acoustic parameters* of speech production. Treatment often requires selecting and training the patient to use an augmentative communication system or device.

5. **Assessment and treatment of cognitive status.** In acute care settings, the speech-language pathologist's evaluation of cognitive status may be a routine part of the "pathways" of care. Speech-language pathologists are usually involved in the standard assessments made with particular populations, such as strokes and head injuries, or SLP services may be ordered when there has been an acute change in cognitive status. Treatment of cognitive disorders is a part of the scope of care provided by the speech-language pathologist. Services range from direct cognitive rehabilitation and reorganization to family and staff education for the cognitively impaired person.

6. **Organic and functional voice and resonance disorders.** Speech-language pathologists in medical settings work in close affiliation with otolaryngologists when conducting diagnostic evaluations and determining a treatment approach for *organic and functional voice and resonance disorders*. Diagnostic evaluations require familiarity with physiologic and acoustic measurement devices and can require the use of videofiberoptic nasendoscopy and videolaryngostroboscopy. Speech-language pathologists have an understanding of vocal fold physiology and organic vocal fold pathologies and functional or psychiatric conditions associated with inappropriate use of the laryngeal and velopharyngeal mechanisms. Treatment requires familiarity with various forms of palatal surgery, phonosurgery, and vocal fold physiology, as well as skills in achieving behavioral changes in phonation and nasality.

7. **Oral, velopharyngeal, and laryngeal surgery.** Any patient about to undergo a surgery that will affect one or more of the structures for speech should be referred to speech-language pathology staff for *presurgical counseling and postsurgical speech rehabilitation*. Individuals who require laryngectomies are especially in need of pre- and postsurgical attention from the speech-language pathologist. Postlaryngectomy treatment includes determining the most efficacious method for alaryngeal communication (electrolarynx, esophageal speech, tracheoesophageal puncture [TEP] voice prosthesis) and helping the patient achieve a functional level of intelligibility with these modes. Treatment also includes instruction in safety concerns and life style changes as a "neck breather" following laryngectomy. Speech-language pathologists assist the patient with purchasing adaptive equipment (e.g., "shower shields" for showering) and encourage participation in community support groups. In cases where the patient with a laryngectomy is a candidate for a TEP voice prosthesis, speech-language pathologists conduct "air insufflation tests" to

determine esophageal adequacy for the prosthesis; fit the patient with the appropriate type of TEP voice prosthesis; train the patient to insert, clean, and care for the prosthesis; and train the patient to maximize TEP speech skills.

8. **Nonvocal, tracheostomized, and ventilator dependent patients.** It is increasingly common for speech-language pathologists to be consulted with patients, both children and adults, who are *unable to phonate due to severe motor deficits* resulting from a neuromotor disease, or injury, or the presence of an *endotracheal tube*. The ward or the Intensive Care Unit staff are usually anxious to assist the patient to communicate optimally, because improved communication allows the staff to provide better care for the patient. Medical speech-language pathologists must be familiar with how the respiratory status is managed with the tracheostomized and ventilator dependent patient. They can examine the patient's mental status and motor abilities as they relate to alternative communication modes. In concert with the respiratory therapist, primary nurse, or physician, they can determine the patient's potential for using a *"speaking trach"* or a mode of *augmentative communication*.

9. **Functional improvements with pharmacologic, surgical, or rehabilitation therapies.** In some medical settings, the speech-language pathologist is asked to make baseline and follow-up assessments of speech, language, or swallowing to evaluate the *efficacy of drug therapies, surgeries*, or other *rehabilitation therapies*. This request is frequent in settings where experimental therapies are being tested, such as in university-affiliated teaching hospitals. (See Chapter 2 for a discussion of teaching hospitals.)

10. **Interdisciplinary team conferences.** The speech-language pathologist is often a key member of various interdisciplinary teams in a medical setting. These teams can include Rehabilitation Medicine and Intermediate Care teams; Extended Care (nursing home) Rehabilitation teams; Dysphagia Evaluation and Management teams; the Geriatric Evaluation team; and special treatment protocol teams, such as the Tumor Board or Otolaryngology/Head and Neck Surgery Indications team.

11. **Staff education.** The medical setting provides frequent opportunities for teaching. Speech-language pathology staff are often asked to provide in-services on selected topics such as communication with the severely aphasic person, the use of nonvocal

communication devices, understanding the communication problems of the patient with dementia, considerations for managing the patient at-risk for aspiration, methods for nonvocal communication with the tracheostomized patient, methods of alaryngeal speech following laryngectomy, and ways to reduce communication barriers in long-term care facilities.

12. **Research.** Facilities and programs vary with regard to the time allowed for "nonbillable" clinical activities; thus, the clinician's ability to conduct research (or even to be a consumer of published and presented research) is often limited to off-duty hours. In the United States, speech-language pathologists working in private settings, university-affiliated teaching hospitals, and, most notably, in Veterans Affairs Medical Centers have made substantial contributions to the research literature in Medical Speech Pathology. Indeed, the majority of tests, assessment procedures, diagnostic instruments, therapy materials, and many of the assistive devices used in medical settings were conceived, designed, and tested by speech-language practitioners.

13. **Continuing education.** In most states, speech-language pathologists working in medical settings are required to have licensure, and the majority of licensure laws mandate continuing education for licensure renewals.

14. **Securing reimbursements.** Medicare, Medicaid, and insurance reimbursements require written evidence (documentation) of appropriate and efficacious treatment. To secure reimbursement for services, speech-language pathologists must provide adequate descriptions of their findings, plans and progress reports, and recertification forms. Clinicians must know how to make appropriate use of the terminology and protocols required for medical reimbursement forms.

15. **Risk management.** "Risk management" is increasingly demanded in hospital care. The concept of risk management includes a systematic approach to identifying and reducing the occurrence of factors that put the patient or the provider at some risk. Reducing risk factors should, ultimately, reduce the costs and improve the quality of care.

16. **External and internal reviews.** Like any other member of the staff in a medical facility or program, speech-language pathologists participate in *internal* reviews (within the facility or pro-

gram) and *external* reviews (by an accrediting agency or commission) of their clinical records and activities.

17. **Cost-containment.** Clinicians contribute data to the facility's cost-containment studies, or "utilization reviews," to participate in determining the most cost-effective way to provide services without diminishing the quality of patient care.

18. **Quality performance and improvement.** Like other staff members, speech-language pathologists are expected to maintain ongoing program evaluation monitors to identify problems in patient care, to evaluate outcomes, and to take effective, remediative actions.

19. **Professional involvement.** Involvement in professional affairs is a special concern for speech-language pathologists in medical settings. Policies affecting funds for reimbursements and payment for services have a major influence on the "what, when, who, where, how, and how much" of clinical services in medical settings. Participation in professional affairs helps to ensure that patients who might benefit from speech-language pathology services will have access to them. Participation in intra- and interdisciplinary professional organizations helps to guide policies affecting the education, research, and practice needs of clinicians.

I. HEALTH CARE PERSONNEL

A. Professional, Technical, and Clerical Staff

There are well over 200 different disciplines or work titles related to health care professions. The following list introduces the clinician to medical personnel and their specialties and some of the clinical support staff. This list applies to medical personnel typically affiliated with hospitals, training programs, rehabilitation programs, home health, and long-term care facilities in the United States. In the U.S., career preparation, certification requirements, licensures, and registration are administered in a variety of ways across the different professional disciplines. Nearly all health care careers, however, are subject to the training and practice guidelines established by the *state regulatory (licensure) bodies* of the state in which they practice. In addition, some health care professions in the U.S. have independent, national certifying bodies. Occupational therapists (OTRs), for example, are "registered" by a national examining body but may also be required to have state licensure in the state where they practice. National certification currently may be required for physical therapists (PTs), but they must take state qualifying examinations and meet state licensure standards. Physicians are usually, but not always, board certified in their specialty of practice. In some states, nurses' aides are not required to have had a formal training program and may have been trained in the institution in which they work; other states require training (anywhere from 5 weeks to 6 months) in an accredited program. Some professionals, for example, physician assistants-certified (PA-Cs) or Advanced Practice Nurses (APNs) are recognized and licensed (or certified) in some states but not in others.

In addition to national and state credentialing, the health care facility itself will have policies regulating the **clinical privileges** that are extended to each member of its professional staff (see Section V, this chapter). Physicians must receive approval by the hospital's medical director or Chief of Staff to have the *privilege* of admitting patients to and making use of the services in that facility. Health care facilities are required by their credentialing bodies to list the privileges afforded to various members of the professional staff including physicians and nonphysicians.

The following list is intended to provide a review of the personnel and consultants encountered in medical settings. It is not a comprehensive list of all health care careers, and the possible list of nursing subspecialties is only partially elaborated.

B. Health Care Personnel

Anesthesiologist. A physician who specializes in the use of anesthetics and anesthesia.

Attending. The staff physician working in a teaching hospital who is a member of the faculty at a medical-surgical training program and who is designated to be legally responsible for the care of all patients on his or her *"service."* (See Bed Service page 23.)

Audiologist. An individual with a minimum of a master's degree, or equivalent, in Audiology who provides diagnostic and treatment services related to audition, including prescribing, or specifying and distributing amplification requirements and other auditory corrective therapies and devices.

Biomedical Engineer, Biomedical Equipment Technician (BET). An individual who provides technical assistance with the selection, ordering, use, and repair of the adaptive devices, equipment, and instruments found in medical facilities.

Cardiologist. A physician who specializes in diagnosis and treatment of cardiac and circulatory diseases.

Cardiovascular Disease Specialist. A physician who specializes in the diagnosis and nonsurgical management of diseases of the heart and blood vessels.

Cardiovascular Surgeon. A physician who specializes in the surgical treatment of cardiac and circulatory diseases.

Case manager. Individual who coordinates and oversees the continuity of care for a patient, or the person assigned to provide agency oversight in the insurance agency or Workman's Compensation insurer.

Certified Occupational Therapy Aide (C.O.T.A.). An individual who has technical training in Occupational Therapy and who works under the supervision of a Registered and Licensed Occupational Therapist (OTR-L).

Certified Medical Aide. An individual who has completed an accredited training program in basic nursing skills who works under the supervision of a Licensed Practical Nurse or Registered Nurse.

Certified Registered Nurse Anesthetist. A Registered Nurse who has completed advanced training and is certified to assist with anesthesia under the supervision of an anesthesiologist.

Chaplain. A member of the clergy, from any religious denomination or community, who performs religious rites and services and provides spiritual counseling for patients, their families, and friends, or the facility's personnel.

Chief Resident. A resident who is in his or her final year of residency, or has taken an additional year of residency, and was chosen or elected to administer certain aspects of the medical or surgical training program and to participate in teaching more junior residents and students.

Circulating Nurse. Operating room nurse who assists with tasks outside of the sterile field that are necessary during a surgery (obtaining additional instruments and supplies, transferring specimens, clearing contaminated materials, etc.).

Clinical Nurse Specialist. A Registered Nurse with advanced training in a specialty of medical care (e.g., Clinical Nurse Specialist in Oncology).

Clinical Pathologist, Pathologist. A physician who specializes in Pathology (the study of the essential nature of disease especially of the structural and functional changes in tissues and organs that cause disease) with a subspecialty in the use of laboratory methods in clinical diagnosis.

Colon-Rectal Surgeon. A physician who specializes in surgeries of the colon and rectum, the lower portions of the large intestine.

Community Care Coordinator, Discharge Coordinator. An individual, usually a nurse or social worker, who serves as a liaison between the staff in a hospital or rehabilitation program and community health care programs.

Critical Care Registered Nurse (CCRN). A Registered Nurse with training and experience in the nursing management of critically ill patients in Intensive Care Units.

Critical Care Specialist, Intensivist. A physician, normally an Internist, who may have subspecialty training in Pulmonary, Cardiac, or Renal Disease with additional advanced training in Critical Care Management, specializing in the care of patients in Intensive Care Units.

Deglutition Therapist. An individual, usually a nurse, who specializes in the management of disorders of deglutition, including dysphagia and nutritional problems.

Dental Hygienist. An individual with a professional degree in Dental Hygiene who specializes in the prevention of dental and periodontal diseases.

Dentist. An individual with a professional (doctoral) degree in Dental Surgery (DDS) or Medicine (DMD) who diagnoses and treats disorders and diseases of dentition, the oral cavity, and the oral structures.

Dermatologist. A physician who specializes in the diagnosis and treatment of diseases of the skin.

Diagnostic Radiologist. A physician who specializes in diagnostic imaging (e.g., x-ray) procedures.

Diener. Laboratory worker who assists the pathologist with laboratory tasks, such as autopsies.

Dietitian, Dietician, Nutritionist. An individual with professional training in nutrition as it relates to health and disease who manages and implements the food services and dietary therapies in health care facilities.

Diet Technician. An individual with technical skills in dietary management who works under the supervision of a dietitian.

Dosimetrist. An individual with technical training in dosages for radiation oncology therapies.

Dysphagia Therapist. An individual, usually a speech-language pathologist, occupational therapist, or nurse who specializes in the diagnosis and management of swallowing disorders.

Electrocardiography Technician (EKG Tech). An individual with the technical skills necessary to make recordings of the electrical activity of the heart through the use of electrocardiography (EKG, ECG).

Electroencephalography Technician (EEG Tech). An individual with the technical skills necessary to make recording of the electrical activity of the brain

Electromyography Technician (EMG Tech). An individual with the technical skills necessary to make recordings of the electrical activity within muscles through the use of electromyography (EMG).

Emergency Medical Technologist (EMT). An individual who has completed a course of training in emergency medical procedures and, in most cases, has passed a state certifying examination.

Emergency Medicine, Trauma Physician, E.R. Doctor. A physician who specializes in emergency medicine and acute management of traumatic injuries.

Endocrinologist, Metabolism Specialist, Diabetologist. A physician who specializes in the diagnosis and treatment of diseases of metabolism or the endocrine system and who may subspecialize in the management of specific endocrine diseases or disorders, such as diabetes, growth disorders, and endocrine-related osteopathies.

Environmental Safety Engineer. An individual who ensures that health care facilities maintain a healthy, safe environment and comply with the standards of the regulatory bodies.

Epidemiologist. An individual who specializes in the study of the relationship between various environmental and behavioral factors and the frequency and distribution of infection or disease in a given population or community. Epidemiologists are often a part of the faculty at Health Science Universities.

Exercise Physiologist. An individual, usually with at least an undergraduate degree in physiology, who has expertise in the use of exercise to promote health and fitness.

Extern. A fourth-year medical student working outside of his or her normal clinical training rotations, usually in private hospitals, as a physician's assistant.

Family Practitioner, General Practitioner (GP). A physician who provides general medical care and some minor surgical treatment for patients from birth through adulthood.

Fellow. A physician who has completed his or her residency program training and is selected for 2 to 3 years of additional training and research in a medical or surgical specialty or subspecialty. Non-physician fellows will also be found in medical training facilities (e.g., Psychology Post-Doctoral, Clinical Fellows in Speech-Language Pathology or Audiology).

Forensic Pathologist. A physician who specializes in pathology with emphasis on medical-legal issues and the adjudication of death due to criminal and other unnatural causes.

Gastroenterologist (G.I.), Hepatologist. A physician who specializes in the diagnosis and treatment of diseases of the gastrointestinal tract and its organs, especially the liver.

General Surgeon. A surgeon who specializes in those surgeries not requiring subspecialty technical training.

Geneticist. An individual who specializes in the study of genetics and genetic diseases.

Geriatrician. A physician who specializes in internal medicine with the aged. A **Gerontologist** specializes in the social, psychological, and physical (including medical) conditions associated with aging.

Gynecologist/Obstetrician. A physician who specializes in urito-genital diseases of women and the science of contraception, conception, fetal and maternal care, and birth.

Hand Surgeon. A physician who specializes in the plastic, neurologic, orthopedic, and vascular surgeries of the hand.

Hand Therapist. An Occupational Therapist or Physical Therapist who specializes in rehabilitation of structures of the hand, arm, and shoulder.

Head and Neck Surgeon. A physician who specializes in surgeries to the oral, nasal, pharyngeal, laryngeal, and esophageal structures.

Hematologist. A physician who specializes in diseases of the blood and blood-forming processes.

Home Health Nurse. A Registered Nurse or Licensed Practical Nurse who practices nursing in the patient's home.

House Staff, House Officers. The residents and interns in a teaching hospital.

Immunologist. A physician who specializes in the diagnosis and treatment of diseases of the immune system.

Infectious Control Nurse. A Registered Nurse with special training in infectious disease and hospital infection prevention and control who assists the Infectious Disease Officer (an infectious disease physician) in preventing and controlling the occurrence of infections and the spread of contagious diseases within the medical facility

Infection Disease Specialist (I.D. Doctor). A physician who specializes in the diagnosis and treatment of infectious and communicable diseases.

Intern. A physician who is in his or her first year of training after graduation from medical school; in most training programs the intern is called a First Year Resident.

Internist. A physician who specializes in the diagnosis and treatment of diseases of the organs of the body.

Kinesiotherapist (K.T.). An individual who specializes in treatment of disease by movement or exercise.

Licensed Practical Nurse (LPN), Licensed Vocational Nurse (LVN). An individual who has, typically completed at least a one year course in nursing techniques and skills and works under the supervision of a Registered Nurse.

Locum Tenens. A physician who temporarily takes the place or takes over the practice of another physician.

Maternal and Fetal Medicine Specialist. A physician who specializes in gestational care of the mother and fetus and at-risk pregnancies and deliveries.

Medical Librarian. An individual, usually with a degree in Library Science, who has had advanced training in the use and access to medical education and library research resources.

Medical Media Technician. An individual with skills in preparation of graphic and audiovisual materials for medical displays, presentations, and publications.

Medical Records Clerk, Medical Records Librarian. An individual who manages the facility's medical records, including controlling access to records and ensuring the records contain the appropriate documents and signatures.

Medical Student. An individual who is in postgraduate (postbaccalaureate) academic and clinical training in preparation for the practice of medicine or surgery. During their clinical rotations (sometimes called "clerkships") medical students may be referred to as "subinterns," indicating that they work under the supervision of house staff.

Medical Technician. An individual who has completed a training program in laboratory techniques and performs laboratory procedures and studies under the supervision of a medical technologist

Medical Technologist. An individual who has completed a professional training program and certification in laboratory sciences and interpretation of laboratory studies.

Medical Supply Clerk. An individual responsible for ordering, maintaining appropriate inventory, and/or distributing medical-surgical supplies.

Microbiologist. An individual, usually with a doctoral degree (Ph.D.) in Microbiology or Bacteriology, who specializes in laboratory studies dealing with microorganisms.

Neonatologist. A physician, usually with specialty training in Pediatrics and Neonatology, who specializes in critical care management of newborns and infants.

Nephrologist, Renal Physician. A physician who specializes in the diagnosis and treatment of kidney diseases and related conditions.

Neurologist. A physician who specializes in the diagnosis and treatment of diseases of the nervous system.

Neuroradiologist. A radiologist who specializes in neurologic imaging procedures and their interpretation.

Neurosurgeon. A physician who specializes in surgeries involving the structures of the nervous system. Subspecialties may include Back (or Spine) Surgeons, Skull Base Surgeons, Neck Surgeons, and Neuro-oncologic Surgeons.

Nuclear Medicine Specialist. A physician who specializes in the therapeutic uses and interpretation of radioisotope studies.

Nurse Practitioner (N.P.). A Registered Nurse with a bachelor's or master's degree in a specialty of nursing whose practice is limited to that specialty (e.g., Pediatric Nurse Practitioner). Nurse practitioners are permitted (credentialed) to write some orders and, in consultation with the patient's physician, can perform certain duties or procedures normally conducted by a physician. (See Clinical Nurse Specialist, page 10.)

Nurses' Aide (N.A.). An individual with training in basic nursing skills who assists and works under the supervision of LPNs and RNs.

Occupational Therapist (Registered-Licensed) (O.T.R./L). An individual with a minimum of a bachelor's degree in Occupational Therapy who specializes in the functional or adaptive restoration of physical disabilities and rehabilitation for visuoperceptual, perceptuomotor, and cognitive disorders.

Officer of the Day (O.D.). The most senior house officer (resident).

Oncologist. A physician who specializes in the diagnosis and treatment of tumors and systemic malignancies.

Operating Room Technician (O.R. Tech). An individual who has completed a training program in operating room skills and who assists during surgeries.

Ophthalmologist. A physician who specializes in the diagnosis and treatment, including surgeries, of diseases of the eye.

Oral Surgeon. An individual who has a professional (doctoral) degree in Dental Surgery and specializes in surgery limited to the oral cavity and its structures.

Orderly. An individual who performs duties assigned by physicians, nurses, and other hospital staff.

Orthopedist, Orthopaedist (Orthopod). A physician who specializes in surgeries to the bony and connective structures of the body.

Osteopathic Physician (O.D.). A physician who has received his or her medical school training in a professional, degree-granting, medical program and utilizes generally accepted medical, physical, and surgical methods of diagnosis and therapy with emphasis on normal body mechanics and manipulative methods.

Otolaryngologist/Head and Neck Surgeon. A surgeon who specializes in the medical and surgical treatment of ear, nose, and/or throat diseases (sometimes referred to as an Ear, Nose, and Throat doctor, *ENT*, or Eye, Ear, Nose, and Throat doctor, *EENT*.

Pediatric Neurologist. A physician who specializes in the diagnosis and treatment of neurologic disorders and diseases in children.

Pediatrician. A physician who specializes in developmental disorders and medical diseases of children (usually from birth to age 21).

Pharmacist. An individual who has completed a professional training program in the study of pharmacology and who is registered (R. Ph.) and licensed to dispense drugs. In most settings, the Pharmacy Service will be directed by a **Pharmacologist**, who has postgraduate education (usually a doctoral degree) in Pharmacology (Pharm. D., D.Ph.).

Phlebotomist. An individual with skilled training in incision techniques for the treatment of blood and circulatory diseases who provides treatment under the supervision of a physician.

Physiatrist/Physical Medicine and Rehabilitation (P.M. & R.) Specialist. A physician who specializes in rehabilitation medicine.

Physical Therapist (P.T.), Physiotherapist. An individual with a minimum of a bachelor's degree in Physical Therapy who specializes in physical rehabilitation methods to achieve functional and adaptive restoration of movement in individuals physically disabled by disease, injury, or developmental disabilities.

Physical Therapist Assistant (P.T.A.). An individual with technical training in Physical Therapy skills who works under the supervision of a physical therapist.

Physician Assistant (P.A.), Physician Assistant–Certified (P.A.–C.), Advanced Practice Nurse (APN). A Registered Nurse with advanced professional training in clinical procedures who may have privileges to write orders and perform medical procedures normally conducted by physicians.

Plastic and Reconstructive Surgeon. A physician who specializes in cosmetic or reconstructive surgeries.

Podiatrist. An individual with a professional (doctoral) degree (D.P.M.) who specializes in Podiatry, the treatment of disorders of the feet, including orthotic therapies.

Post-Anesthesia Nurse. A Registered Nurse with advanced training in postsurgical recovery nursing management who works in the surgical recovery room.

Primary Care Physician (PCP). The patient's primary physician (G.P., Internist, Pediatrician) who has oversight and "gatekeeping" control over specialty referrals and other orders in managed care.

Proctologist. A physician who specializes in the diagnosis and management of diseases of the rectum.

Prosthetist. An individual with technical training in the fabrication and fitting of artificial limbs and other prosthetic devices (e.g., breast prostheses, artificial limbs, eyes, noses, etc.).

Prosthodontist. A dentist who specializes in the fabrication and fitting of oral prosthetic devices (e.g., obturators and palatal lifts).

Psychiatrist. A physician who specializes in the diagnosis and treatment (medical and behavioral) of cognitive, emotional, and mental disorders.

Psychologist, Child Psychologist, Clinical Psychologist, Medical Psychologist, Neuropsychologist, Geropsychologist. An individual with a master's or doctoral degree (Ph.D.), or equivalent, and professional training in Clinical Psychology and its subspecialties. Psychology includes the practices dealing with the mind and mental operations especially as they relate to behavior. Psychologists specialize in the assessment, diagnosis, and (nonmedical) treatment of cognitive, emotional, and mental disorders.

Psychometrist. An individual with training in test administration.

Psychology Assistant. An individual with technical skills in testing and clinical-clerical procedures used in psychology who assists and works under the supervision of a psychologist.

Public Health Specialist. An individual who has completed a master's or doctoral degree (M.P.H., D.P.H., Sc.D., M.S., Ph.D.) in the study of environmental/public health principles, epidemiology, and the behavioral and biological basis of diseases.

Pulmonary Disease (P.D.) Specialist. A physician who specializes in Pulmonology, the diagnosis and treatment of diseases of the respiratory system.

Radiation Safety Specialist. An individual with training in nuclear science who oversees the hospital's program for radiation protection of employees and patients.

Radiologist. A physician who specializes in methods of body structure imaging and the use of radiotherapies.

Radiology Technologist. An individual who has completed a training program (typically 2 years) in radiology techniques and procedures and who assists the radiologist by preparing the patient, equipment, and instruments and processing the films or tapes from radiology studies.

Registered Nurse (R.N.). An individual who has completed a comprehensive professional training program leading to a degree in Nursing (which may or may not include a bachelor's degree) and who may have a variety of roles in patient care, including administering medication, monitoring vital signs, educating patients and families, and implementing the physician's orders.

Resident. A physician in a 3- to 6-year clinical training in a specialty area (Medicine, Surgery, Pediatrics, Psychiatry, Neurology, Radiology, etc.) who is responsible for providing care for patients in teaching hospitals and their clinics and who practices medicine or performs surgeries under the supervision of, fellows and attending physicians.

Respiratory Therapist (R.T.). An individual with professional training in the ventilator management and respiratory therapies for pulmonary disease.

Rheumatologist. A physician who specializes in the diagnosis and treatment of diseases affecting the joints and connective tissues.

Scrub Nurse. Registered Nurse who assists surgeons in the operating room.

Social Worker. An individual having a degree and licensed in Social Work who assists the patient with financial arrangements, serves as a liaison to other community agencies and services, and provides counseling therapies.

Speech-Language Pathologist (SLP). An individual with a minimum of a master's degree, or equivalent, in Speech-Language Pathology who provides diagnostic and rehabilitation services for communication disorders, cognitive problems, learning problems, and dysphagia.

Stoma Therapist, Enterostomal Therapist. An individual, usually a nurse, with expertise in patient and family training for stoma management.

Surgical Assistant, First Assistant. A physician or an individual trained in particular surgical techniques who assists the primary surgeon during an operation.

Teratologist. An individual who specializes in the relationship between the environment and disorders of embryologic-fetal development.

Therapeutic Radiologist. A radiologist who specializes in the therapeutic uses of x-ray.

Thoracic Surgeon, Cardiothoracic Surgeon, Chest Surgeon. A physician who specializes in heart and lung surgeries.

Transplant Surgeon. A physician who subspecializes in organ transplantation surgery and the medical management of patients with transplanted organs.

Transportation Aide, Escort Aide. An individual who transports patients between various locations within the facility.

Ultrasound Technician. An individual (usually a radiology technician) with training in conducting ultrasound studies for interpretation by the radiologist.

Urologist. A physician who specializes in surgeries of the urinary tract.

Vascular Surgeon. A physician who specializes in surgical repairs and anastomoses of blood vessels.

Volunteers. Individuals who work in various capacities within the facility to assist patients and professional, technical, and clerical staff.

Ward Secretary, Clinic Secretary, Medical Secretary. An individual with training in medical terminology and medical administrative-clerical skills who is typically responsible for relaying doctors' orders, scheduling special procedures and therapies, preparing and maintaining charts and files, filing reports, and answering telephone inquiries.

C. Preparation in Health Care Careers

Most physicians, nurses, dentists, and specialty technologists in health care professions who are trained in the United States receive their training in either "Health Sciences Universities," or university-affiliated Schools of Medicine, Dentistry, or Nursing. These institutions offer professional degrees, such as a Doctor of Medicine (M.D.), Doctor of Dental Surgery/Medicine (D.D.S./ D.M.D), Medical Technologist (Med. Tech.), or Registered Nurse (R.N.) degrees. Other health care personnel, such as physical therapists, occupational therapists, dietitians, audiologists, and speech-language pathologists usually receive their training in colleges or universities having schools or departments with professional programs leading to bachelor's, master's, doctoral, or professional doctorate degrees (e.g., Doctor of Optometry, D.O.; Doctor of Public Health, P.H.D.) in their disciplines. Some health care professionals, such as a microbiologist or a pharmacologist, could receive their career preparation either from a Basic Science Department within a medical school or from the Science Department in a university with no direct health career training affiliations. Hospitals, both private and teaching hospitals (see below), may have in-house training programs for assistants, aides, or technicians such as radiology technicians, operating room technicians nurses, practical nurses, or nurses' aides.

Physicians trained in the United States normally have completed medical school (4 years of postgraduate academic and clinical training in medicine leading to the M.D. degree) and a minimum of 1-year of residency, or internship. The physician planning to enter a nonspecialized, general practice might take a residency in Family Medicine or could enter practice as a General Practitioner (G.P.) after completing a degree in medicine and a year of internship and obtaining state licensure. Internists are physicians who, following medical school, have completed at least a 3-year residency training program in diseases of the internal organs and structures. Physicians who practice any one of the dozen or so subspecialties of Internal Medicine usually have had 3 years of residency and have taken a national board-certifying examination in Internal Medicine before entering a 2- or 3-year Fellowship program in their subspecialty. Surgeon subspecialists are usually required to have taken 1 or more years of General Surgery before they begin their subspecialty training. Some subspecialties require more than one residency; for example, the pediatric urologist usually has studied general surgery, urology, and pediatric urology.

D. Aides, Assistants, and Technicians

Among health care professions, a wide variety of job titles that reflect specialized technical skills are designated as "aides," "assistants," and "'technicians." These are individuals who, usually, have completed a relatively brief training course ranging, for example, from a few weeks for nurses, aides to 2 years for Physical Therapist Assistants. Aides, assistants, and technicians usually work under the supervision of a member of the licensed staff. The "First Assistant" surgeon, however, is typically another surgeon who assists with the surgery.

Aides and assistants help the professional staff with routine tasks. In some professions, there are notable differences between a *technician* and a *technologist*. Technologists, such as medical technologists, usually have had longer specialized training and certification programs and have greater independence and responsibility. Similarly, one sometimes finds aides and assistants designated to have a hierarchical relationship. For example, Physical Therapist Assistants,

(P.T.A.s), and Certified Occupational Therapy Assistants (C.O.T.A.s)
have completed an accredited training program.

E. Administration

Hospitals and most other health care facilities are organized under
administrative structures for **direct patient care services** and **indirect patient services**. The direct patient care services are usually the
medical, surgical, dental, laboratory, pharmacy, rehabilitative, and
nursing services the hospital provides to the patient. The indirect
patient services include the financial operations, physical management of the facility, and the support personnel (clerical, engineering,
housekeeping, security, voluntary, and supply services). Direct
patient care services are usually administered by a physician who is
selected to permanently, or for a designated tenure, serve as the
Medical Director, or **Chief of Staff**. Reporting to the Chief of Staff
are the Department Chiefs. In the Veterans Affairs Medical Centers,
the Service Chiefs, Associate Chief of Staff for Education, and
Associate Chief of Staff for Research and Development report to the
Chief of Staff. Hospital Administration is typically directed by the
Chief Executive Officer (CEO) who oversees the Chief Operating
Officer (COO) and the Chief Financial Officer (CFO).

The extent to which a system of elaborated tiers and subordinations
exists within the facility's administration depends on the nature and
size of the facility and its programs. In most settings, the CEO, or
Hospital Director, is responsible to a Board of Governors or Trustees.
The Board of Governors or Trustees is ultimately responsible for all
aspects of the facility's operations and all fiduciary concerns.

III. HEALTH SERVICES ORGANIZATIONS

In the United States, health services care organizations provide services
directly and indirectly to patents in a number of ways. **Primary care
provider organizations** can include group practices, multispecialty
groups, government health services, or single specialty groups. **Acute
care provider organizations** are typically hospitals and ambulatory
surgery centers. **Rehabilitation care provider organizations** are home
health agencies and rehabilitation centers. **Maintenance care provider
organizations** include nursing homes and hospice programs. **Supplier
organizations** are pharmaceutical companies, biotechnology companies, and multipurpose medical and laboratory supply providers. Other

important organizations involved with the provision of health services include **insurers** (Blue Cross-Blue Shield, Aetna, Prudential, managed care groups, and self-insurance), **professional and trade organizations, educational and research organizations, employers**, and **government payers** (Medicare and Medicaid) and **regulators** (such as state health departments or JCAHO). Increasingly, certain aspects of these health service organizations are linked into a "system" of health care. In such settings, acute care, recuperative care, rehabilitation, and home health programs all a part of one health system, or provider "network." Health services organizations also may be "networked" through the facilities' managed care contracts. Managed care places restrictions on payment for services to encourage keeping patients "within the network" of those providers and facilities attached to the managed care group.

IV. HEALTH CARE SETTINGS

The following is a list of many of the locations and facilities, and relevant abbreviations, where health care services are provided.

A. Locations and Settings

Admitting Office/Area. The area of the facility where payment status and eligibility for services at that facility are determined and the facility's admission forms are completed.

Ambulatory Care/Outpatient Clinic. The area where outpatients are seen.

Bed Service, Service. The hospital beds designated for inpatient admissions to a particular specialty (e.g., Neurology bed service, Cardiology bed service).

Blood Bank. The area in the hospital's laboratory service where blood and blood products are kept and blood typing takes place. Often hospitals share blood and other laboratory facilities or a private facility will serve several hospitals.

Burn Care Unit (B.C.U.). An intensive care unit devoted to patients with burns; these units are found only in specially designated hospitals.

Cardiac Care Unit (C.C.U.). An intensive care unit devoted to patients with acute or critical cardiac disease.

Cardiac Rehabilitation Unit/Center/Program. An inpatient or outpatient rehabilitation program devoted to patients who have undergone heart surgery and/or have chronic cardiac disease.

Comprehensive Outpatient Rehabilitation Facility (CORF). An outpatient facility providing, at a minimum, physician services, physical therapy, and social or psychological services. Typically, CORFs also have speech-language pathology services and occupational therapy services for patients requiring comprehensive rehabilitation.

Day Surgery Center. A free-standing facility or part of a hospital facility where relatively minor, elective surgeries are performed.

Day Treatment Center (DTC), Day Treatment Facility (DTF). A medical program or facility providing comprehensive therapies for patients who do not require hospital or nursing facility admissions. DTCs and DTFs include programs providing comprehensive outpatient treatment for targeted groups (e.g., alcohol and drug abuse, Alzheimer's day care programs, etc.).

Dialysis Unit. The area of the hospital or an outpatient clinic devoted to hemodialysis. Some hospitals have an inpatient unit ("acute unit") for patients admitted to the hospital and a "chronic unit" for outpatient hemodialysis.

Endoscopy Unit/Endo Lab. Usually the location for GI endoscopy and bronchoscopy studies.

Episodic Care Centers. Facilities or programs providing limited emergency and on-call physician services. These centers are sometimes referred to condescendingly as "doc-in-the-box."

Extended Care Facility. Nursing home or residential center for individuals requiring nursing care and/or supervision.

File Room/Record Room. The area in the facility where medical records are kept. Access is usually restricted. Incomplete files (files which are missing signatures or documents) are usually kept separately in a "signature room" or medical records room.

Geriatric Medicine Unit. The Geriatric Unit is a bed service (see above) or ward devoted to admissions and transfers of elderly patients with problems. These units are found where the facility has a geriatric program or geriatrician on its staff.

Home Health Program. Programs and agencies providing nursing, social, and rehabilitation services to the patient in his or her home.

Hospice Program. Programs providing brief inpatient treatment, day treatment, and/or home health nursing, counseling, social, and other support services to patients with terminal illnesses.

Inpatient Rehabilitation Unit. A bed service (see above) or ward devoted to patients requiring physical and other rehabilitation therapies. These units are found in facilities where there are rehabilitation therapists and physiatrists on staff.

Intensive Care Unit (I.C.U.). A ward equipped with special monitoring instruments and staffed with specially trained nurses and support staff for the purpose of managing acute and critical illness.

Isolation Bed/Ward. A room or ward designated for admission or transfer of patients with contagious diseases, especially when the infectious process is airborne or when the patient has a susceptibility for infections from others.

Laboratory. The area in a medical facility where laboratory studies, such as blood and tissue analyses, are conducted upon the request of a physician or individuals with clinical privileges for ordering laboratory studies.

Medical Intensive Care Unit (M.I.C.U.). An intensive care unit devoted to the management of patients with acute or critical medical problems involving the internal organs.

Medical and Surgical Hospital (Med-Surg Hospital). Hospitals with personnel and facilities to provide basic medical and surgical services.

Morgue. The area in the hospital where postmortem anatomical examinations are made by the pathologist. Postmortem pathologic studies (autopsies) are sometimes required to determine the cause of death or factors leading to the patient's demise.

Neonatal Intensive Care Unit (N.I.C.U.). An intensive care unit devoted to critically ill neonates and infants.

Nurses' Station. The area in an Intensive Care Unit, hospital ward, or clinic where medical records and the nurses' "Kardex" are kept. This is the area where nurses write progress notes and other documentation, access computerized records and data, and monitor a patient's status with central monitors.

Operating Room (O.R.). The area or suite of rooms devoted to surgical procedures.

Pain Center. The bed service or outpatient program devoted to interdisciplinary management of chronic, debilitating pain syndromes.

Post Anesthesia Care Unit (PACU). Recovery room.

Private Office. The clinical facility where health care professionals with private practices treat outpatients.

Pulmonary Function Laboratory (PFL). The area of the hospital equipped with instruments and staffed with personnel trained to evaluate pulmonary status and functions. Invasive pulmonary studies, such as bronchoscopy, are performed in the operating room, outpatient surgical suite, or specially designed area within the PFL.

Radiology Department/Unit/Clinic. An area in a hospital or freestanding clinic specially equipped with instruments and staffed with personnel trained in the use of various imaging techniques to diagnose disease.

Recuperative Care Unit. A ward or bed service for patients who require a less acute level of care, but are not quite ready for transfer to a rehabilitation, home care, or other program.

Respite Care. Referring to the brief inpatient or day treatment program providing time-limited nursing and rehabilitation services mainly for the purpose of providing caregiver respite.

Skilled Nursing Facility (S.N.F.). An extended care facility, or nursing home, for patients whose medical status requires continuous monitoring and skilled nursing services.

Surgical Intensive Care Unit (S.I.C.U.). An intensive care unit for patients who are critically ill following surgery or who need to have their vital signs monitored and to have intensive nursing care before transferring to a room or ward.

Surgical Recovery. The area adjacent to the operating room or day surgery suite where patients, vital signs are monitored while they recover from anesthesia following surgery.

Tertiary Care Facility. Facility capable of providing care to the critically ill.

Transitional Care Unit (T.C.U.), "Step Down Unit." In some hospitals a Transitional Care Unit is available for patients who no longer require the degree of continuous monitoring and nursing supervision found in an Intensive Care Unit, but are not yet stable enough to be transferred to a ward.

Ward. A single, large room with multiple patient beds or designated sections of a hospital floor with several adjacent patient rooms.

Ward Administration Desk. Ward secretary's desk.

B. Abbreviations for Health Care Settings and Personnel

AuD. Doctor of Audiology

B.C.U. Burn Care Unit

C.C.U. Cardiac Care Unit

C.M.H.C. Community Mental Health Clinic

C.N.H. Community Nursing Home

C.O.R.F. Comprehensive Outpatient Rehabilitation Facility

C.O.T.A. Certified Occupational Therapy Assistant

D.O., O.D. Doctor of Optometry, Doctor of Osteopathy

D.O.N. Director of Nursing

E.M.T. Emergency Medical Technologist

E.R. Emergency Room

H.H. Home Health

I.C.U. Intensive Care Unit

L.P.N. Licensed Practical Nurse

M.I.C.U. Medical Intensive Care Unit

M.D. Doctor of Medicine

M.S.I, II, III, IV. First-year, second-year, third-year, and fourth-year medical students, respectively

N.I.C.U. Neonatal Intensive Care Unit; Neurologic Intensive Care Unit

O.D. Officer of the Day

O.T. Occupational Therapist/Therapy

P.A.-C. Physician's Assistant-Certified

P.M.D. Private M.D.

P.M. & R. Physical Medicine and Rehabilitation

P.T. Physical Therapist/Therapy

P.T.A. Physical Therapist Assistant

R.N. Registered Nurse

R.R. Recovery Room

R.T. Respiratory Therapist/Therapy, Recreation Therapist/Therapy

S.I.C.U. Surgical Intensive Care Unit

S.L.P. Speech-Language Pathologist

S.N.F. Skilled Nursing Facility

S.W., M.S.W. Social Worker, Master of Social Work

T.C.U. Transitional Care Unit

V. ROUNDS AND CONFERENCES

In training program hospitals, conferences for the purpose of discussing the care of patients are called "rounds." **Morning rounds**, sometimes called "work rounds," are attended by residents, interns, and medical students and take place on the hospital wards in the early morning. During morning rounds, the residents who were assigned care of patients the previous night inform the rest of the team of the status of their patients. **Attending rounds** are scheduled by the staff physician overseeing the care of patients on a given service. Laboratory findings, pertinent history, and vital signs are presented to the attending physician. **Evening rounds** take place in the early evening during which time the plans for any procedures or special monitoring orders are discussed and conveyed to the house staff on call for that evening. In most training programs, the entire house staff and attending physicians also meet daily for a "Morning Report" and weekly for a **Morbidity and Mortality (M & M)** conference during which any deaths, iatrogenic problems, medical, or surgical complications are discussed. In training facilities, **Clinicopathologic Conferences (CPCs)** are formal teaching conferences during which the clinical data from an interesting "teaching case" are presented to an expert or panel of experts for discussion of the management options.

Grand rounds are teaching conferences held in medical school affiliated hospitals (teaching hospitals). Most teaching hospitals will have Surgery Grand Rounds, Medicine Grand Rounds, Neurology Grand Rounds, Pediatric Grand Rounds, and so forth. These teaching conferences present specific topics, research, or interesting teaching cases.

Change of shift conferences occur at each nursing shift change (Day, Evening, and Night). The primary care nurses will either dictate or discuss in conference with incoming nurses what has transpired during the previous shift and what needs to occur during the next shift. It is not advisable to interrupt nurses during this conference, because it causes the nurses going off-shift to be delayed. It may be helpful to discuss with the day shift nurse any special requests or plans that need to be communicated to the evening and night nurses so that he or she can convey these requests during the shift change conferences. Nurses or social workers usually conduct **Discharge Planning Conferences** and welcome input from any discipline that has been involved in a patient's care.

Team Conferences for special purposes are often scheduled on a regular basis depending on the needs of the facility. These multidisciplinary conferences can include **Neuropathology Rounds, Pathology Rounds, Tumor Board** or **Cancer Team Rounds, Rehabilitation Team Rounds, Cardiac Care Rounds, Dysphagia Management Team Conference**, and the like.

VI. MEDICAL STAFF CATEGORIES AND PRIVILEGES

Medical staff in most hospitals usually are categorized according to the extent of their **clinical** and **administrative privileges**. *Clinical privileges* refer to the procedures that can be performed without prior authorization. Clinical privileges can be general, for example, a surgeon may have privileges to admit patients, order tests, and perform surgeries. Privileges can also be *limited* or *specific*, for example, a Clinical Nurse Specialist maybe able to write orders with the exception of medications. *Administrative privileges* refer to participation on hospital boards and voting in staff elections.

A. Medical Staff

Physicians who are fully eligible for all medical privileges and administration privileges. Certain other nonphysician staff (dentists, psychologists, and other doctoral level professional staff) are sometimes elected to the medical staff, but they do not receive full medical privileges, such as the privilege to admit patients to the hospital.

B. Associate Staff

Physicians who have not met all the requirements for full staff privileges and have limited administrative privileges.

C. Provisional Staff

Physicians who are newly appointed to the staff and are still under review. Provisional staff typically do not have full clinical or administrative privileges.

D. Courtesy Staff

Physicians who are given privileges for occasional admissions but do not have administrative privileges.

E. Temporary Staff

Physicians who are given certain clinical privileges for a limited period of time.

VII. STATES OF ILLNESS

A. Acute Illness

Acute illness refers to conditions characterized by an abrupt or life-threatening change in vital signs or mental status. Examples of such conditions are cardiac arrest, acute psychosis, stroke, sudden fever, or respiratory arrest. The term *subacute* is sometimes used to refer to a condition with an abrupt presentation that has not yet reached a critical or life-threatening state.

B. Critical Illness

Critical illness includes conditions that are potentially life-threatening and require treatment in intensive or critical care units. Critically ill patients require special monitors, therapies, and personnel. Patients with critical illness can have conditions that are reversible, such as pneumonia, or irreversible. The term *gravely ill* is used to refer to patients who are critically ill and potentially near death.

C. Serious Illness

Patients described to be *seriously ill* are those whose conditions have stabilized, but continue to require life support therapies, such as oxygen support, or I.V. therapies.

D. Chronic Illness

Patients with chronic illness, or chronic disease, are those who have irreversible conditions affecting their physical and/or mental well-being. Patients with heart disease, stroke residuals, pulmonary disease, or diabetes, as examples, require ongoing pharmacologic and other medical therapies and generally live with some limitations secondary to their chronic condition.

E. Subclinical Illness

Medical conditions that have not yet been revealed to be significant or in need of treatment, conditions too mild to be found on examination, or conditions the patient is not aware of having may be called *subclinical* conditions.

F. Clinically Significant Illness

Medical conditions sufficiently severe to require treatment or monitoring are referred to as *clinically significant*.

G. Factitious Illness, Functional Disorders

A faked or nonorganic condition (see Chapter 9, Neurologic and Psychiatric Disorders) may be called *factitious*, or *functional*.

VIII. NOTES

_____

_____

_____

_____

_____

_____

_____

_____

_____

_____

_____

_____

_____

_____

NOTES *(continued)*

_____

_____

XI. REFERENCES

Avery, M., & Imdieke, B. (1984). *Medical records in ambulatory care.* Rockville, MD: Aspen.

Gray, B. H., & Field, M. J. (Eds.). (1989). *Controlling costs and changing patient care?* Washington DC: National Academy Press.

Haller, R. M., & Sheldon N. (1976). *Speech pathology and audiology in medical settings.* New York: Stratten International Medical Book.

Miller, R. M., & Groher, M. E. (1990). *Medical speech pathology.* Rockville, MD: Aspen.

Nicolosi, L., Harryman, E., & Kresheck J. (1983). *Terminology in communication disorders* (2nd ed.). Baltimore: Williams & Wilkins.

Wolper, L. F., & Pena, J. J. (Eds.). (1987). *Health care administration.* Rockville, MD: Aspen.

CHAPTER

2

Communicating Information and Record-Keeping

Communication is enhanced by an understanding of the medical terminology found in the patient's medical files and how medical conditions are described in ward or team conferences. The patient's medical record is the primary vehicle for communication within medical facilities, including communication among the health care personnel actively caring for the patient, between the health care providers and the patient, and between the health care providers and third party payers. The use of **abbreviations, acronyms,** and **eponyms** is necessary for quick documentation in handwritten medical records and their use is encouraged when completing reimbursement forms.

Abbreviations are letters standing for a word or phrase, such as P.T. for physical therapy. **Acronyms** are words formed from the initial letters of a compound term. For example, the word *laser* is an acronym for *l*ight *a*mplification *s*timulated *e*mission of *r*adiation. The word *rads* refers to *r*adiation *a*bsorbed *d*oses. **Eponyms** are words or phrases derived from the name of a person, as in the Babinski sign.

Any health care professional reading and writing notes in medical charts should be comfortable with the language and format appropriate for those documents. This chapter introduces basic concepts in medical terminology and discusses the purposes and types of medical notations including prescriptions and other notations. Abbreviations and symbols commonly found in progress notes and in doctors' orders are included. Issues such as confidentiality protections and informed consent, as well as guidelines for appropriate entries in medical records, and other methods of communicating in medical settings are also discussed.

I. SOURCES FOR MEDICAL TERMINOLOGY

Speech-language clinicians in hospital practice should have at least one comprehensive textbook on medical terminology and a medical dictionary in their professional libraries. These texts provide explanations on word origin, spelling, and pronunciation, and definitions of medical terms. It is often helpful to define the suffixes and prefixes and the meanings of the root words to understand the polysyllabic language of medicine. The majority of medical terms are derived from Greek or Latin; thus, knowing etymologic features of medical terms will help to determine both their meaning and pronunciation.

Throughout this book are lists of terminology and abbreviations likely to appear in medical records, reports, and progress notes. In cases where the word is entirely unfamiliar to the clinician, a *medical dictionary should be consulted to determine pronunciation.* The preparation of this *Sourcebook* required consulting and comparing several comprehensive books on medical terminology as well as medical dictionaries and terminology in critical care, medical manuals, and nursing care handbooks. The sources consulted in preparation of this text are listed collectively at the end of each chapter. These references and similar texts would be useful additions to the clinician's departmental or personal libraries. Most facilities will have a medical library with comparable resource texts. In addition to published texts on medical terminology, medical centers are required to have a list of "acceptable abbreviations," or legends, for their facility which can usually be obtained from the Transcription Office, Medical Records Department, Medical Administration Office, medical library, or Ward Administration Office.

II. SELECTED MEDICAL TERMINOLOGY

A. Terms for Direction

Afferent. Going toward a body or center

Efferent. Going away from a body or center

Superior. Above or in an upward direction

Inferior. Below or in a downward direction

Posterior. Toward the back or behind

Anterior. Toward the front or before

Medial. Toward the midline

Intermediate. Between the medial and lateral parts

Lateral. Toward the side

Cephalad. Toward the head

Proximal. Toward the body or nearest point of attachment

Distal. Away from the point of attachment

Ventral. In front or anterior

Dorsal. In back of or posterior

Superficial. Near the surface

Deep. Away from the surface

B. Terms for Spatial Orientation or Planes

Apex, apical. Referring to the top or tip of a body organ or part

Base, basal. Referring to the foundation or lowest part

Midsagittal. Vertical division of the body through the midline to make a left and a right half

Frontal, or coronal. Vertical plane parallel to the coronal suture of the cranium, dividing the body's front from the back at right angles to the midsagittal plane

Transverse, or horizontal. Dividing superior (upper) from inferior (lower) portions of the body

Longitudinal. Any plane parallel to the long axis of a structure

C. Terms Used to indicate Regions

[Figure 3–1, in Chapter 3, illustrates some of these regions.]

Axillary. In the armpit

Cervical. Area involving the neck

Perianal. Around the anus.

Perineal. Between the anus and genitalia

Peritoneal. Pertaining to the membranous sac lining the abdomi-no-pelvic cavity containing the viscera (internal organs)

Flank. Part of the side of the body extending below the ribs to the ilium

Lumbar. Mid-lateral regions of the back

Sternal. Near the sternum

Clavicular. Near the clavicle

Umbilical. Near the navel

Inguinal. Lower pelvic regions; groin area

Hypogastric. Abdominal; below the stomach

Epigastric. Lower mid chest; above the stomach

III. ROOTS, PREFIXES, SUFFIXES, PLURALS, AND PRONUNCIATIONS

A. Roots

Aden– Gland	**Arterio–** Artery
Adip– Fat	**Arth–** Joint
Aer– Pertaining to air	**Athero–** Fatty substance
Angio– Vessel	**Blephar–** Eyelid

Cardi– Heart

Cerebro– Brain

Cephal– Head

Cerv– Neck

Cheil–, **chil**– Lip

Chol– Bile

Chondr– Cartilage

Cost– Rib

Crani– Skull

Cysto– Bladder

Cyt– Cell

Dactyl– Finger, toe

Enter– Intestine

Gastr– Stomach

Gloss– Tongue

Glyco– Sweet

Hem– Blood

Hepa– Liver

Histo– Pertaining to tissue

Hyster– Uterus

Ile–, **elie**– Ileum (small intestine)

Ili– Ilium (pelvis)

Inguino– Groin

Leuk– White

Lipo– Fat

Lith– Stone

Mening– Membrane

Metr– Uterus

Morph– Form, shape

Myel– Marrow

Myo– Muscle

Nephr– Kidney

Ophthalm– Eye

Oro– Mouth

Ortho– Straight

Osteo– Bone

Pneum– Lung

Proct– Rectum

Psych– Mind

Pyel– Pelvis

Pyo– Pus

Radi– Ray

Spondyl– Vertebral

Trache– Neck

Viscer– Organ

B. Prefixes

a–, **an**–without

ab– from, away from

ad– increase, near, toward

ana– up, increase

ante– before

anti– against

bi– two, both

cata– down, decrease

con– together

contra– opposite, against

cost– rib

cysto– sac, bladder

dia– through, between

dys–bad, poor

ecto– outside

em–, **en**– in

ed– out of or from

endo– within

epi– upon, in addition

ex– out

eu– good, normal

hemi– half

hyper– above, excessive

hypo– beneath, deficient

iatro– related to medicine or a physician

intra– within

leuko– white

mega– large

meta– beyond, change

micro– small size

neutr– neutral

pan– all, total, wide

para– beside, near, abnormal

per– through, by

peri– around

poly– much, excessive

pre– before

pro– in front of, forward

pseudo– false

retro– backward, behind

semi– half

sub– below, under

super–, **supra**– above, beyond, superior

sym–, **syn**– with, together, beside

trans– across

C. Suffixes

–**algia.** Pain

–**cele.** Herniation, tumor, protrusion

–**centesis.** Puncture

–**cyte.** Cell

–**dynia.** Pain

–**ectomy.** Excision

–**edasis.** Expansion, dilatation

–**emesis.** Vomiting

–**emia.** Blood

–**genic.** Origin, caused by

–**iasis.** Condition, formation of

–**itis.** Inflammation

–**lysis.** Breaking down, destruction

–**malacia.** Softening

–**megaly.** Enlargement

–**oma.** Tumor

–osis. Condition, disease

–pathy. Disease

–penia. Deficiency

–pexy. Suspension, fixation

–plasty. Surgical correction or repair

–plexy. Fixation

–ptosis. Falling, drooping

–ptysis. Spitting

–rrhage. Gushing, flowing

–rrhaphy. Suture

–rrhea. Discharge, flow

–rrhexis. Rupture

–scopy. Inspection

–stalsis. Contraction

–stasis. Stopped

–staxia. Dripping

–stomy. Creation of a new opening

–tomy. Incision into

–tripsy. Crushing

–trophy. Development, nourishment

D. Plurals

Singular		Plural
a as in bursa	to	**ae** as in bursae
us as in incus	to	**udes** as in incudes
us as in alveolus	to	**i** as in alveoli
um as in datum, or ovum	to	**a** as in data, or ova
ex as in apex	to	**ices** as in apices
ix as in appendix	to	**ices** as in appendices
ax as in thorax	to	**axes** as in thoraxes
nx as in larynx, or phalanx	to	**nges** as in larynges,[1] or phalanges
oma as in adenoma, or stoma	to	**omata** as in adenomata, or stomata[1]
u as in cornu	to	**ua** as in cornua
ur as in femur	to	**ura** as in femura
us as in nucleus	to	**i** as in nuclei

---

[1]"Stomas" and "larynxes" are also acceptable and conventional.

is as in crisis	to	**es** as in crises
is as in iris	to	**ides** as in irides
er as in tuber	to	**era** as in tubera
en as in foramen	to	**ina** as in foramina
on as in criterion	to	**a** as in criteria

E. Pronunciation

1. ae– When the **ae** ending is a plural of a Latin word, it is pronounced like the diphthong "i," for example, the plural word "petechiae," referring to small hemorrhages, is pronounced as /pe–**ti**-ki-aɪ/. Words beginning with the letters **aer** are derivatives from Greek or combined forms using Greek and Latin. These letters are pronounced "ehr" (for example, /ərobɪks/).

2. cn–, gn–, kn–, mn–, pn– Words beginning with **cn, gn, kn, mn,** and **pn,** as in cnemical, gnathic, knot, mnemic, and pneumonia, are pronounced as though they began with "n."

3. ps– Words beginning with **ps**, as in psychology, are pronounced as though they began with "s."

4. phth– Words beginning with **phthir** are pronounced as though they began with "thir"; words beginning with **phthis** are pronounced as though they began with "tiz."

5. pt– Words beginning with **pt**, as in ptosis, are pronounced as though they began with "t "

6. –gm. Words ending in **gm**, as in diaphragm, are pronounced as though they ended with "m" (the "g" is silent).

IV. PURPOSES AND TYPES OF MEDICAL RECORDS

As an ongoing log of health care, the medical record helps to reduce the risk for duplication or omission of medications and other therapies.

The medical record is:

- *A documentation procedure protecting the patient's safety;*
- *A means for health care personnel to communicate their observation and plans;* and

> • *A legal document* that is "discoverable" evidence in legal proceedings.

The primary purpose of the medical chart is to provide a *permanent record* of the patient's health status and the interventions that have been administered. Hospitals keep medical charts pertaining to the patient's current admission and an integrated file of any previous care at that facility. These records are organized and labeled for easy accessibility.

The most common organizational formats for medical records include:

- *Flowsheets* and *Clinical* (Critical) *Pathway Documentation;*

- *Source-Oriented* (SO) or *Source-Indexed* (SI) medical records;

- *Problem-Oriented Medical Records* (POMR);

- *Standards-Based Documentation* or *Documentation by Exception;*

- *Problem-Intervention-Evaluation Format;* and

- *Chronologic Records.*

A. Flowsheet and Pathway Documentation

Most health care facilities are making efforts to move to "paperless" systems of documentation to the fullest extent possible; however, some sort of paper record will probably be needed, especially at the patient's bedside. The type of documentation that is most commonly found at bedside is the **flowsheet.** Flowsheets typically span 24 hours and contain spaces, or "cells," for the most common parameters recorded (vital signs, ins and outs, nutrition, mental status, respiratory therapy treatments, and rehabilitation therapy treatments). Similar to the flowsheet documentation are the **clinical (or critical) care pathways documents**. Care pathways are "maps" of the care plan for particular diagnoses or conditions spanning the entire event of care from admission (in some cases preadmission data are included) through the projected day of discharge. The care pathways are typically documented in individual booklets, or flowsheets, with cells for recording the completion of the all of the elements in the plan. In an acute care setting, for example, the clinical care pathway for the patient undergoing a total hip replacement will include cells to document such things as presurgical teaching and training, x-ray and laboratory studies, the physical examination, and surgeon's and anesthesiologist's presurgical visits prior to or during the first hours/day of admission. The pathway will map out the course and schedule of care and each of the expected elements of care. A clinical pathway for treatment in a rehabilitation center will map out the expected course of care and expected outcomes across the days and weeks of treatment through the anticipated date of discharge.

B. Source-Oriented Medical Records

Source-Oriented (SO) or *Source-Indexed* (SI) records contain separate sections for physicians' orders, progress notes, nurses' notes, x-ray reports, laboratory findings, and so forth. SO records are often written in a narrative format documenting the problem, or reason for visit; the duration of the problem; physical findings; laboratory and other study findings; diagnosis and secondary conditions; therapeutic and preventive services or medications prescribed; and the follow-up plan. Entries may also be made in a **"S.O.A.P.," or "S.O.A.P.I.E.,"** format, described in the next section.

C. Problem-Oriented Medical Records

Problem-Oriented Medical Records (POMRs) are organized relative to the patient's "Problem List," including both the reason for the admission or visit and pre-existing or active diseases. The patient's medical problems are listed and numbered and might include medical, surgical and previous surgeries, and psychiatric and social problems. Previously treated problems or surgeries are sometimes listed with the word "resolved" next to them. The problem list can also include the need to "R/O," or rule out, a questionable diagnosis.

In general, POMRs are organized with the following sections:

- Introductory section, or the *Data Base;*
- *Problem List;*
- *Initial Plan;* and
- *Progress Notes.*

The latter are itemized, or headed, relative to each problem. For example, the speech-language pathologist's notes might be headed "Problem #1: Aphasia, secondary to left CVA" followed by "Speech-Language Pathology Initial Plan." Progress notes may be organized in a format termed "S.O.A P.," or "S.O.A.P.I.E.," or notes may be brief written narratives. The S.O.A.P.I.E. format allows quick access to pertinent information following the outline below.

D. S.O.A.P.I.E. Format in Medical Progress Notes

S *Subjective* observations (what you notice about the patient, the mental status or patient's complaints), for example,
  S — "Pt. said 'I'm feeling sick all over.' " or
  "Pt. c/o (complains of) fatigue."

O *Objective* observations (data and facts), for example,
  O — "Pt. reliably indicated yes and no to 10 orientation questions."

A *Assessment* (your analysis and formulation), for example,
  A — "Mental status has improved from yesterday."

P *Plan* (steps and measures to be taken or recommended), for example,
  P — "Standardized testing is scheduled to begin tomorrow."

I *Implementation* (interventions taken and progress made)

E *Evaluation* (efficacy of the interventions)

E. Problem-Intervention-Evaluation (P.I.E.) Format

A documentation format used occasionally in nursing notes is referred to as Problem-Intervention-Evaluation, or P.I.E., format. This system consists of a running list of nursing diagnoses, each with a progress note and divided into three components: "P," statements of the *problems*; "I," *interventions* made; and "E, "*evaluation* of the outcomes of the interventions.

F. Standards-Based Documentation or Documentation by Exception

Standards-Based Documentation, or Documentation by Exception, is a method of documentation of care that refers to predefined norms, protocols, and standards of care. If care is provided in accordance to these prestated standards and the patient's response is the expected response, then only symbols, such as check marks, or notations such as "P" for *progressing* or "E" for *evaluation* are required for noting. If there are variations in the typical plan or in the patient's response, then a *focused note* will be written. Focused notes are one or two phrase narrative notes. Usually, the Standards-Based, Documentation by Exception format uses a 24-hour flowsheet that will refer to predetermined standards. For example, if the facility has established a standard of care for "Laryngectomy," the SLP's Laryngectomy Communication Protocol will be referenced. The flowsheet will contain a place for the clinician to note that the standard protocol is being followed; consequently, daily, long narrative notes will not be needed unless there is some variation from the protocol due to a complication or abnormal response.

G. Chronologic Records

Chronologic records place all notes, laboratory findings, reports, and so forth in the file *sequentially* as they are written or received. This sort of file might be found in some outpatient clinic records, such as a Voice Clinic, where there is a single problem, followed longitudinally and involving relatively few visits.

H. Computerized Flowsheets and Electronic Data and Order Entries

Bedside computer terminals are increasingly available with software to input complex parameters into the hospital's data bases. Most bedside equipment uses either a touch sensitive pad or screen, or a keyboard. Computerized flowsheets and data have some disadvantages (with systems breaking down occasionally) and can be expensive to maintain. Some of the advantages to computerized systems for documentation are increased **confidentiality** (if managed properly), **legibility**, **standardization** of information, and **data base development**. Computerized orders are also a time saver. For example, when multiple disciplines are needed for an evaluation, such as the Dysphagia Team, the computer can generate the orders simultaneously.

V. GUIDELINES FOR ENTRIES IN PROGRESS NOTES

Medical chart notes and reports should always be signed with the *name and title of the author* and should state his or her discipline. Some medical record departments require that the nature of the note and the author's discipline also be designated in the note headings. For example, progress notes might be headed as "Speech-Language Pathology Consultation," "SLP-Admitting Note," "SLP-Progress Note," "SLP-Treatment Note," "SLP-Transfer Note," or "SLP- Discharge Plan." Because the styles and procedures for medical charting will vary between institutions, speech-language pathologists should determine the local format and follow it.

A. Guidelines for Entries in Medical Records

When making medical chart entries you should:

- Use a *pen,* preferably with black ink.

- Write *legibly.*

- *Enter the date and time of the note and duration of the visit* (some facilities require entering the time of the note and may prefer a 24-hour clock or "military time", where 6:00 p.m. equals 1800 hours).

- Record only information significant to *your* assessment or plan.

- *Correct all mistakes.* If you make an error or information is omitted do not erase or "white out" the error; draw a line through your mistake or insert the missing information with a caret (∧). Put your initials next to any corrections and write "error" above the mistake.

- Avoid phrases such as "seems to," "appears to," or "apparently."

- Avoid *assigning* blame.

- Avoid leaving excessive spacing within and between notes.

- *Use descriptions in place of labels.*

- Use conventionally accepted *abbreviations* and omit words such as "an," "a," and "the" whenever possible.

- Be *brief.*

- Sign all notes with your name and professional title.

VI. PATIENT AND FAMILY EDUCATION

Regardless of the documentation format used in patient care, one important area that must be addressed is patient and family education. In the current standards for health care facilities, an assessment of the patient's and caregiver's needs for education is mandatory. This assessment must take into account language, cultural/religious, sensory, or cognitive barriers to learning, as well as the preferred learning method (i.e, demonstration versus spoken, written, videotaped instruction), and the motivation level of the learner. Anyone providing patient education must document the topic instruction, the teaching method and materials used, and the recipient's response to the instruction (demonstrated level of learning/knowledge gained from the instruction). In most cases a standard form will be provided for education documentation or the flow-sheets and clinical pathways will contain grids for noting education.

VII. SOURCES OF INFORMATION

A. Medical Chart Organization

Medical charts are generally organized to contain the following information:

1. **Admitting History and Physical.** An outline of the medical history and current physical status of the patient.

2. **Doctors' Orders.** Section containing specific tests, procedures, therapies, and medications ordered by the physician.

3. **Progress Notes.** Narrative or problem-oriented notes of observations, data, and plans for treatment. Occasionally, charts will contain separate sections for Physicians' Progress Notes and the progress notes made by other staff. This is obviously not preferable since it discourages physicians from reading other staff notes.

4. **Nurses' Progress Notes.** A separate section of notes made by the patient's primary nurse(s) at the end of each shift or whenever a notable change or problem arises.

5. **Nutrition Care Plans.** Diet histories, nutritional status notes, and nutrition plans prepared by the dietitians, dietary techs, or nurses.

6. **Consultation Reports.** Written responses to requests for consultation from various disciplines.

7. **Lab Findings.** Data summaries of laboratory studies ordered by the physician (usually containing the laboratory findings and indicating whether these findings are within normal limits for that laboratory).

8. **EKG.** Section containing selected electrocardiograph strips.

9. **X-Ray Studies.** Reports from any radiology studies.

10. **Op. Notes.** The dictated narrative summary describing details of the patient's surgeries.

11. **Miscellaneous Data and Notes.** Special administrative forms.

12. **Discharge Summaries.** The physician's narrative summary of the hospital course and discharge plan.

13. **Patient Data.** Patient's address, phone number, next-of-kin contact, insurance plan, and employer.

14. **Research Releases, Special Protocol Forms, and Informed Consents.** The original copies of any special consent forms or waivers will be filed with the patient's medical record. These forms will be reviewed and approved by the Medical Records Committee, Human Subjects Committee or Institutional Review Board, or the facility's attorneys. Consent forms must adhere to rigorous guidelines that are intended to inform the patient fully of the risks and benefits of the study and to protect the patient. In some cases it may be necessary to use alternative communication methods, assistive devices, or interpreters to make sure the patient or the patient's representative understands the informed consent. In cases when the speech-language pathologist or another member of the hospital staff has assisted with an explanation of the consent form (due to a communication handicap or some other barrier to communication), the procedures taken to ensure that the patient, or the patient's representative, was fully informed and his or her behavioral responses demonstrating knowledge should be documented.

B. Physician's Chartwork

The format used for the physician's admitting medical notes and orders will vary according to the preferences of the physician and the facility. One charting format often used by house staff is known by the mnemonic **"A.D.C. VAAN DIML,"** referring to the following:

Admit (to a stated ward, team, doctor, or service);

Diagnosis (admitting medical diagnoses);

Condition (stating if the patient is critical or stable);

Vitals (listing temperature, heart rate, respiration rate, blood pressure, height, and weight);

Activity (indicating degree of allowable activity);

Allergies (drug, food, environmental, reactions);

Nursing (stating bed positioning, preps, wound care, etc.);

Diet (stating the method for nutritional support);

Ins and outs (listing the tubes and drains that are to be inserted);

Medications (listing therapeutic drugs and any drugs for pain, bowel management, or sedation); and

Labs (indicating which studies and special tests need to be made and the times they should be done).

Further discussion of the physical examination and its findings is found in Chapter 3. An illustration of a commonly used method for recording laboratory values as part of the physician's chart work is provided in Figure 2–1. The top diagram shows how the "blood work," or hematologic analysis, will be noted. The other two diagrams indicate how fluid and electrolyte parameters will be noted. Chapter 5 discusses the significance of fluid and electrolyte findings, and Chapter 7 describes the meaning of certain hematologic parameters. The values for a normal range in these laboratory analyses are provided in Appendix C.

C. Computerized Records

It is becoming increasingly common for portions of a patient's medical record, especially laboratory data and medication histories, to be kept in a computerized record. Access to this information is always limited and obtained by permission from the Medical Records Department or Medical Administration office according to hospital policies. Usually, access requires a coded entry, or *user key,* from the user who agrees to adhere to the facility's rules for confidentiality. Inputting information in the patient's computerized record is restricted to appropriate, designated personnel, normally including the ward secretaries, physicians, nurses, laboratory personnel, dietitians, and so on. Some facilities use a computerized form of the Problem-Oriented Medical Record Information System, referred to as **"PROMIS."**

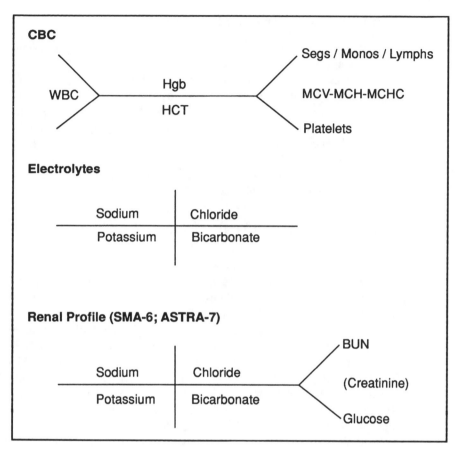

Figure 2–1. Common methods for noting laboratory values in medical charts

D. Nurses' Kardex

In acute care facilities a Kardex is kept on the ward to provide a "hard" (not computerized) record of the current orders and key parameters of the patient's care. The Kardex has plastic covered index cards with pertinent information for each patient affixed to a holder in a series according to the room and bed numbers for each ward. The Kardex sometimes contains information not retrievable from the patient's medical chart, such as an unlisted telephone number for the patient's closest relative. The most current diet and medication orders are also noted in the Kardex. In some facilities there is one Kardex for medications and another Kardex for procedures. The Kardex can be especially useful when the computer is not operational or is unavailable.

E. Incident and Variance Report Forms

Some system for the reporting and facility's oversight of accidents or variances in care of patients will be in place in health care facilities as part of the risk monitoring processes. Usually, there is a requirement that a formal report of any accident, incident, or variance in care be made within 24 hours of its occurrence, and occasionally an investigation by Risk Management personnel may be needed. The facility will have policies and procedures for reporting these events. If the incident or variance involved a medical device, then the reporting guidelines for compliance with the Safe Medical Devices Act will be followed.

VIII. CHART NOTES IN TRAINING PROGRAMS

Hospitals affiliated with physician training programs, or *teaching hospitals,* require notes written by medical students, house staff (residents), fellows, and attendings (staff physicians) be headed to designate the author's status. Notes written by students are co-signed by the supervising staff member and the attending physicians will often write an addendum stating they were present during the examination and/or they concur with the plans. The medical students' notes may be headed "MS III AN," meaning it was written by a third-year medical student and the note is his or her "Admitting Note." The notation "RAN" denotes a "Resident Admitting Note," and "IPN" denotes an "Intern Progress Note" and so forth. Consultation requests to specialists and subspecialists for their opinions will usually receive a response from either the attending staff physician in a particular subspecialty or the "Fellow" from that specialty (see Chapter 1). Thus, one might find consultation reports and notes headed, for example, as "Cardiology Fellow."

IX. SYMBOLS AND PRESCRIPTION NOTATIONS

Medical abbreviations, acronyms, eponyms, symbols, and prescription notations can be difficult to interpret, although one can frequently surmise the meaning from the context. Some abbreviations are idiosyncratic to the user or a given facility and some notations are used inappropriately or mistakenly by medically trained personnel, especially medical students. Chapter 3, Vital Signs and the Physical Examination, contains a list of terminology and abbreviations commonly encountered in progress notes and reports.

Table 2–1 provides a summary of prescription order notations. Table 2–2 lists common medical chart symbols. For discussions of the effects of drugs on communicative abilities and disorders, see Vogel and Carter (1995) and Poon (1995).

A. Medical Administrative Terminology

Access. The ability to obtain medical care.

Advanced medical directives. Living will.

Ambulatory Patient Groups (APGs). Outpatient "DRGs."

Ancillary services. Hospital services provided in conjunction with medical care (e.g, physical therapy, radiology, laboratory services).

TABLE 2–1. Abbreviations used in prescriptions

Abbreviation	Derivation	Meaning
aa	ana	of each
a.c.	ante cibum	before meals
ad	ad	to, up to
ad lib	ad libitum	as desired
alt. dieb.	alternis diebus	every other day
alt. hor.	alternis horis	every other hour
aq.	aqua	water
b.i.d.	bis in die	two times a day
b.i.n.	bis in nocte	twice at night
c.	cum	with
Cap.	capiat	let him take
Det.	detur	let it be given
Ft.	fiat	make
o.d.	omni die	every day
o.h.	omni hora	every hour
o.m.	omni mane	every morning
o.n.	omni nocte	every night

(continued)

TABLE 2-1. *(continued)*

Abbreviation	Derivation	Meaning
os	*os*	mouth
p.c.	*post cibum*	after meals
per	*per*	through or by
p.o.	*per os*	by mouth
p.r.n.	*pro re nata*	when needed
q.d.	*quaque die*	each day
q.h.	*quaque hora*	every hour
q. 2 h		every 2 hours
q. 4 h		every 4 hours
q. 6 h[a]		every 6 hours
q.i.d.[a]	*quarter in die*	four times a day
q.l.	*quantum libet*	as much as desired
q.n.	*quaque nocte*	every night
q.p.	*quantum placeat*	as much as desired
q.v.	*quantum vis*	as much as you please
q.s.	*quantum suffcit*	as much as required
q/s	*quaque*/shift	each shift
Rx	*recipe*	prescription
s	*sine*	without
Sig. or S	*signa*	write on label
s.o.s.	*si opus si*	if necessary
ss	*semis*	a half
stat.	*statim*	immediately
t.d.s.	*ter die sumendum*	to be taken three times daily
t.i.d.	*ter in die*	three times a day
t.i.n.	*ter in nocte*	three times at night
ut dict	*ut dictum*	as directed
via	*via*	by way of

[a]Note that *q.i.d.* and *q. 6 h* are not the same orders. *Q.i.d.* means the medication will be administered every 4 hours; *q. 6 h* means it will be administered by designated clock intervals (12 noon, 6 p.m., 12 midnight, 6 a.m.).

TABLE 2–2. Common medical symbols

Symbol	Meaning
ī; īī; īīī	one; two; three (drops)
#	Number; pounds; size
+	Plus; excess; positive; acid reaction
−	Minus; deficiency; negative; alkaline reaction
↑	Increase; increasing
↓	Decrease; decreasing
⇄	Reversible reaction
□, ♂	Male
○, ♀	Female
>	Greater than
<	Less than
≯	Not greater than
≮	Not less than
Δ	Change
°	Degree
≅	Approximately equals
=	Equals
≠	Not equals
::	As; equal ratios of
2°	Secondary to
∴	Therefore
c̄	With
s̄	Without
→	Yields; causes; leads to; leading to
:	Ratio
n, N̶	Negative
p̄	Post; after

Appropriate. Medically justified and necessary.

Beneficiary. Insured person.

Capitation. A fixed rate of payment to cover specifically designated services.

Claim. A reimbursement application or bill submitted to a health benefits plan.

Coinsurance. The percent of medical costs that the beneficiary (insured person) must pay after the deductible is satisfied.

Common Procedural Terminology (CPT). Referring to 5-digit codes with modifiers as a standard for identifying services or procedures for third party payers.

Consolidated Omnibus Budget Reconciliation Act. Federal legislation enacted in 1985 containing amendments to the Medicare and Medicaid entitlements.

Cost Center. The facility's program or department budgeted for particular costs (e.g., a SLP salary may be paid by the Rehab Department's "cost center").

Criteria. Stated guidelines for determining the necessity and appropriateness of a health care service.

Deductible. The amount of a medical expense that must be incurred and paid by the beneficiary before the third party payer becomes liable for payment.

Diagnosis-Related Groups (DRGs). Under Medicare payment procedures for hospitals, DRGs refer to categories of reimbursement for care based on the patient's diagnosis(es). This payment system assumes that patients with certain diagnoses will require more expensive and extended services than others.

Effectiveness. Probability of benefit.

Encounter. Outpatient visit.

Enrollee. Insured person; person covered by a health benefit plan.

Fee-for-service. Method for payment for treatment on an event basis rather than by salary or through a capitation plan.

Health Care Financing Administration (HCFA). The branch of the U.S. Department of Health and Human Services that administers Medicare and Medicaid programs.

Managed Care. Refers to various cost containment systems put in place with the expressed goal of delivering cost-effective care without compromising the quality. Managed care plans include limits on inpatient hospitalization coverage by prospective payments (see Diagnosis Related Groups, or DRGs), encouraging the hospital to reduce the lengths of stays as much as possible, and limit the services to only those essential for quality care. Outpatient services are usually provided through a "gatekeeper" mechanism, which requires that certain steps be followed in the referral processes and places limits on the number of visits covered for various conditions. Medications will also have restrictions, so that less expensive drugs are encouraged and stockpiles of several months of any medications are discouraged.

Medicare Part A. Referring to the schedule of payment in Medicare benefits covering nonspecific institutional expenses incurred by inpatients in hospitals, in skilled nursing facilities, home health care, and hospice care requiring skilled services. Eligibility for Part A is automatic for U.S. citizens over the age of 65.

Medicare Part B is the optional medical insurance for people over the age of 65 that covers services rendered by physicians and other practitioners in outpatient hospitals and clinics, nonskilled nursing settings, rehabilitation agencies, and similar settings.

Medicare Title XVIII of Social Security Act. A federal health insurance program for people age 65 or older and for individuals with certain disabilities.

Outcome. The result of treatment.

Outliers. Cases that fall outside of normal statistical predictions.

Performance Improvement. The term that has replaced "Quality Assurance" to refer to an organized program within a facility for identifying and correcting problems and monitoring outcomes to improve the quality of health care services.

Practice guidelines. Standard recommendations for patient care.

Practice pattern. Data illustrating the characteristics of a given practitioner's use of medical resources.

Preadmission review. A review of the justification for procedures prior to admission.

Premium. The amount paid to purchase health insurance.

Prior authorization. A review by the third party payer of the justification of a given service before it is provided to a beneficiary.

Product Line. In health service administration, a *product line* refers to the revenue or cost center for a particular "line" of service. For example, Head and Neck Cancer rehabilitation can be a line of service and all aspects of care required to provide that health service "product" would fall under that cost center. Thus, the speech-language pathology costs attached to head and neck cancer rehabilitation team or unit would be included in calculating the costs for that program, or product line. There are a couple of advantages to having product line revenue and cost centers, one being the ease of determining costs for particular programs. Additionally, it organizes multiple providers into a unit, or team, whose members are responsible for its costs, revenues, and outcomes.

Provider. An entity providing health care services.

Quality assessment (Q.A.). An evaluation of the interpersonal and technical aspects of health care.

Reasonable cost basis. A method that determines the Medicare reimbursement amount based on the operational expenses of the provider.

Resource-Based Relative Value Scale (RBRVS). Referring to a valuation or rating of Medicare Part B services on the basis of relative resource inputs (work and other practice costs) required to provide services.

Retrospective utilization review. An examination of the appropriateness, cost, and outcome of medical services in a retrospective review of medical charts.

Third party payer. An entity providing health care financing on behalf of the patient (first party) to the health care provider (second party).

Total quality improvement (TQI), Continuous Quality Improvement (CQI). A quality assurance process directed toward continually improving services to meet the needs of the customer or client and preventing defects or deficiencies in the provision of services. (See Performance Improvement).

Unbundle. A charging practice where individual services are billed separately rather than under one procedure code.

Upcode. Billing for a procedure that reflects a higher level of care than was provided.

Utilization review. A method to manage health care costs through a case-by-case evaluation of the justification for clinical services.

B. Administrative Medical Abbreviations

AEP. Appropriateness evaluation protocol

A & H. Accident and health (insurance)

BCBSA. Blue Cross and Blue Shield Association

C.A.R.F. Commission on Accreditation of Rehabilitation Facilities

CHAMPAS. Civilian Health and Medical Program for Armed Services

CHAMPVA. Civilian Health and Medical Program for Veterans Affairs

CME. Continuing medical education

COBRA. Consolidated Omnibus Budget Reconciliation Act

CPR. Customary, prevailing, and reasonable

CPT. Common procedural terminology; current edition is CPT-4

DHHS. (U.S.) Department of Health and Human Services

DME. Durable medical equipment

DMERC. Durable Medical Equipment Regional Carrier

DRG. Diagnosis-related group

FFS. Fee for service

FMG. Foreign medical graduate

FY. Fiscal year

GAO. General Accounting Office (Federal Government)

HCFA. Health Care Financing Association

HCPCS. HCFA Common Procedural Coding System

HICN. Health insurance claim number

HMO. Health Maintenance Organization

ICD-9 (CM); ICD-10 (PCS). *International Classification of Disease* (Clinical Modification); *International Classification of Disease—* 10th Version (Procedural Coding System)

IPA. Individual practice association

I.R.B. Institutional Review Board

ISD-A. Intensity of service, severity of illness, discharge and appropriateness (screenings)

JCAHO. Joint Commission on the Accreditation of Healthcare Organizations

LOS. Length of (hospital) stay

MAC. Maximal allowable charge

MFS. Medicare fee schedule

MHB. Maximum hospital benefits

OBRA. Omnibus Budget Reconciliation Acts

PCP. Primary care physician

PN. Provider number

POC. Plan of care

PPRC. Physician Payment Review Commission

PPS. Prospective payment system

PRO. Peer review organization

RBRVS. Resource-based relative value scale

RVU. Relative value unit

SNF. Skilled nursing facility

SOC. Start of care

SS. Social Security

SSI. Supplemental Security Income

SSN. Social Security number

TQI. Total quality improvement

VAMC. Veterans Affairs Medical Center

X. PRESCRIPTIONS

In the United States, most pharmacologic therapies are *regulated* in that they are *prescribed* by physicians who are licensed by the Medical Licensure Boards in the states where they practice and are duly registered with the **Drug Enforcement Agency** (**DEA**). Prescriptions are not required for "over-the-counter" medications. The federal **Food and Drug Administration** (**FDA**) determines whether a drug may be distributed and sold and if a physician's prescription is required for its use. The *United States Pharmacopeia (U.S.P.)* sets standards for purity and determines if the drug is indeed a useful therapy. Licensed pharmacists dispense drugs in accordance with the physician's verbal (by telephone) or written orders (by signed prescription or written request in the "Doctor's Orders" section of the medical chart). In medical progress notes, telephone orders are noted as *T/O* and verbal orders are noted as *V/O*. Table 2–1 defines some of the abbreviations used on written prescriptions and orders.

XI. ADMINISTRATION OF MEDICATIONS

A. Drug Names

A drug can have three different names:

- The *chemical name,* which is its chemical formula,

- The *brand name* or trade name, which will usually be followed by a superscript® notation to indicate it is registered; and

- The *generic,* or official name, the name of the drug that is its legal and scientific name.

Example: *Alpha-aminobenzyl P* (chemical name), *Amcap, Amcill, D-Amp, Omnipen, Pfizerpen A, Polycillin, Principen, SK-Ampicillin, Supen, Totacillin* (brand names), and *ampicillin* (generic name).

The hospital library or pharmacy will have two large listings of drugs: the **Hospital Formulary** and the **Physicians' Desk Reference (PDR)**. The latter is published privately and updated yearly.

B. Administration of Drugs

The method of drug administration will vary depending on how the medicine is best absorbed. Drugs given **orally** are absorbed into the bloodstream through the intestinal wall. Drugs administered **sublingually** are dissolved by the saliva and absorbed rapidly through the mucous membranes of the mouth. Some drugs are applied **topically**, on the skin, and some are **inhaled** as vaporous gases, or aerosols. **Rectal administration** through suppositories is usually done when the patient is too nauseated to tolerate oral intake. Direct injection of a drug may be done through a syringe (needle) into the muscle tissue *(intramuscular,* I.M.); under the skin *subcutaneously* ("sub Q"); into the skin, *intradermally;* or into a vein *intravenously* (I.V.).

XII. INFORMED CONSENT AND CONFIDENTIALITY

Very strict policies are in force in all health care facilities to ensure that patients give "Informed Consent" to any procedures posing a risk or of an experimental nature. Surgeries or special invasive x-ray studies, for example, will require written permission. Patients or their representatives will be requested to sign a consent form describing in "lay language" the procedures that are planned and delineating the risks for those procedures. Any patient who is to be included in a research project is required, with rare exceptions, to have agreed to that participation by signing a consent form. Health care facilities have Human Studies Committees, or **Institutional Review Boards (IRBs),** that review research projects and examine the wording of consent forms to ensure they meet legal criteria and ethical guidelines.

There are also strict policies in health care facilities regarding the *confidentiality* of the medical record. Generally, legal guidelines maintain that, although the medical record itself does not belong to the patient, the *information contained* in the record does. The patient's medical file is a document belonging to the facility and should **never** be removed from the facility. Sending photocopied medical chart notes or data and even reading such information over the telephone to anyone outside of the treatment facility *requires a release of information* form signed by the patient or his or her representative. Releasing information *to the patient* in the form of copies of notes or reports also requires a release of information. Any photocopies of pages from the document that contain any type of identifying information should be limited to inhouse use, unless explicitly released by the patient or his or her representative.

XIII. BIOMEDICAL ETHICS AND ETHICAL REVIEWS

Most professions have codes of ethics that direct professional conduct. These codes are not mere guidelines, they are the ethical practices directives of the profession. Usually, adherence to both legal restrictions and codes of ethics are sufficient to make appropriate decisions in patient care, business practices, and so forth, but occasionally dilemmas arise. Consequently, most facilities have an Ethics Committee, which will include clergy members, facility attorneys, social workers, physicians, nurses, and "lay" community representatives.

XIV. NOTES

_____

_____

_____

_____

_____

_____

NOTES *(continued)*

_____

_____

_____

_____

_____

_____

_____

_____

_____

_____

_____

_____

_____

_____

_____

_____

_____

XV. REFERENCES

Avery, M., & Imdieke, B. *Medical records in ambulatory care*. Rockville, MD: Aspen.

Burke, L. J., & Murphy, J. (1988). *Charting by exception*. New York: John Wiley & Sons.

Fromberg, R. (1990). *Medical records review*. Oak Brook Terrace, IL: Joint Commission of Healthcare Organizations.

Kelly, W. J. (Ed.). (1992). *Clinical skillbuilders: Better documentation*. Springhouse, PA: Springhouse Publishers.

Lewis, L. W., & Timby, B. K. (1988). *Fundamental skills and concepts in patient care* (4th ed.). Philadelphia: J. B. Lippincott.

University Hospital Pharmacy Service. (1992). *Hospital formulary*. Little Rock: University Hospital of Arkansas.

Vogel, D., & Carter, J. E. *The effects of drugs on communication disorders*. San Diego: Singular Publishing Group, Inc.

Wolper, L. F., & Pena, J. J. (Eds.). (1987). *Health care administration*. Rockville, MD: Aspen.

CHAPTER

3

Vital Signs and the Physical Examination

This chapter outlines features of the physician's medical history interview, or "review of systems," the physical examination, and vital signs. Terminology related to the findings of the physical examination and vital signs and a list of commonly ordered laboratory tests are provided.

Temperature, pulse and respiratory rates and characteristics, weight, and blood pressure are the vital signs essential for determining an individual's state of health. Deviations from normal vital parameters usually indicate illness. The objective of this chapter is to provide terminology, abbreviations, and a description of the physical examination to aid the medical speech-language pathologist in appreciating the patient's medical status. Additional terminology and further elaboration of diseases and procedures specifically related to respiration and circulation are found in Chapter 7. The mental status and neurologic examination are described in detail in Chapter 4.

I. VITAL SIGNS AND THE PHYSICAL EXAMINATION

A. Terminology Describing Vital Signs and Physical Findings

ABO blood group incompatibility. Hemolytic anemia in which maternal antigen-antibody reaction causes fetal blood cell destruction.

Acrocyanosis. Peripheral cyanosis (blue discoloration) involving the hands, feet, and lips.

APACHES scores. Referring to a computerized evaluation system for scoring severity of illness used in the ICU to predict survival outcomes. APACHES scores take into account the acute condition and chronic illness variables. APACHES is an acronym for **A**ctivity, **P**hysiology **A**nd **C**hronic **H**ealth **E**valuation **S**ystem.

Apical rate. The number of heartbeats occurring in 1 minute as monitored by auscultation (listening by stethoscope) over the apex (upper tip) of the heart.

Apical-radial pulse rate (A/R). The pulse rate obtained by two listeners when one obtains the apical pulse rate and the other obtains the radial (wrist) pulse rate.

Apnea. A period when there is no breathing.

Apnea monitor. Device for monitoring heart beats and respiration.

Arrhythmia. An irregular pattern of heartbeats and pulse.

Arteriosclerosis. A loss of arterial wall elasticity.

Ascites. Severe effusion (collection) of serous fluid into the abdominal cavity.

Atherosclerosis. A narrowing of the inside of the arteries due to fat accumulations.

Auscultate. To examine by way of listening with a stethoscope.

Axilla. Armpit.

Axillary temperature. The measurement of body heat obtained from a thermometer placed in the axilla.

Babinski sign. Extension, instead of the normal flexion, of the large toe on stimulation of the plantar surface of the foot indicative of pyramidal disease (see Chapter 4 for further discussion of neurologic findings).

Barrel chest. Expanded chest cavity sometimes seen in association with severe pulmonary disease.

Battle's sign. Ecchymosis (swelling due to a bruise) behind the ear associated with basilar skull fractures.

Bifurcation. Forking into two divisions; Y-shaped.

Blood gases. Blood gas analysis or, more accurately, arterial blood gas (ABG) analysis provides the best means for establishing acid-base imbalances. Blood gases are abbreviated as PaO_2 (the level of dissolved arterial oxygen in the blood, with a normal range of 95–100 mm Hg); $PaCO_2$ (the level of dissolved arterial carbon dioxide in the blood, with a normal range of 35–45 mm Hg); HCO_3 (the level of bicarbonate in the blood, with a normal range of 23 to 25 mEq/L); SO_2 (the level of oxygen saturation, with a normal range of 90–100%); and pH (the acidity of the blood, with a normal range of 7.35–7.45).

Blood pressure (BP). The force of blood within a vessel or chamber.

Bounding, full pulse. A pulse that feels strong to the touch.

Bradycardia. Slow pulse; pulse that is below 60 beats per minute in adults.

Bradypnea. A slow respiratory rate.

Brazelton Neonatal Behavioral Assessment Scale (BNBAS). Tool used to assess a neonate's interactive and behavioral capabilities.

Bruit. An abnormal murmur heard on auscultation of a vessel.

Cachexia. State of malnutrition, emaciation, debilitation, and anemia. (See Chapter 5 for further discussion of malnutrition.)

Cardinal signs. Measurements of body temperature, pulse, respiration, and blood pressure; synonymous with *vital signs*.

Carina. Ridge at the bifurcation to the main bronchi from the trachea.

Cellulitis. An inflammation that has spread within tissues.

Chemosis. Connective tissue swelling near the cornea.

Chest tube. Drainage tube for removing fluid from the chest cavity after thoracentesis.

Cheyne-Stokes respirations (CSR). A gradually increasing then gradually decreasing depth of respirations, followed by a period of apnea.

Chvostek's sign. Facial spasm brought on by tapping over the facial nerve, indicative of hypocalcemic states.

Circumcision. Surgical removal of the *prepuce* (foreskin) of the glans penis.

Coloboma. Congenital incomplete development of the eye structures.

Congestive heart failure (CHF). A condition in which the heart is unable to pump adequately, thus allowing blood to accumulate in the lungs and liver.

Constant fever. Fever that is consistently elevated.

Crisis (in body temperature monitoring). A dramatic return of an elevated body temperature to normal.

Crock. Condescending reference to a patient felt to have imagined, nonphysical, insignificant, factitious illness; malingering patient.

Cullen's sign. Ecchymosis (swelling due to a bruise) in the flank associated with retroperitoneal hemorrhage.

Cyanosis. Generalized blue discoloration of the skin or mucous membranes due to a reduced hemoglobin concentration.

Diaphoresis. Profuse perspiration.

Diaphragmatic breathing. Respirations performed mainly by the diaphragm.

Diastole. The phase of a heartbeat when the ventricular heart muscle relaxes.

Diastolic pressure. The least amount of pressure detectably present in arteries when the heart muscle is in a relaxed state (the bottom number in a blood pressure recording).

Dubowitz assessment. System for examining physical and neurologic development of neonates to assess gestational age.

Ecchymosis. Extravasation of blood under the skin; swelling due to a bruise.

Epididymitis. Inflammation of the excretory duct of the testes.

Epulis. Nodular enlargement of the gums.

Erythema. A redness in areas of the skin or mucous tissues.

Erythema toxicum. A pink papular rash usually present in the first or second day of life in newborns.

Eschar. Slough of skin cells.

Etiology. Cause.

Exacerbation. Increased in severity.

Febrile. Having an elevated body temperature.

Feeble, or thready pulse. Description of an abnormal weak pulse volume to touch.

Fibrillation. Rapid, random, ineffectual, and irregular heart contractions.

Fissure. A crack split or groove in the skin or mucous membrane.

Fistula. A communication between two normally separated spaces.

Flutter. Rapid, regular but ineffectual heart contractions.

Fontanelle. "Soft spots" on the skulls of infants.

Fox's Law. A three-part maxim in which one predicts that: 10% of patients have 90% of diseases; individuals with no redeeming qualities will survive, while nice people get terminal illnesses.

Gallop. A pathologic extra heart sound, producing the auditory effect of a galloping horse. A gallop may be heard with severe myocardial disease. A *ventricular gallop* is indicative of congestive heart failure.

Gomer. A reference made to patients who refuse or are unable to comply with medical management, making medical care difficult. The term may be an acronym for "**G**et **O**ut of **M**y **E**mergency **R**oom," or may have come from the word "gummer," referring to the characteristic lesions in later-stage syphilis.

Hemangioma. Referring to a group of benign blood vessel tumors visible on the skin, including *spider hemangiomas, port wine hemangiomas,* and *strawberry hemangiomas.*

Hematemesis. Vomiting red blood or "coffee ground" appearing blood.

Hematochezia. Bright red blood coming from the rectum.

Hemodynamic parameters. *Peripheral arterial pressure, central venous pressure, pulmonary artery pressure, pulmonary capillary wedge pressure, left atrial pressure, cardiac output, cardiac index,* and *mixed venous oxygen saturation* are hemodynamic parameters commonly used to assess and monitor critically ill patients.

Hemoptysis. Coughing up blood.

Hepatojugular reflex. Referring to pressure on the liver causing an increase in cervicovenous pressure in patients having right side heart failure.

Hoffmann's sign. A neurologic sign elicited by flicking of the palm surface of the end of a finger causing the fingers to flex, indicative of pyramidal disease.

Hydroma. Fluid-filled sacs or cysts.

Hypertension. Abnormally high blood pressure.

Hyperthermia. Abnormally high body temperature.

Hyperventilation. Abnormally rapid, deep, and prolonged respirations.

Hypotension. Abnormally low blood pressure.

Hypothermia. An abnormally low body temperature.

Hypoventilation. Abnormally low amount of air entering the lungs.

Idiopathic. Disease of unknown origin.

Induration. Hardened area.

Inspiration. Inhalation.

Intermittent fever. High body temperatures broken by periods of normal or subnormal temperatures.

Intermittent pulse. Periods of normal pulse rhythm broken by periods of irregular rhythms.

Interstitial edema. Collection of fluid within spaces in an organ or within tissues.

Invasion. The point at which fever begins.

Janeway lesion. Erythematous or hemorrhagic lesion on the palm or sole seen in association with subacute bacterial endocarditis.

Jaundice. A yellow tint or coloration to the skin resulting from excessive bilirubin.

Korotkoff's sounds. The blood flow sounds heard through a stethoscope when obtaining blood pressure readings.

Kussmaul's respiration. Deep, rapid respiration seen in some cases of coma or metabolic acidosis.

Lanugo. Thin, downy fine hair covering the infant's body.

Loculated. Enlarged small space or cavity; most often refers to fluid trapped in chambers that are difficult to drain.

Lymphadenopathy. Abnormal enlargement of the lymph glands due to infection or neoplasm.

Lysis (in body temperature monitoring). The gradual return of body temperature to normal; the term *lysis* may also refer to destruction or rupture of cells. Drugs or immune responses that cause tumors to break down are said to *lyse* tumors.

Melena. Black tarry stool, usually indicative of an upper gastrointestinal hemorrhage.

Milia. Tiny, white papules usually on the chin, nose, and forehead in newborns.

Mucopurulent. Containing pus and mucus.

Murphy sign. Severe pain and inspiratory arrest occurring with palpation (touching) of the right upper quadrant, associated with cholecystitis (gall bladder inflammation).

Neonate. Infant less than 28 days old.

Neurodermatitis. A skin lesion of neurologic origin.

Neutropenia. Abnormally low number of neutrophiles (leukocytes that stain easily).

Nodal. Referring to lymph nodes.

Orchitis. Inflammation of the testes.

Orthopnea. A condition in which breathing is easier when the patient is in a sitting or standing position.

Orthostatic hypotension. A fall in blood pressure when a person sits or stands too quickly; synonymous with *postural hypotension.*

Pallor. Pale skin.

Palpate. To examine by touch or feel.

Palpitation. Awareness of one's own heartbeat.

Patent. Open.

Patent ductus arteriosus. A congenital heart defect in which a small duct between the aorta and pulmonary artery, which normally closes at the time of birth, remains open.

Pathognomonic. Specifically associated with a given disease.

Pedal circulation. Circulation in the foot.

Percussion. A physical diagnostic procedure involving short, sharp blows to a body part.

Perineum. Space between the anus and the genitalia.

Peripheral pulses. Pulse readings taken from sites distant from the heart.

Peritoneum. Membranous sac enclosing the abdominal and pelvic organs.

Petechiae. Small, pinpoint, nonraised, round purplish-red spots on the skin; small cutaneous hemorrhages.

Pleural effusion. Presence of fluid in the pleural space.

Polypharmacia. The use of multiple medications, prescribed and/or over-the-counter medications, which has caused drug interaction effects.

Premature contraction. A heart pulsation that occurs sooner than previous contractions.

Prostatism. Urinary difficulty caused by obstruction of the bladder by an enlarged prostate gland (in males).

Pulse. A circulatory wave through the blood vessels set up by a contraction of the heart.

Pulse deficit. The difference between an apical (at the apex of the heart) and radial (at the wrist) pulse rate.

Pulse pressure. The difference between diastolic and systolic blood pressure.

Pulse rate. The number of pulsations felt per minute.

Pulse rhythm. The pattern of pulsations and pauses.

Pyrexia. Fever.

Quincke's sign. Alternating blushing and blanching of the fingernail following compression, seen in aortic regurgitation.

Rales. Crackling sounds heard with a stethoscope indicative of fluid in the respiratory passages.

Raynaud's phenomenon. Short episodes of pallor (whitening) followed by cyanosis (bluing) then erythema (reddening) associated with numbness in the fingers and toes due to temporary constriction of the arterioles in the skin.

Remittent fever. A fever that fluctuates but does not come within the normal range.

Rhonchus. A low-pitched breath sound heard on auscultation indicating narrowed respiratory passages.

Rigors. Chills.

Rub. The scratchy, grating sound made when two internal surfaces rub against one another.

Sanguinous. Containing blood.

Sepsis. When infection is present; a patient is said to be *septic* when he or she has an infection.

Serum. The clear, noncellular component of blood after removal of the clotting proteins.

Serum enzyme tests. Tests for enzymes released in the blood following myocardial infarction; these tests include *creatine kinase* (CK), *lactic dehydrogenase* (LD), and *aspartate aminotransferase* (AST). The latter is also known as the *serum glutamic-oxaloacetic transaminase test* (SGOT).

Sign. An observation made by an examiner.

Sinus arrhythmia. An irregular pulse rhythm characterized by slowing on exhalation and increasing on inhalation.

Smith's minor anomalies. Physical abnormalities (such as abnormal dermal ridges) in newborns.

Sphygmomanometer. An instrument used to measure blood pressure.

Stertorous respirations. Noisy breathing; snoring.

Stethoscope. An instrument used to carry sounds from the body to the ear of an examiner.

Stool. Feces.

Stridor. Noisy breathing due to an obstruction in the upper (laryngeal) airway.

Symptom. An observation felt or described by the patient.

Systole. The phase in which the ventricular heart muscle is contracting.

Systolic pressure. The maximum pressure exerted on arterial walls when the ventricle is contracting (the top number in a blood pressure recording).

Tachycardia. A rapid heart rate.

Tachypnea. A rapid respiratory rate.

Tampanade (cardiac). Accumulation of excessive fluid in the pericardium (flbrous sac that surrounds the heart).

Telangiectasias. Hemangiomas that are flat, red, localized areas of capillary dilation.

Teratology of Fallot. A congenital malformation of the heart with the following distinct defects: *pulmonary artery stenosis, ventricular septal defect, shift of the aorta to the right,* and *hypertrophy of the right ventricle.*

Thoracic respiration. Using primarily the thoracic and intercostal muscles for respiration.

Thrill. A vibration perceptible on palpation (touch) due to surfaces rubbing together, or to blood flow; for example, a thrill of the chest wall can be felt if there is friction between surfaces of the pericardium (fibrous sac surrounding the heart).

Tissue respiration, internal respiration. The exchange of oxygen and carbon dioxide between the body and blood cells.

Trousseau's sign. Carpal spasm produced when inflating the blood pressure cuff around the arm to a pressure above the systolic pressure. Trousseau's sign may indicate hypocalcemia.

Very low birth weight. Neonate weight between 500–1,500 grams.

Vital signs (VS), cardinal signs (CS). Measurements of body temperature, weight, pulse rate, blood pressure, and respiratory rate.

B. Abbreviations Used in Vital Signs Descriptions and the Physical Examination

AA. Aortic aneurysm

AAA. Abdominal aortic aneurysm

AAO. Awake, alert, and oriented

AAS. Acute abdominal series

A&B. Apnea and bradycardia

ABGs. Arterial blood gases

AXR. Abdominal X ray

ACG. Angiocardiography

ACLS. Advanced cardiac life support

AD. Right ear; *auris dexter*

AE (BE). Above the elbow (below the elbow)

AEIOU TIPS. Mnemonic for Alcohol, Encephalopathy, Insulin, Opiates, Uremia, Trauma, Infection, Psychiatric, Syncope (in coma diagnosis)

AF. Afebrile, aortofemoral, or atrial fibrillation

AFB. Acid fast bacilli

AFP. Alpha fetoprotein

AFVSS. Afebrile and vital signs are stable

AI. Aortic insufficiency

AIF. Aorto-ileo femoral (graft)

AK (BK). Above the knee (below the knee)

AKA (BKA). Above the knee amputation (below the knee amputation)

AMA. Against medical advice

AMI. Acute myocardial infarction

AN. Admitting note

ante. Before

AO. Admitting office

A & O. Alert and oriented

AOB. Alcohol on breath

AODM. Adult onset diabetes mellitus

AOR. At own risk

A-P. Anterior-posterior

A & P. Auscultation and percussion

ARD. Acute respiratory disease

ARDS. Adult respiratory distress syndrome

ARF. Acute renal failure

AS. Aortic stenosis, or left ear (*auris sinister*)

ASA. Aspirin

ASAP. As soon as possible

ASD. Atrial septal defect

ASH. Asymmetrical septal hypertrophy, synonymous with the older term idiopathic hypertrophic subaortic stenosis (IHSS)

ASHD. Arteriosclerotic heart disease

AST. Aspartate aminotransferase

ATC. Around the clock

AV. Atrioventricular

AVSS. Afebrile and vital signs are stable

A & W. Alive and well

AWOL. Absent without leave

BAL. Blood alcohol level

BBB. Bundle branch block

BM. Bowel movement, bone marrow

BM/BF. Black male/ black female

BMT. Bone marrow transplant

BOT. Base of tongue

BP. Blood pressure

BPH. Benign prostate hypertrophy

BPM. Beats per minute

BRB. Bright red blood

BRBPR. Bright red blood per rectum

BS. Breath sounds, bowel sounds, blood sugar

BUN. Blood, urea, nitrogen

BW. Birth weight

BX. Biopsy

CA. Cancer, carcinoma

CABG. Coronary artery bypass graft

CAD. Coronary artery disease

CAN. Cord around neck

Cath. Catheter

CBC. Complete blood count

CBG. Capillary blood gases

CC. Chief complaint

cc. Cubic centimeter

CF. Cystic fibrosis

CFx. Compound fracture

Ch. Chloride

CHF. Congestive heart failure

CHI. Closed head injury

CK. Creatine kinase

CN. Cranial nerve

CO. Cardiac output

c/o. Complains of

COAD. Chronic obstructive airway disease

COLD. Chronic obstructive lung disease

COPD. Chronic obstructive pulmonary disease

CP. Chest pain, or cerebral palsy

CPK, CK, CPMB. Creatine phosphokinase, creatinine kinase, creatine phosphokinase-myocardial band

CPR. Cardiopulmonary resuscitation

Cr. Cl. Creatinine clearance

C-R. Crown-to-rump (newborn measurement)

CRF. Chronic respiratory failure, or chronic renal failure

Crit. Hematocrit

CSF. Cerebrospinal fluid

CT; CAT. Computed tomogram; computed axial tomography

CT w C. Computed tomogram with contrast

CTA. (Lungs) clear to auscultation

CVA. Cerebrovascular accident

CVD. Cerebrovascular disease

CVL. Central venous line

CVP. Central venous pressure

c/w. Consistent with

CXR. Chest X ray

DAT. Diet as tolerated

DC. Discontinue

D/C. Discharge (from the facility)

DD. Developmental delay

DDx. Differential diagnosis

Decub. Decubitus

DI. Diabetes insipidus

DIC. Disseminated intravascular coagulation

DJD. Degenerative joint disease

DM. Diastolic murmur; diabetes mellitus

DM-I. Diabetes mellitus Type I

DM-II. Diabetes mellitus Type II

DMFT. Decayed, missing, and filled teeth

DNR. Do not resuscitate (per family's or patient's request)

DNT. Did not test

DOB. Date of birth

DOE. Dyspnea on exertion

DP. *Dorsalis pedis*

DPT. Diphtheria, pertussis, tetanus

DTRs. Deep tendon reflexes

DTs. *Delirium tremens*

DU. Diagnosis unknown

D & V. Diarrhea and vomiting

DVTs. Deep vein thromboses

D/W. Discuss with

Dx. Diagnosis

EAHF. Eczema, asthma, hay fever

EBL. Estimated blood loss

EC-ASA. Enteric coated aspirin

ECC. Extracorporeal circulation

ECG. Electrocardiogram

Edent. Edentulous

EKG. Electrocardiogram

EMT. Emergency medical technologist

EMV. Eyes, motor, verbal (Glasgow Coma Scale)

eod. Every other day

EOM. Extraocular movements/ muscles

ERV. Expiratory respiration volume

ET. Endotracheal

ETC. Emergency treatment completed

ETOH. Ethanol (alcohol)

FB. Foreign body

FBS. Fasting blood sugar

FD. Forceps delivery

Fem-pop. Femoral-popliteal

FEV. Forced expired volume

FHR. Fetal heart rate

FHS. Fetal heart sounds

FLK. Funny looking kid

FME. Full mouth extraction

FOB. Fecal occult blood

FOM. Floor of mouth

FP. Floor procedure (done at bedside), full plate (denture)

FRC. Functional residual capacity

FTA-ABS. Fluorescent treponemal antibody-absorbed

FTR. Failed to report

FTT. Failure to thrive

F/U. Follow up

FUO. Fever of unknown/ undetermined origin

Fx. Fracture

G. Gravida

GA. Gestational age.

G1, G2, G3, G4, G5, G6. Grade one, two, etc. (extra heart sounds)

Grade I, II, III, etc. Grade one, two, etc. (tumor histologic grades)

GC. *Gonococcus* (gonorrhea)

G.I. Gastrointestinal

G.O.K. God only knows

G.O.R.K. God only really knows

GSW. Gunshot wound

gt. Drops ("gutta")

GU. Genitourinary

HA. Headache

HAA. Hepatitis associated antigen

HAV. Hepatitis A virus

HBc. Hepatitis B core (antigen)

HBeAg. Hepatitis B e antigen

HBsAg. Hepatitis B surface antigen

HCO$_3$. Bicarbonate

HCT. Hematocrit

HD. Hospital day

HDL. High density lipoprotein

HEENT. Head, eyes, ears, nose, throat

HepB. Hepatitis B.

Hgb. Hemoglobin

HIV. Human immunodeficiency virus

HJR. Hepatojugular reflex

H & L. Heart and lungs

HO. History of

HOB. Head of bed

HPF. High power field

HPN, HPT. Hypertension(ive)

HR. Heart rate

HSV. Herpes simplex virus

Ht. Height

HTLV-III. Human lymphotropic virus, type III (AIDS agent, HIV)

HTN, HPT; HBP. Hypertension(ive); high blood pressure

Hx. History

Hyperal. Hyperalimentation

I & O. Intake and output

I.A.O. Immediately after onset

IDDM. Insulin dependent diabetes mellitus

IPPB. Intermittent positive pressure breathing

IR. Inspiratory reserve

IRDM. Insulin resistant diabetes mellitus

IRDS. Infant respiratory distress syndrome

IRV. Inspiratory reserve volume

IV. Intravenous

IVC. Intravenous cholangiogram

IVP. Intravenous pyelogram

JODM. Juvenile onset diabetes mellitus

K. Potassium

KOR. Keep open rate

K.U.B. Kidneys, urethra, bladder

LA. Left atrium

LAG. Large for gestational age

LBBB. Left bundle branch block

LD. Lactic dehydrogenase

LDL. Low density lipoprotein

LE. Lupus erythematosus

LFTs. Liver function tests

L (R) LE. Left (right) lower extremity

L (R) LL. Left (right) lower lobe

L (R) LQ. Left (right) lower quadrant

LOC. Loss of consciousness

L (R) UE. Left (right) upper extremity

L (R) UL. Left (right) upper lobe

L (R) UQ. Left (right) upper quadrant

LV. Left ventricle

MAS. Meconium aspiration syndrome

M1, M2. Mitral valve sounds

MBC. Minimum bacterial concentration

MCH. Mean cell hemoglobin

MCHC. Mean cell hemoglobin concentration

MCV. Mean cell volume

Mets. Metastases

MFC. Measure for coffin

MHB. Maximal hospital benefits

MI. Myocardial infarction

MIC. Minimum inhibiting concentration

mL. Milliliter

MODY. Maturity onset diabetes of youth

MOSF. Multiple organ systems failure

M & R. Measure and record

MRGT. Murmur, rub, gallop, thrill

MRSA. Methicillin resistant *Staphylococcus aureus*

MS. Mitral stenosis, mental status, medical student, multiple sclerosis

MVA. Motor vehicle accident

MVC, MCH, MCHC. Mean cell volume, mean cellular hemoglobin, mean cellular hemoglobin concentration

MVit. Multivitamin

MVP. Mitral valve prolapse

Nl. Normal

Na. Sodium

NAD. No acute distress; no active disease

N.A.N.D.A. North American Nursing Diagnosis Association

NBC. Non bed care

NED. No evidence (of recurrent) disease

NIDDM. Non-insulin dependent diabetes mellitus

NKA. No known allergies

NKDA. No known drug allergies

NOK. Next of kin

NPD. No pathologic diagnosis

NPO. Nothing by mouth (*nil per os*)

NSAID. Nonsteroidal anti-inflammatory drugs

NT/ND. Nontender/ nondistended (abdomen)

NTG. Nitroglycerin

N & V. Nausea and vomiting

OD. Officer of the day, overdose, right eye (*oculus dexter*)

OM. Otitis media

OOB. Out of bed

O & E. Observation and examination

O×3. Oriented times 3

OS. Left eye (*oculus sinister*)

OU. Both eyes

p. Post, para per

PaCO₂. Arterial carbon dioxide (blood gases)

PaO₂. Arterial oxygen (blood gases)

PAT. Paroxysmal atrial tachycardia

PB. Piggy back

PDx. Primary diagnosis

PEEP. Positive end expiratory pressure

PEERLA. Pupils are equal (in size) and equally reactive to light and accommodation.

PERLA. Pupils are equal and reactive to light and accommodation.

PERRLDAC. Pupils are equal, round, and reactive to light directly and accommodation consensually.

PHC. Post hospital care

PI. Present illness

PKU. Phenylketonuria

PMH. Past medical history

p MN. After (post) midnight

P-MVA. Pedestrian in a motor vehicle accident

PND. Postnasal drip, paroxysmal nocturnal dyspnea

POC. Plan of care

POD. Post operation (surgical) day

PP. Partial plate (denture), pulsus paradoxus, or postprandial

P & PD. Percussion and postural drainage

PPD. Purified protein derivative

ppd. Packs (of cigarettes) per day

PRN. As needed (*pro re nata*)

Pr. Tx. Prior treatment (or therapy)

PSH. Past surgical history

P.Sz. Paranoid schizophrenia

Pt. Patient

PTA. Prior to admission

PTH. Parathyroid hormone

PUD. Peptic ulcer disease

PVC. Premature ventricular contraction

PVD. Peripheral vascular disease

Px. Physical

Q. Each (*quaque*)

q/s. Each shift

QNS. Quantity not sufficient

RA. Right atrium

RBBB. Right bundle branch block

RBC. Red blood cell, red blood count

REP. Renal electrolyte profile

RIND. Resolving ischemic neurologic deficit

RLW. Routine lab work

RO. Renew order

R/O. Rule out

ROP. Retinopathy of prematurity

ROS. Review of systems

RRR. Regular rate and rhythm (heart)

RTC. Return to clinic

RV. Right ventricle, residual volume

Rx. Recipe, prescription

Rx'd. Prescribed

S1, S2, S3. Sound one, two, etc. (heart sounds)

SA. Sinoatrial

SBE. Subacute bacterial endocarditis

SBFT. Small bowel follow through

SCD. Sudden cardiac death

SDx. Secondary diagnosis

SG. Swan-Ganz

SGA. Small for gestational age

SGOT. Serum glutamic-oxaloacetic transaminase

SIDS. Sudden infant death syndrome

sl. Sublingual

SMA. Sequential multiple analysis

SO. Significant other

SO$_2$. Oxygen saturation

SOB. Shortness of breath; short of breath

SOC. Start of care

S/P. Status post

Ss. Half

SS. Soap suds, Social Security

Stat. Immediately (*statim*)

STD. Sexually transmitted disease

Sub ling. Sublingual

Sub q. Subcutaneous

SVT. Sinoventricular tachycardia

Sz. Seizure

T & A. Tonsillectomy and adenoidectomy

TAA. To all areas

TB, LC. Term birth, living child

TBSB. Total body surface burn

TENS. Transcutaneous electrical nerve stimulator

TIA. Transient ischemic attack

TIBC. Total iron binding capacity

TKO. To keep open

TM. Tympanic membrane

TNJ. Tongue, neck, jaw

T/O. Telephone order

TPO. Time postonset

TPR. Temperature, pulse, respiration

TSH. Thyroid secreting hormone

TTN. Transient tachypnea of the newborn

TURB. Transurethral resection of the bladder

TURP. Transurethral resection of the prostate

TV. Tidal volume

Tx. Treatment, therapy, traction

U. Units (of)

UA. Urine analysis, urinalysis

UCD. Usual childhood diseases

UFN. Until further notice

USOH. Usual state of health

VC. Vital capacity

VDRL. Venereal Disease Research Laboratory

VF. Visual field

Viz. Namely

VLDL. Very low density lipoproteins

Vol. Volume

V/O. Verbal order, or voice order

VS. Vital signs

VSD. Ventricular septal defect

V-tach. Ventricular tachycardia

WBC. White blood count, or white blood cell

WC. Wheelchair

WD. Well-developed

Wk. Week

WN. Well-nourished

WM/WF. White male/white female

WNL. Within normal limits

Wt. Weight

W/U. Work up

×. Times (multiplied by)

XRT. X-ray therapy

XX. Female chromosomes

XY. Male chromosomes

YO. Years old

II. MEDICAL HISTORY, REVIEW OF SYSTEMS, AND PHYSICAL EXAMINATION

When patients are admitted to the hospital they normally undergo a thorough H & P, or history, which includes a review of systems (ROS) and physical examination.

The medical history interview reviews the following areas:

- *Chief Complaint* (CC) (a statement in the patient's own words describing the current problem);
- *History of the Present Illness* (HPI);
- *Past Medical History* (PMH);
- *Family Medical History* (FMH); and the
- *Psychosocial History.*

A. Review of Systems

After the medical history has been taken, the physician interviews the patiet with questions about various organ systems. This review of systems normally follows a standard interview format similar to that outlined below:

1. **General.** Queries about any recent weight gain or loss, complaints of fatigue, fever, chills, nocturnal sweats, or appetite changes.

2. **Skin.** Queries about any rashes, pruritus, lesions, or bruising noted by the patient.

3. **Head.** Queries regarding trauma, headache, tenderness, or dizziness.

4. **Eyes, ears, nose, and throat.** Queries regarding vision and hearing changes, tinnitus, pain, discharge, vertigo; sinus problems, polyps; teeth, tongue, gums, dentures, hoarseness, or sore throat.

5. **Respiratory.** Queries regarding cough, dyspnea, or history of pulmonary problems.

6. **Cardiovascular.** Queries regarding chest pain, dyspnea on exertion, claudication (pain when walking), and edema.

7. **Gastrointestinal (GI).** Queries regarding dysphagia, heartburn, nausea, vomiting, hematemesis, indigestion, diarrhea, abdominal pain, melena, red blood in the stool, hemorrhoids, change in stool appearance, and jaundice.

8. **Genitourinary (G.U.).** Queries regarding urinary frequency, urgency, hesitancy, hematuria, dysuria, nocturia, incontinence, discharge, or sexually transmitted diseases.

9. **Gynecological.** Queries regarding birth and deliveries, including gravida, abortions, age of menarche, dysmenorrhea, and forms of contraception.

10. **Endocrine.** Queries regarding polyuria, polydipsia, polyphagia, temperature intolerance, hormone therapy, or changes in skin or hair.

11. **Musculo-skeletal.** Queries regarding arthritis, trauma, and bony deformities.

12. **Hematologic.** Queries regarding anemia, bleeding tendency, easy bruising, or lymphadenopathy.

13. **Neuropsychiatric.** Queries regarding seizures, memory problems, syncope, weakness, dyscoordination, problems with mood, sleep disorders, emotional problems, or substance abuses.

B. Physical Examination

Following the medical history and the review of systems, the physician's physical examination will follow a format similar to the following for infants, children, and adults. Abdominal quadrants and region referents are illustrated in Figure 3–1.

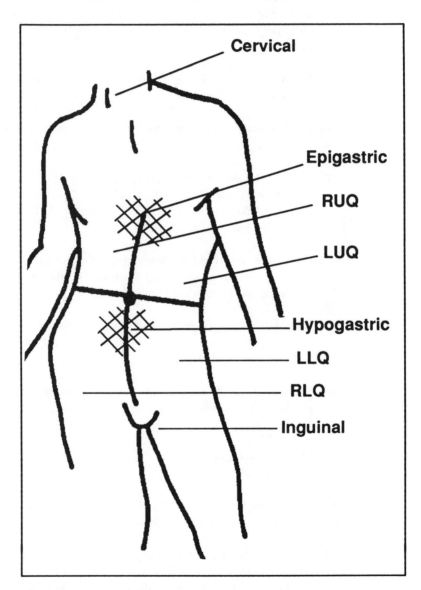

Figure 3–1. Body site referents used in the physical examination

1. **General.** Race, sex, development, mood and mental status, remarkable characteristics, and state of distress.

2. **Vital signs.** Temperature, pulse, respirations, blood pressure, weight, and height.

3. **Skin.** Rashes, scars, moles, hair distribution and pattern, and eruptions.

4. **Nodes.** Location of any enlarged nodes (cervical, supraclavicular, axillary, inguinal) and their size, mobility, and tenderness.

5. **Head, Eyes, Ears, Nose, and Throat.** *Head*—Fontanel suture line in pediatric patients, size, shape, tenderness, trauma, and bruits (pronounced "brew-eez," referring to sounds or murmurs in blood flow with auscultation of head and neck vessels). *Eyes*—Pupil size, relative shape of the pupils of both eyes, reactivity to light and accommodation, extraocular muscular movements, acuity, fields, conjunctive, sclera, eyelids, enophthalmos/exophthalmos positioning of the eyeball, and fundus (disc color, size, margins, cupping, venous patterns, and pulses). *Ears*—Hearing, discharge, tinnitus, external auditory canal, tympanic membrane appearance, position of the ears and appearance. *Nose*—Symmetry, tenderness, lesions, obstructions. *Throat*—Lips, teeth, gums, tongue, tonsils, and pharynx; noting the appearance, swelling, lesions, symmetry, shape of the palatal vault, and clefts.

6. **Neck.** Range of motion, jugular venous distention (JVD), tenderness, nodes, masses, thyroid, larynx (vocal fold movement), bruits (see above), and hepatojugular reflex.

7. **Chest.** Shape, movement during respiration, and breath sounds.

8. **Heart.** Regularity of rate and rhythm, thrill, auscultation at the apex, lower sternal border, right and left second intercostal spaces (listening for murmurs, rubs, gallops, and clicks).

9. **Breast.** Surgeries, shape, nipple, discharge, masses, dimpling, or tenderness.

10. **Abdomen.** Shape (flat, distended, obese, scaphoid), scars, bowel sounds, tenderness, masses, guarding, rebound, span of the liver, tenderness, and adenopathy.

11. **Genitals (male) and pelvic (female).** Swelling, lesions, drainage, or masses.

12. **Rectum.** Fissures, skin tags, hemorrhoids, sphincter tone, masses, prostate, presence of stool, and presence of occult (hidden) blood.

13. **Extremities.** Range of motion, deformities, joint tenderness or swelling, amputations, hair pattern, pulses, cyanosis, clubbing, and edema.

14. **Neurologic and mental status examination.** Orientation, memory, speech and language, cranial nerves, motor functions of extremities, cerebellar functions, sensory functions, reflexes, and neurologic tests and studies. (See Chapter 4 for further information on neurologic examinations.)

C. Characteristics of Masses

Abnormal body masses are described by their *mobility* (fixed or mobile); *shape* (irregular, round, tubular, ovoid); *consistency* (nodular, granular, spongy, hard, or edematous); *tenderness*; and *size* (indicated in centimeters).

D. Disease Staging

Some diseases, particularly forms of cancer, are ranked by the stages of the disease. These are a part of the taxonomy of medical conditions and are especially important when clinical treatment trials are tested and outcomes compared. In staging some types of cancer (see Chapter 11, TNM system) disease staging is included in the description, but other disorders (diabetes, AIDS, appendicitis) also will be "staged" as follows: *Stage I*, No complications; *Stage 2*, Local complications limited to a single organ or system; and *Stage 3*, Multiple site involvement or systemic involvement and complications.

III. COMMONLY ORDERED TESTS, STUDIES, AND PROCEDURES

The physical examination will provide indicators as to which laboratory tests should be ordered. This section summarizes tests commonly ordered as part of the diagnostic workup or as tests for changes in medical status. Typically, normal laboratory values and the range for normal values are printed on the patient's laboratory report data form. **Laboratory data should be compared to the range of values that are normal for the reporting laboratory.** Acceptable levels for "normal" can be adjusted according to several factors, such as the patient's sex, age, body mass, medications taken, and existing diseases. The clinical significance of findings outside of the normal range is interpreted by the patient's physician. Some laboratory tests are affected by factors that need to be considered in their interpretation, such as recent immunizations, current drugs, the foods recently ingested, the age of the patient, and pregnancy status. Figure 2–1, in the previous chapter, illustrates one of the shorthand methods used to record laboratory values in the patient's progress notes (refer to the normal values listed in Appendix C).

Standard laboratory tests include a **complete blood count** (white blood count, hemoglobin, hematocrit, platelets, types of cells, and the volume and concentration of hemoglobin), **electrolytes** (sodium, chloride, potassium, and bicarbonate ratios), and a **standard blood chemistry panel**, which provides an analysis of renal function. The latter series may or may not include a creatinine analysis and may be labeled in various ways depending on the facility and the laboratory it uses. Typically, renal electrolyte findings are profiled as: ASTRA-7, *sequential medical analysis* (SMA-6), or *renal electrolyte profile* (refer to Figure 2–1 on page 49).

A. Laboratory Tests and Assays and What They Diagnose

Acid-fast bacilli stain (AFB smear). Test for microorganisms, specifically mycobacterium, of which tuberculosis is the most common.

Acid phosphatase. Indicators for carcinoma of the prostate.

ACTH (adrenocorticotrophic hormone). Adrenal gland function, pituitary insufficiency.

Albumin. Nutritional status, renal disease, Hodgkin's disease, leukemia, alcoholic cirrhosis, inflammatory bowel disease, hyperthyroidism, collagen disease.

Aldosterone. Adrenal and pituitary function.

Alkaline phosphatase. Hyperparathyroidism, hyperthyroidism, bone tumors, osteomalacia, liver disease, malnutrition, excessive ingestion of vitamin D.

Alpha-fetoprotein (AFP). Spina bifida (when found in the mother's serum), testicular tumor, hepatoma.

Ammonia. Reye's syndrome, liver disease.

Amylase. Pancreatitis or duct obstruction, alcohol ingestion, liver damage, renal disease, mumps, parotiditis, gall bladder disease, peptic ulcers, intestinal obstruction, mesenteric thrombosis.

Antinuclear antibody (ANA). Systemic lupus, lupus-like syndromes, scleroderma, rheumatoid arthritis.

Antistreptolysin O. Streptococcal infections, rheumatoid arthritis.

Aspartate aminotransferase (AST). Myocardial infarction; see SGOT.

B12. Polycythemia rubra vera, malabsorption, pregnancy, pernicious anemia, leukemia.

Bilirubin. Liver damage, obstruction, or dysfunction; biliary obstruction; hemolytic anemia; jaundice of the newborn.

Bleeding time. Thrombocytopenia, defective platelet function in aspirin therapy.

Blood serum test. Analysis of certain proteins to determine if cancer synthesis is present.

Blood urea clearance. Renal function.

Blood urea nitrogen (BUN). Renal failure, decreased renal profusion due to congestive heart failure and other causes, starvation, drugs, overhydration or dehydration.

C. Peptide. Diabetes.

Calcitonin. Anemia, chronic renal sufficiency, carcinoma of the thyroid.

Carbon dioxide, bicarbonate. Acidosis and ketoacidosis (from various causes), dehydration, severe diarrhea, drugs, adrenal insufficiency, starvation.

Carboxyhemoglobin. Smoke or exhaust exposure.

Catecholamines. Neural crest tumors, pheochromocytoma.

Cholesterol. Hypercholesterolemia, biliary obstruction, nephrosis, hypothyroidism, diabetes, malnutrition, anemia, steroid therapy.

Cold agglutinins. Atypical pneumonia, cirrhosis, infections.

Complement C3. Rheumatoid arthritis, rheumatoid fever, systemic lupus, glomerulonephritis, sepsis, subacute bacterial endocarditis, hepatitis.

Complement C4. Rheumatoid arthritis, systemic lupus, hepatitis, cirrhosis, glomerulonephritis.

Complete Blood Count (CBC). A complete blood count includes *a white cell count, red cell count, hemoglobin, hematocrit, mean corpuscular hemoglobin* (MCH), *mean corpuscular hemoglobin concentration, mean corpuscular volume* (MCV), and *red cell distribution width* (RDW). These studies are made as a part of routine assessment, for diagnostic assessment with multiple medical conditions, and prior to surgeries.

Coombs' test. Incompatible blood transfusion.

Cortisol. Adrenal adenoma, adrenal carcinoma, Cushing's disease, ACTH-producing tumor, pituitary insufficiency.

Creatine phosphokinase (CPK, CK, CKMB). Muscle damage due to acute myocardial infarction, myocarditis, muscular dystrophy trauma; brain trauma, rhabdomyolysis, hypothyroidism.

Enzyme-linked immunosorbent assay (ELISA). Screening assay for Human Immunodeficiency Virus (HIV) and other viruses; this assay is confirmed by a Western Blot Test.

Ferritin. Iron deficiency.

Fibrin degradation products (FDP). Deep vein thrombosis, pulmonary embolism, myocardial infarction.

Fibrinogen. Sepsis, amniotic fluid embolism, surgery, hematological conditions, snake bite, acute severe bleeding, burns.

Fluorescent treponema antibody absorbed (FTA-ABS). Syphilis.

Fungal serologies. Antibodies to various fungi.

Gastrin. Pyloric stenosis, pernicious anemia, atrophic gastritis, renal insufficiency, ulcerative colitis.

Glucose, glucose tolerance test. Diabetes mellitus, Cushing's syndrome, pancreatitis, glucagonoma and other pancreatic tumors, liver disease, endocrine disorders, hypothyroidism, hypopituitarism, malnutrition, sepsis, infant born to a diabetic mother, prematurity, and other inborn metabolic disorders.

Glycosolated hemoglobin. Diabetes mellitus, renal failure.

Gonococcal (GC) cultures. Gonorrhea.

Gram stains. Tests for types of bacterial growth.

Guiac test. Blood in the feces, gastrointestinal bleeding.

Haptoglobin. Liver disease.

Hemoccult. Gastrointestinal bleeding.

Hemogram. Referring to an order for a standard blood chemistry study.

Hepatitis HBsAG, anti-HBc, anti-Hbclgm, HbeAg, anti-HBe, anti-HBs, anti-HAV, anti-HAV IgM. Tests for antigens and antibodies to hepatitis viri.

High density lipoprotein-cholesterol (HDL). Obesity, diabetes, liver disease, uremia, assessment for coronary artery disease risks.

HIV. Human Immunodeficiency Virus.

Iron, iron-binding capacity (TIBC). Anemia, hemochromatosis.

Kline test. Blood test for syphilis.

Lactate dehydrogenase (LDH). Acute myocardial infarction, anemia, malignant tumors, pulmonary embolus, renal infarction, muscle injury, liver disease.

Lactic acid. Hypoxia, hemorrhage, shock, cirrhosis, carcinoma, and sepsis.

Lee-White clotting time. Plasma clotting factor deficiency, heparin therapy.

Leukocyte alkaline phosphatase (LAP) score. Leukemia, nephrotic syndrome, acute inflammation, Hodgkin's disease.

Lipase. Acute pancreatitis or duct obstruction, fat embolus syndrome.

Low density lipoprotein-cholesterol (LDL). Endocrine disease (hypothyroidism, diabetes), excessive saturated fats in the diet, biliary cirrhosis, liver disease, malabsorption, hyperlipoproteinemia.

Lupus erythematosus (LE) preparation. Systemic lupus erythematosus, rheumatoid arthritis, scleroderma.

Magnesium. Renal failure, severe dehydration, lithium intoxication, hypo- or hyperthyroidism, malabsorption, alcoholism, hypophosphatemia, respiratory or metabolic acidosis, response to chronic dialysis or diuretic use, response to hyperalimentation or nasogastric suctioning, acute pancreatitis.

Mantoux. Skin test for detecting tuberculosis exposure.

Methylene blue test. Test for kidney function in which an injection of blue dye is expected to appear in the urine after 30 minutes, if the kidneys are functioning normally.

Monospot. Lymphoma, viral hepatitis, rheumatoid arthritis, mononucleosis.

Myoglobin (urine analysis). Acute myocardial infarction, severe hyperthermia, electrical burns, crushing injury, severe muscle injury.

5' Nucleotidase. Liver disease.

Parathyroid hormone (PTH). Hyper- or hypoparathyroidism.

Partial thromboplastin time (PTT). Heparin therapy, defect in blood clotting mechanisms.

Phosphorus. Hyper- or hypoparathyroidism, renal failure, alcoholism, diabetes, response to hyperalimentation, gout, vitamin D deficiency, acidosis, alkalosis, response to diuretics, hypokalemia, hypomagnesemia.

Prostate-specific antigen (PSA). Prostate cancer.

Protein electrophoresis. Nutritional disorders, liver disease, collagen disease, hypo- or macroglobulinemia, alpha-1 antitrypsin deficiency, cancer.

Prothrombin time (PT). Blood clotting mechanisms.

Retinol-binding protein (RBP). Malnutrition, vitamin A deficiency, chronic liver disease.

Rheumatoid factor. Rheumatoid arthritis, systemic lupus erythematosus, chronic inflammation, subacute bacterial endocarditis, pulmonary disease, syphilis.

Sedimentation rate (ESR). Infections, inflammation, rheumatic fever, myocardial infarction, neoplasm.

Serum calcium. Hyper- or hypothyroidism and hyper-/hypoparathyroidism, metastatic bone tumors, response to thiazides, Paget's disease, chronic renal failure, acute pancreatitis, insufficient vitamin D, hypomagnesemia.

Serum chloride. Diabetes with ketoacidosis, renal disease with sodium loss, excessive vomiting, diarrhea, renal tubular acidosis, response to hyperalimentation.

Serum creatinine. Renal failure, acromegaly and gigantism, loss of muscle mass.

Serum foliate. Malabsorption, malnutrition, neoplasm, anemia.

Serum gamma-glutamyl transpeptidase (SGGT). Liver disease, pancreatitis.

Serum glutamic-oxaloacetic transaminase (SGOT). Acute myocardial infarction, brain damage, liver disease, muscle trauma, pancreatitis, burns, renal failure, Reye's syndrome, burns, severe diabetes with ketoacidosis. This test is now referred to as aspartate aminotransferase (AST).

Serum glutamic-pyruvic transaminase (SGPT). Liver disease, pancreatitis.

Serum osmality. Alcohol ingestion, hyperglycemia, response to mannitol, response to diuretics, poor fluid balance management, disorders of sodium and water balance.

Serum potassium. Renal failure, acidosis, massive tissue damage, vomiting, nasogastric suctioning, diarrhea, metabolic alkalosis.

Serum protein. Myeloma, macroglobulinemia, hypergammaglobulinemia after an acute inflammatory process, sarcoidosis, malnutrition, inflammatory bowel disease, leukemia, Hodgkin's disease.

Serum sodium. Nephrotic syndrome, congestive heart failure, cirrhosis, renal failure, response to antidiuretic hormone, response to mannitol, excessive sweating, Cushing's syndrome, vomiting, diarrhea, pancreatitis, hyperlipidemia, hyperglycemia, multiple myeloma.

Sputum cytology. Abnormal (cancerous) cells in the bronchi and lungs.

Stool cultures. Infections, Crohn's disease, G.I. hemorrhages, ulcerative colitis, tuberculosis.

Sweat chloride. Cystic fibrosis.

T3 triiodothyronine (RIA). Thyroid functions.

T3 resin uptake (RU). Thyroid functions.

T4 total thyroxine. Thyroid functions.

Thrombin time. Response to heparin therapy, fibrinogen deficiency.

Thyroglobulin. Grave's disease, thyroid carcinomas, nontoxic goiter, testosterone, steroids.

Torch battery. Herpes viruses, cytomegalovirus, rubella, toxoplasmosis.

Transferrin. Iron deficiency, poor nutritional status, acute inflammation, liver disease.

Thyroid-stimulating hormone (TSH). Thyroid functions.

Uric acid. Gout, renal failure, response to diuretics, anemia, toxemia, hypothyroidism, lactic acidosis, Wilson's disease.

Urinalysis (UA) studies. The urinalysis studies commonly made include an examination of the appearance, specific gravity, and pH of the urine and tests for bilirubin, blood, acetone, glucose, protein, nitrite, leukocyte esterase, urobilinogen, epithelial cells, hyaline cases, bacteria, and crystals. Like the CBC, the UA is done for routine and preoperative assessments and as a part of the diagnostic workup with multiple medical conditions. The UA is used to detect the presence of urinary tract infections, renal disease, drugs, and diabetes. Creatinine clearance and urine output are indicators of renal disease and fluid imbalances.

Venereal Disease Research Laboratory (VDRL) screen. Syphilis.

Viral cultures and serology. Viral infections (such as herpes simplex).

Wayson stain. Bacterial infections.

Western blot analysis for AIDS. Confirmation following positive antigens for Acquired Immune Deficiency Syndrome.

B. Commonly Ordered Diagnostic Procedures

This section lists some of the commonly ordered special examinations and procedures. (Also see Chapter 4 for descriptions of neurologic studies, Chapter 5 for procedures related to nutrition and hydration, and Chapter 8 for more detailed descriptions of x-ray and other imaging studies.)

Angiography. Radiologic examination of blood vessels.

Barium enema. A lower G.I. x-ray study using both air and barium (double contrast) introduced through an enema to examine for obstructions, growths, and abnormalities on the surface of the lower intestine lining.

Biopsy. Excision and removal of a tissue specimen for microscopic analysis. An *excisional biopsy* involves removing a piece of tissue from a suspicious mass; an *incisional biopsy* refers to a surgical incision to remove a wedge of tissue from a suspicious tumor. A *needle biopsy* removes a core of tissue through a special needle lumen. A *punch biopsy* removes a plug of tissue, usually from the skin. A *stereotaxic needle biopsy* involves a precise placement of a needle for aspiration of tissue, a methodology used in some brain tumor biopsies.

Bronchoscopy. Examination of the trachea and bronchi with either a rigid or a flexible (fiberoptic) endoscope.

Chemstick. Examination for levels of sugar in blood.

Chest X ray (CXR). A still x-ray film of the chest to examine the lungs, heart, ribs, and upper spine.

Cholecystography. Examination of the gall bladder with x-ray.

Cystoscopy. Examination of the urethra and bladder with an endoscope.

Echoradiography. Ultrasound imaging procedures in which deep body structures are visualized from reflections of sound pulses.

Endoscopy. Examination with an *endoscope,* which can be a rigid instrument or a flexible (fiberoptic) tube, introduced into a hollow cavity, tube, or duct.

Gastric analysis. Examination of secretions aspirated (suctioned) from the stomach.

Intravenous pyelography (IVP). An x-ray examination of the urinary tract using a contrast medium to delineate the structures.

Kidneys, ureters, and bladder (KUB). A plain x-ray film of the kidneys, ureters, and bladder.

Laparoscopy. Endoscopic examination of the abdomen.

Lumbar puncture. A procedure in which a needle is inserted below the arachnoid layer of the meninges between the fourth and fifth or third and fourth lumbar vertebrae to remove cerebrospinal fluid for analysis.

Panendoscopy. Endoscopic examination with a complete exploration of the cavity.

Paracentesis. Removal of fluid from the abdominal cavity through a procedure that uses a piercing instrument (trocar) or needle with an outer cannula for draining fluids into rubber tubing. The fluids are removed to reduce pressure and for microscopic analysis.

Sigmoidoscopy and proctoscopy. Examination of the lower colon with a flexible (fiberoptic) scope.

Thoracentesis. Removal of fluid from the plural cavity for the purpose of examining for infection, tumor cells, and pulmonary diseases.

Thyroid scan. A radiology study using a radioactive iodine administered to the patient orally or by injection. After allowing time for absorption by the thyroid gland, a scanning device is used to detect any alterations in the rate or symmetry of absorption.

Upper G.I. series. An x-ray study using barium to study the esophagus, stomach, and duodenum for evidence of dysmotility, tumors, strictures, ulcers, and reflux.

IV. MONITORING AND RECORDING VITAL SIGNS

Nurses monitor vital signs and record findings graphically at the patient's bed. Vital signs are usually recorded at least once per shift (day, evening, and night shifts). Unless specifically ordered, weight is measured at admission and discharge, and blood pressure is usually measured once a day. Measurements and recordings are made of temperature, pulse, and respiration three times a day. In addition, nurses note the patient's level of activity, appetite, and urine and stool elimination.

A. Pulse and Heart Sounds

Pulse rate ranges decrease with age (see Table 3–1). Pulses can be taken from different peripheral sites (see Figure 3–2) and are record-

Table 3–1. Normal Pulse Rates

Age	Average Range (heartbeats/min.)
Neonate	120–160
2 year old	80–140
5 to 12 years old	75–100
Adolescent and adult	60–100

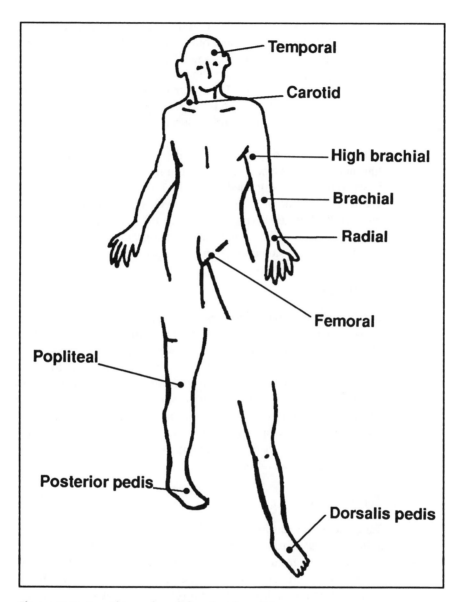

Figure 3–2. Locations of peripheral pulse sites

ed by noting the site(s) used (e.g., "femoral pulse," "carotid pulse," brachial pulse," etc.)

The sounds heard during auscultation of the beating heart itself will be described using four basic heart sound types: **S1** (sound occurring at the onset of systole when the mitral and bicuspid valves close); **S2** (sound attributed to the closure of the aortic and pulmonary valves); **S3** (difficult to hear sound associated with ventricular filling); and **S4** (nearly impossible to hear sound associated with ventricular filling and atrial contraction). Usually only the S1 and S2 sounds are described (the "lub dub" sounds, respectively). The notation **M1** and **M2** denotes a "split" sound heard during S1.

Extra heart sounds are also described, usually as snaps, clicks, murmurs, and rubs (see above). The timing and intensity of the extra heart sounds will be graded as **grade 1** (softest audible murmur); **grade 2** (murmur of medium intensity); **grade 3** (loud murmur without thrill; **grade 4** (murmur with thrill); **grade 5** (loudest murmur requiring a stethoscope to hear); and **grade 6** (murmur that is audible without a stethoscope on the chest).

B. Respiration

In ICUs, respiration may be monitored with special devices; however, when special devices are not used, respiration is monitored by observing breathing characteristics. Respiratory rates, like pulse rates, tend to decrease with age. Newborns have a respiratory rate ranging from 30 to 80 respirations per minute, whereas adult respirations range from 14 to 20 per minute. Adult patients who are breathing quietly (with an average tidal volume of 500 mL) at the average rate of 16 respirations per minute will breathe about 8 liters of air per minute. Chapter 7 contains descriptive terminology used for respiration observations.

C. Temperature

Temperature is measured with a clinical thermometer (oral, rectal, or axillary). Heat sensitive paper, tape, or patches are sometimes used to obtain temperature. Electronic thermometers with disposable probes are preferred by most hospitals. Most thermometers will display temperature in degrees *Celsius* (C) and *Fahrenheit* (F). Celsius temperature refers to a centigrade scale referenced by the freezing point for water (0° C) and the boiling point for water (100° C). Fahrenheit scale, in which the freezing point for water is 32° F and the boiling point for water is 212° F, is not commonly used in medical settings. To compute Celsius from Fahrenheit temperatures, subtract 32 from the Fahrenheit temperature, multiply that number by 5, and divide by 9.

D. Weight

In medical settings, weight is more commonly measured in kilograms (kg) than pounds (lb) and height in centimeters (cm) rather than inches (in.). Table 3–2 provides a translation table for kilograms and pounds.

E. Blood Pressure

The force produced by the volume of blood pressing on the walls of the arteries is termed *blood pressure*. Blood pressure measurements reflect the elasticity of the arteries, the volume of the blood circulating in the body, and the efficiency of the heart's pumping action. Blood pressure is measured in millimeters of mercury (mmHg), with the *systolic* pressure (representing ventricular contraction) as the top number and the *diastolic* pressure (representing the ventricular relaxation) as the bottom number. The average normal ranges for blood pressure readings increase with age. Children at 1 year of age have an average normal blood pressure of around 95/65 mmHg, whereas adults over age 18 have an average blood pressure of around 120/80 mmHg. With aging, the normal range will increase.

Table 3–2. Comparison of kilograms to pounds

Kilograms (kg)	Pounds (lb)
1	2.2
5	11
10	22
15	33
20	44
25	55
30	66
40	88
50	99
60	132
70	154
80	176
90	198
100	220

F. I.C.U. Monitors

Patients in ICUs require continuous human and electronic monitoring of vital signs. Vital signs are monitored with *hemodynamic and cardiovascular monitors, respiratory and pulmonary function monitors, spectrometry and capnography, blood gas monitoring*, and *assessment of nutritional status* by measuring the production of carbon dioxide (CO_2) and consumption of oxygen (O_2) Patients with neurologic dysfunction related to increased intracranial pressure will require intracranial pressure (ICP) monitoring, described below.

The following list describes some of the procedures for monitoring and managing ICU patients.

Arterial catheters. Catheters used for continuous monitoring of blood gases and blood pressure. *Pulmonary artery catheters* (balloon-tipped catheters inserted through the right side of the heart into the pulmonary artery for cardiac monitoring) are frequently referred to as Swan-Ganz catheters.

Cardiac Monitors. On-line cardiac rhythm and conductivity monitoring equipment for cardiac functions will be at each bedside in the l.C.U. Cardiac monitoring will include a central console at the nurses' station, slave oscilloscopes for visualization of the patient's heart rhythms, rhythm strips at a central station and at bedside, and memory and alarm circuitry with visual and auditory signals.

Central venous pressure (CVP) catheters. Manometric measures of right atrial pressure.

Dobbhoff feeding tube (DHFT). Virtually any nasogastric tube can be used as a feeding tube, but usually the physician will use one of the mercury-weighted tubes, such as the Dobbhoff feeding tube, DHFT, or similar tube (Keogh tube, Duo-tube) for *enteral feeding.* This variety of feeding tube is inserted when feeding is the main requirement for a gastrointestinal tube insertion (there is no need for gastric aspiration or decompression). Since the DHFT is a small bore tube, it is less irritative to the pharynx, and the weighted tip makes it easier to pass beyond the pylorus into the duodenum or through to the small intestine (jejunum). Placing the feeding tubes further into the gastrointestinal tract is sometimes felt to be preferable for reduced aspiration risks (also see NGTs and NITs, below) or when there is concern for gastric pooling.

Drains. Surgical drains or catheters to remove unwanted body fluids may be in place. Drain types include: Penrose drains, the cigarette drain, Foley catheters, and double lumen sump catheters.

Intracranial pressure (ICP) monitoring. ICP monitors are placed with a subarachnoid screw and inserted by way of a burr hole through the cranium and dura into the subarachnoid space. In some cases, a fiberoptic device with a pressure transducer-tipped catheter will be used instead of the subarachnoid screw. Other methods for intracranial monitoring include an *Ommaya reservoir* (a mushroom-shaped capped tube placed into one of the lateral ventricles that can be left in place to sample cerebrospinal fluid) and a *ventricular drain* (No. 8 pediatric feeding tubing placed into the lateral ventricles for drainage).

Nasogastric (NG) tubes. Nasogastric tubes are used mainly for aspiration and gastric decompression, as well as administration of medications, gastric lavage, or feedings. **Nasointestinal tubes (NITs)** are sometimes preferred as they are felt to have lower risks for aspiration (see Dobbhoff feeding tubes, above).

Nasotracheal, orotracheal (endotracheal), or tracheostomy tubes and obturators. These devices will be in place for patients requiring airway or air supply support.

Oximeters. These devices provide continuous measurements of oxygen saturation and may be either indwelling intravascular devices or less invasive devices worn on the finger, earlobe, or foot (in infants) in which monitoring of oxygen levels is done *transcutaneously*, by way of a light shining through the body part. Problems reported with the reliability of oximetry include ambient light interferences in the measurements and skin breakdowns.

Oxygen therapy. Patients with conditions requiring oxygen therapy will be given some sort of oxygen delivery system. This can include a *Venturi mask*, which is driven by pure oxygen, or a *nasal cannula*, which has nasal prongs and allows oral breathing augmented by oxygen.

Pacemakers. External pacemakers provide temporary or permanent correction of cardiac arrhythmias.

Pulmonary artery catheters. These are manometric monitors of left heart filling pressures and cardiac output.

Sengstaken-Blakemore tubes. This tube has a balloon and lumen for aspiration of stomach contents and is used to treat bleeding esophageal or gastric varices.

Ventilator monitoring. Patients on mechanical ventilators (respirators) will have *suction equipment* at bedside, and the ventilator will be equipped with alarms for *oxygen, apnea, low pressure, high pressure*, and *tidal volume*. The ventilator will have settings for *tidal volume; ventilatory rate; positive end-expiratory pressure (PEEP)*; and *mode of function* (intermittent mandatory ventilation [IMV] and controlled mandatory ventilation [CMV] or synchronous intermittent mandatory ventilation [SIMV]).

V. APGAR SCORES AND ESTIMATION OF GESTATIONAL AGE

A. Apgar (APGAR) Scores

Apgar scores are the numerical rating of the vital signs of infants observed at 1 minute and 5 minutes following delivery. Although "Apgar" is an eponym referring to Virginia Apgar, who introduced the scoring system in the early 1950s, the five areas examined are often listed by use of the acronym APGAR (see Table 3–3). This is

Table 3–3. Apgar scores

| Sign | Scores | | |
	0	1	2
Appearance	Blue or pale	Blue extremities	Pink
Pulse	Absent	Less than 100/min	More than 100/min
Grimace	No response	Grimace	Cough or sneeze
Activity	Limp	Some flexion	Active
Respirations	Absent	Slow, irregular	Good, crying

a slight modification of Apgar's original terminology, but the categories are essentially the same. Apgar ratings are made at 1 minute post delivery, because that is considered the time of maximal stress to the infant. Newborns with Apgar scores of 4 to 6 will usually require resuscitation. Scores of 0 to 3 indicate acute distress.

B. Gestational Age Estimates

Estimating gestational age and neonatal development is important for determining risk for post-delivery complications. Figure 3–3 illustrates the neurologic maturity examination, and Table 3–4 explains the ratings. Higher scores indicate a greater gestational maturity. The neurologic maturity ratings also may be applied in post-neonates when there is a question of delayed neurologic development.

VI. NORMAL PEDIATRIC BLOOD PRESSURES AND RESPIRATORY RATES

In neonates, respirations are typically abdominal and range from 30 to 50 per minute. Respiratory rates gradually slow through the age of 16 when adult rates are reached (16 per minute at rest). Blood pressure measures will be taken immediately after birth and followed to detect cardiac abnormalities. Normal blood pressures for infants and children are variable, and physicians typically take measurements over time to look for trends toward high or low ranges. The normal ranges for young children, aged 2 to 6, will be considerably lower than that of adults. A systolic pressure between 80 and 110 mmHg and diastolic pressure of 50 to 80 mmHg would be considered normal in very young children. Normal ranges gradually increase through adolescence and teenaged years to adult values.

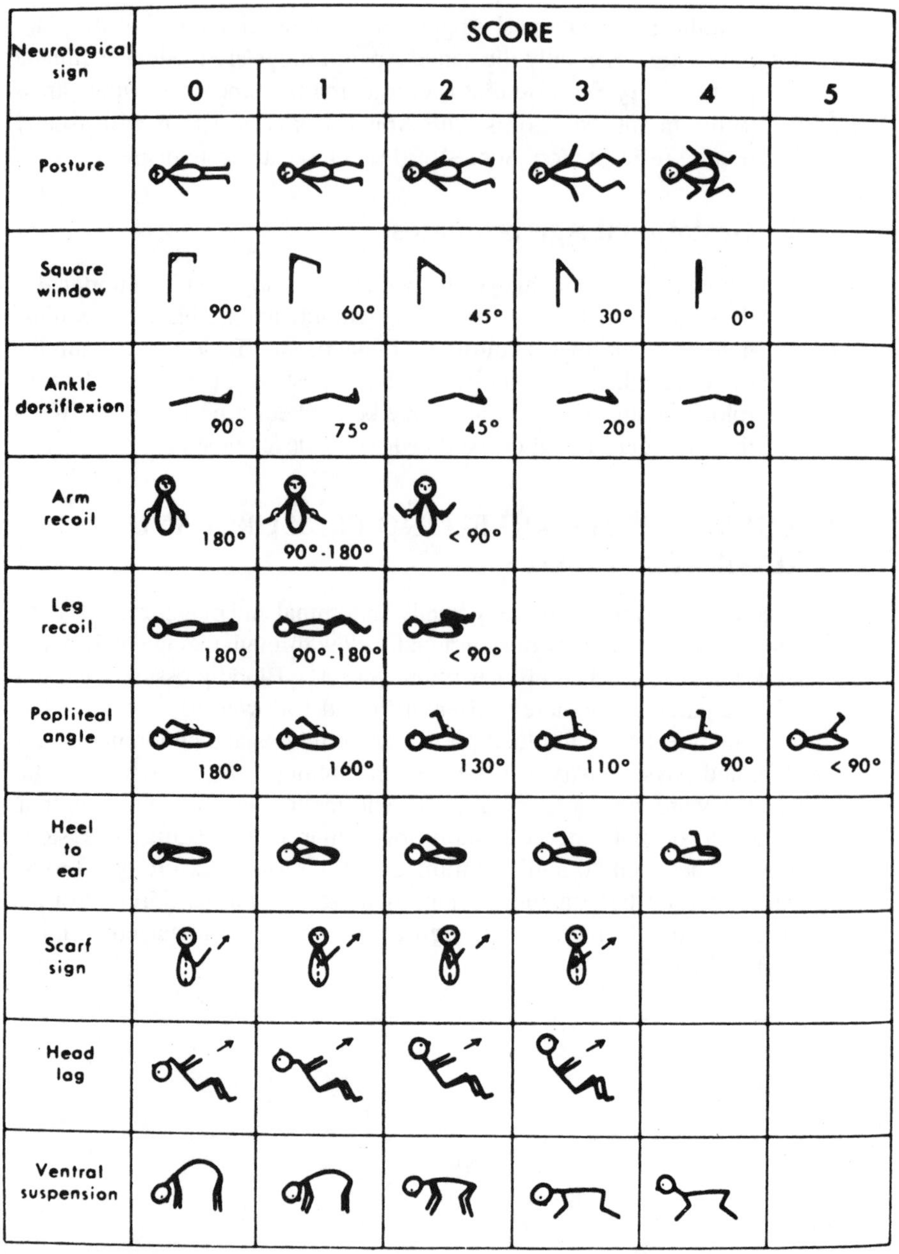

Figure 3-3. Illustration of neurologic scoring system (From Dubinowitz, L. M. S., Dubinowitz, V., & Goldberg, C. 1977. Clinical assessment of gestational age in the newborn infant. *Journal of Pediatrics, 77,* 1–6, with permission; and Amiel-Tison, C. 1968. Neurologic examination of the maturity of newborn infants. *Archives of Diseases in Childhood, 43,* 89–91, with permission.)

Table 3–4. Newborn neurologic maturity assessment[a]

Sign	Score	Findings
Posture	0	Arms and legs extended
	1	Slight to moderate flexion of LEs
	2	Strong flexion of LEs
	3	Slight flexion of UEs, strong flexion of LEs
	4	Full flexion of arms and legs
Square window	0	Flexing the hand at the wrist produces a 90° angle
	1	60° angle
	2	45° angle
	3	30° angle
	4	0° angle
Ankle dorsiflexion	0	Flexing the ankle produces a 90° angle
	1	75° angle
	2	45° angle
	3	30° angle
	4	0° angle
Arm recoil	0	Flexing the arm for 5 seconds followed by pulling the arms and releasing produces a recoil posture at 180°
	1	90 to 180°
	2	less than 90°
Leg recoil	0	Flexing the legs and hips for 5 seconds then pulling the legs to a full extension produces no response recoil
	1	90 to 180° recoil
	2	less than 90° recoil
Popliteal angle	0	Fully flexing the thigh produces a 180° angle
	1	160° angle
	2	130° angle
	3	110° angle
	4	90° angle
	5	less than 90° angle

(continued)

Table 3-4 *(continued)*

Sign	Score	Findings
Heel to Ear Maneuver	0	Movement of the infant's foot toward the head is fully possible
	1–4	See Figure 3-3
Scarf sign	0	Infant's hand can be drawn across its neck and shoulder fully to the opposite side
	1–3	See Figure 3-3
Head lag	0	When lifting infant by the arms the head shows no evidence of support
	1	Slight support
	2	Partial support
	3	Fully supported
Ventral suspension	0	When lifting the infant by the hand under the chest from a prone position, there is no truncal support
	1–4	See Figure 3-3

[a] Refer to Figure 3-3.

VII. NOTES

_____

_____

_____

_____

NOTES *(continued)*

VIII. REFERENCES

Amiel-Tison, C. (1968). Neurologic examination of the maturity of newborn infants. *Archives of Disabled Children, 43*, 89–91.

Andreoli, T. A., Carpenter, C. J., Plum, F., & Smith, L. H. (1990). *Cecil essentials of medicine* (2nd ed.). Philadelphia: W. B. Saunders.

Apgar, V. (1953). A proposal for a new method of evaluation of the newborn infant. *Anesthesia and Analgesia, 32*, 260–264.

Ballard, J. L., Novak, K. K., & Driver, M. (1979). A simplified score for assessment of fetal maturation of newly born infants. *Joumal of Pediatrics, 95*, 770.

Berkow, R. (Ed.). (1990). *The Merck manual* (I5th ed.). Trenton, NJ: Merck Sharpe, and Dohme.

Boggs, R. L., & Wooldridge-King, M. (1993). *AACN procedure manual for critical care (3rd ed.).* Philadelphia: W. B. Saunders.

D'Angelo, H. H., & Welsh, N. P. (1988). *The signs and symptoms handbook.* Springhouse, PA: Springhouse Corporation.

DeGowin, E. L., & DeGowin, R. L. (1987). *Bedside diagnostic examination* (4th ed.). New York: Macmillan.

Detmer, W. M., McPhee, S. J., Nicoll, D., & Chou, T. M. (1992). *Pocket guide to diagnostic tests.* Norwalk, CT: Appleton-Lange.

Dubinowitz, L. M. S., Dubinowitz, V., & Goldberg, C. (1977). Clinical assessment of gestational age in the newborn infant. *Journal of Pediatrics, 77*, 1–6.

Gomella, L. G. (Ed.). (1989). *Clinician's pocket handbook* (6th ed.). East Norwalk CT: Appleton & Lange.

Gomella, L. G. (Ed.) (1993). *Clinician's pocket reference (7th ed.). East* Norwalk, CT: Appleton & Lange.

Kelly, W. J. (Ed.). (1992). *Clinical skillbuilders: Better documentation.* Springhouse, PA: Springhouse Publishers.

Kenner, C. A. (1992). *Nurse's clinical guide: Neonatal care.* Springhouse, PA: Springhouse Corporation.

Melonakos, K. (1990). *Saunders pocket reference for nurses.* Philadelphia: W. B. Saunders Company.

Willett, M. J., Patterson, M., & Steinbock B. (1986). *Manual of neonatal intensive care nursing.* Boston: Little, Brown.

CHAPTER

4

Mental Status and the Neurological Examination

Health care professionals make an assessment of mental status as a routine part of the physical examination of adults, especially when there is some reason to suspect the presence of a psychiatric disorder, delirium, or dementia. Geriatric patients are more likely to undergo a formal mental status examination than younger persons. Patients with notable impairments in mental (cognitive) functions are usually referred to a psychologist or psychiatrist for a consultative evaluation. Any communication deficit should prompt a referral to a speech-language pathologist. When a patient's mental status is impaired, most of the staff caring for that patient are likely to record their observations of the patient's alertness, orientation, memory, or speech (e.g., "Alert and communicative," or "Patient denies having met this examiner yesterday").

Assessment of mental status is a routine part of the neurologic examination and may be as cursory as asking the patient his or her name, current location, and the date. The patient who successfully complies with those requests and is able to provide a seemingly adequate medical history may be said to be, "Oriented × 3, memory O.K.; no speech problems or difficulties with understanding."

This chapter reviews the essential elements of a mental status examination. A detailed outline of the neurologic interview and examination is reviewed, and reference figures are provided. The neurologic examination of newborns and children is not discussed separately; however, differences in the assessment format and normal findings are noted when appropriate. Neonatal neurologic maturity assessment is illustrated in Chapter 3, Figure 3–3. A review of commonly ordered neurologic studies is provided. Brief discussions of coma, delirium, depression, and dementia are also included in this chapter. Specific neurologic and psychiatric disorders are described in Chapter 9, and neuroradiologic studies are discussed in Chapter 8.

I. TERMINOLOGY AND ABBREVIATIONS USED IN THE NEUROLOGIC EXAMINATION

A. Terminology

Abduction. Motion away from the center.

Abulia. Slowness, apathy, psychomotor retardation.

Acalculia. Impaired ability to perform arithmetic operations.

Accommodation. Adjustments in the lens, pupil, and position of the eye in response to objects held close to the eye; near vision reflex.

Achromatopsia. Lack of color vision.

Acrophobia. Fear of high places.

Adduction. Motion toward the center.

Adductor tenotomy and obturator neurectomy (ATON). Surgery performed on children with cerebral palsy to release the adductor muscles of the hips and reduce partial dislocation (subluxation).

Afferent. Impulse traveling toward the nerve body.

Agnosia. An impairment, unrelated to sensory loss, in the ability to recognize a sensory stimulus despite relatively preserved primary sensory input.

Akathisia. The inability to remain still; motor restlessness.

Akinesis. Lack of motor movement not attributable to paresis/paralysis.

Amaurosis fugax. Temporary episode of unilateral visual loss often characterized by a gradual visual field loss from the top-down as if a window shade were being pulled down over the eyes.

Amnesia. A loss of memory.

Amusia. A loss of musical ability and/or recognition of musical features.

Analgesia. Lack of pain.

Anencephaly. Lack of brain and cranium development.

Anesthesia. Loss of sensation.

Aneuploidy. An abnormal number of chromosomes.

Anisocoria. Unequal pupil size.

Anosmia. A loss in the sense of smell.

Anosodiaphoria. Tendency to minimize or joke about the extent of paresis/plegia of an affected limb; occasionally seen in patients with right hemisphere cerebral dysfunction.

Anosognosia. An inability to recognize the presence of one's illness or to exaggerate the residual function of the affected limb.

Aphasia. An acquired loss of language ability.

Apraxia. An inability to initiate, imitate, coordinate, or perform a previously learned skilled movement despite an intact motor and sensory system.

Argyll Robertson pupil. An impairment in the pupillary reflexive reaction to light with a retained near vision (accommodation) reflex. Argyll Robertson pupils are found in chronic degenerative diseases of the nervous system, such as diabetes, late stage Alzheimer's disease, viral encephalitis, Wernicke's encephalopathy, and cerebrovascular disease.

Autonomic dysfunction. Neurologic disorders manifested in dysfunction of autonomic regulations (e.g. orthostatic hypotension, syncope, impotence, pupillary abnormalities or urinary and gastric disorders).

Astereognosis. A type of agnosia characterized by an inability to recognize objects placed in the hand. *Oral astereognosis* refers to the inability to recognize objects or shapes placed in the mouth.

Asterixis. A rapid palmar flapping when the wrists are dorsiflexed, seen in association with metabolic encephalopathies (as in liver or renal failure).

Astrocyte. A star-shaped neuroglial cell.

Asymmetrical tonic neck (ATN) reflex. In infants, as the head is turned the arm and leg extend in the same direction; "fencer's posture."

Ataxia. Broad, jerky, dyscoordinated movements. This is often due to proprioceptive disturbances, causing what is sometimes termed *sensory ataxia*, or to cerebellar lesions (or lesions to its connections), producing a so-called *cerebellar ataxia*.

Atelencephaly. Incomplete development of the cerebral hemispheres.

Atelomyelia. Incomplete spinal cord development.

Athetosis. A movement disorder characterized by slow, writhing movements of the distal extremities, face, or trunk muscles; a feature of chorea, dystonia, and ballismus.

Atrophy. Decrease in muscle mass due to denervation or disuse.

Automatism. Compulsively performed or repetitive behaviors.

Autonomic nervous system (ANS). Pertaining to the nerves that maintain the internal environment of the body including heart rate, digestion, and bowel and bladder control. Breathing is an autonomic function controlled by the central nervous system. The ANS is divided into two divisions, *sympathetic* and *parasympathetic*, which have counteractive functions serving to maintain the body's homeostasis.

Autotopagnosia. A form of agnosia in which there is a failure to recognize a body part.

Axon. Long fiber extending from the neuron carrying messages away from the cell body.

Babinski sign. An abnormal reflexive response to stroking the plantar surface of the foot in which there is extension of the great toe and fanning of the toes instead of the normal flexion response. This sign usually indicates an abnormality of the central nervous system involving the pyramidal tracts (upper motor neurons).

Ballismus. A movement disorder characterized by an abrupt flinging motion of a body part, usually associated with lesions of the subthalamic nucleus.

Basal ganglia, basal nuclei. Referring to the subcortical gray masses (caudate and lentiform nuclei of the corpus striatum, the amygdaloid body, and the claustrum) deep within each hemisphere.

Bell's palsy. Weakness of the upper and lower hemiface caused by irritation to the facial nerve or nerve sheath.

Biogenic animes. Neurotransmitters (epinephrine, norepinephrine, acetylcholine, dopamine, and serotonin).

Bite reflex. A jaw closing reflex elicited with stimulation of the teeth or surfaces within the mouth.

Blood-brain barrier. A neurophysiologic mechanism regulating the entry of certain serum substances to brain tissues. The blood-brain barrier is a physical barrier formed by the basement membrane of the capillaries of the brain and foot processes of the astrocytes.

Bradykinesia. Movement disorder characterized by slowness or lack of movement independent of rigidity and tremor, often associated with Parkinson's disease and other states, such as drug toxicities and multi-infarct dementia.

Bradyphrenia. Slowed cognitive processes.

Brain stem. Base of the brain consisting of the pons and medulla.

Brain stem auditory evoked responses (BAER, BSER). A computerized, evoked potential study used to detect an interruption in the synapses in the central auditory system to determine a site of lesion.

Broca's aphasia. A type of aphasia (acquired language disorder) usually corresponding to anterior, left, middle cerebral artery lesions characterized by dysfluent (nonfluent) verbal expression with relatively intact auditory comprehension.

Cacogeusia. Sensation of a disagreeable taste. *Ageusia* refers to a loss in taste sensation.

Capgrass syndrome. A visual agnosic disorder in which a familiar person is thought to be an imposter.

Carpal tunnel syndrome. Intermittent numbness and paresthesia of the median nerve distribution in the wrist due to disease or injury causing compression of the nerve.

Cauda equina. "Horse tail," or fanlike, nerve roots exiting from the thecal sac of the spinal cord. In most adults, the spinal cord ends at the second lumbar vertebra, the level where the cauda equina originate.

Causalgia. Burning pain that radiates distally to an injured nerve.

Central nervous system (CNS). Pertaining to the functions and structures of the spinal cord, brain stem, midbrain, and cerebral hemispheres.

Central pontine myelinolysis. Condition occurring mainly in alcoholics, menstruating women, and patients who have had rapidly corrected hyponatremia; manifested by quadriparesis and gaze palsy, dysarthria and obtundation leading to coma.

Cerebellar nystagmus. Although there are several forms of cerebellar nystagmus, if horizontal gaze nystagmus is more obvious when the patient looks laterally toward the lesioned side, the nystagmus is felt to be cerebellar in origin.

Cerebellum. Portion of the brain lying dorsal to the pons and medulla oblongata, consisting of two lateral hemispheres and the vermis, a narrow middle portion, which are attached to the brain stem by three pairs of fiber bundles. The cerebellum controls synergistic skeletal muscle activity and coordination of voluntary movement.

Cerebromalacia. Softening of the brain tissue.

Cerebrum. The largest part of the brain including two hemispheres separated by a deep longitudinal fissure with a surface characterized by **gyri** (folds) and **sulci** (fissures) and containing white matter tracts and deep gray masses (basal ganglia) within the hemispheres. The cerebrum receives sensory information, controls motor activity, and is the center of higher cognitive abilities.

Cervical spondylosis and cervical osteoarthritis. Degenerative diseases of the cervical spine.

Chorea. A movement disorder characterized by abrupt writhing movements.

Chronic pain. Discomfort lasting more than 6 months.

Clonus. Sustained series of rhythmic jerks.

Cogwheel rigidity. Movement pattern in which the fluidity of movement is lacking with intermittent resistance present during passive stretching motions, often associated with Parkinson's disease.

Coma. Condition in which there is little or no evidence of mental or motor response to vigorous, persistent and noxious external stimulation. Although terms such as "stupor," "obtundation," and so forth will be found in medical documents, coma is best *rated* by one of the objective scales, described later.

Conduction aphasia. Type of aphasia (acquired language disorder) characterized by a predominant impairment in verbal repetition with relatively intact auditory comprehension and oral expression, said to be due to a disruption of the sensory-to-motor white matter connections of the language dominant hemisphere.

Confusional state. Clouded state of consciousness characterized by incoherent, inappropriate, or nonmeaningful verbal expression; misperceptions of surroundings and others; and nonpurposeful or inappropriate behaviors.

Conjugate gaze movements. Eye movements occurring in unison are termed *conjugate gaze movements. Dysconjugate gaze devia-*

tions refer to eyes that do not move to one direction. Conjugate gaze deviations can occur *toward the side of a unilateral destructive hemispheric lesion* (opposite the side of the hemiparesis), "looking at the lesion"; *away from the side of a unilateral irritative lesion* (away from the seizure focus); *away from the side of a destructive lesion in the brain stem* (at the occulomotor decussation lesions cause gaze to deviate toward the side of the paralysis); or there may be a *vertical deviation upward with an irritative lesion of the frontal lobes* (e.g., "oculogyric crisis" in post-encephalitic parkinsonism). Impaired voluntary gaze away from the side of the lesion is seen following disease of one frontal lobe. Impaired smooth eye movements in visual pursuit will be seen following diffuse disease of the hemispheres, particularly disorders involving the parietal lobes. Ocular impersistence (inability to sustain gaze on one object) will be seen following diffuse disease of the hemispheres. Upward gaze or loss of gaze in either direction will occur following bilateral involvement of the corticobulbar tracts at the level of the midbrain. Conjugate gaze reflexes may be impaired with pontine lesions and multiple sclerosis. Dysconjugate eye movements may also be present producing *diplopia*. Although not a gaze disturbance, accommodation responses also may be dysconjugate.

Constructional apraxia. Inability to plan and execute the production of designs or three dimensional structures.

Copralalia. Involuntary, scatologic utterances often described in patients with Gilles de la Tourette syndrome.

Corneal reflex. A reflex test in which bilateral blinks are elicited by a light touch to the cornea to examine the ophthalmic division of the Trigeminal (V) nerve and the Facial nerve (VII).

Cortical, or central blindness. Loss of the ability to see resulting from bilateral lesions in the visual sensory cortex. Unlike other forms of blindness, the pupillary reflexes are preserved.

Cortical deafness. Loss of the ability to hear resulting from bilateral lesions to the auditory sensory cortex.

Cranial nerves. Referring to the nerve bodies that provide motor and sensory innervation to head and neck structures and autonomic innervation of visceral organs.

Craniocele. Herniation of brain tissues.

Craniotomy. Opening into the cranium.

Decerebrate posture, decerebrate rigidity. Referring to the posture of a comatose patient in which the legs are stiff and extended, the arms are extended and internally rotated, the jaw is clenched, and the head is retracted. Decerebrate posture is associated with upper brain stem destructive lesions between the red nucleus and the vestibular nuclei (see Figure 4–6 on page 148).

Decorticate posture. Referring to the posture of a comatose patient with a deep, hemispheric lesion at or above the level of the upper brain stem. In decorticate posturing the arms are flexed and adducted, the fists are clenched and the legs extended (see Figure 4–6 on page 148).

Déjà vu phenomenon. Neurologic phenomenon sometimes associated with complex partial (psychomotor) seizures in which an individual has the intense feeling that he or she is reliving a past experience.

Delirium. Clouded state of consciousness characterized by difficulty in sustained attention, sensory misperceptions, disordered thinking, disturbances in sleep-wake cycles, and psychomotor unrest.

Delusion. False belief.

Dementia. Usually referring to a loss of multiple cognitive abilities as a result of diffuse damage or dysfunction of the central nervous system.

Dendrite. Tendrils extending from the neuron carrying input to the cell body.

Dermatome. Region innervated by a single segmental nerve.

Dialysis encephalopathy. A form of dementia characterized by personality changes, dysarthria, myoclonus, and seizures; felt to be a multisystem disorder in dialysis patients with end-stage renal disease.

Diffuse. Multifocal or widespread.

Diplegia. Bilateral lower extremity weakness.

Diplopia. Double vision.

Distant vision. Visual acuity tested from a distance of 20 feet.

Doll's eye phenomenon, oculocephalic reflex. Reflexive conjugate eye movements normally cause the eyes to move opposite to the direction of head movement, maintaining their position in relation to the environment. When present this reflex indicates integrity of the third, fourth, and sixth cranial nerves and their interconnections. No movement of the eyes, or an asymmetry of movement, indicates pontine-midbrain level destructive lesions. Barbiturate poisoning can also abolish this reflex.

Dorsiflexion. Upward flexion, or lifting.

Dysarthria. Speech disorder characterized by neuromotor paralysis, paresis, and/or dyscoordination of movement of the muscle groups supporting speech.

Dysdiadochokinesia. Inability to perform rapidly alternating hand and/or articulatory movements.

Dysesthesia. Abnormal, unpleasant sensation in response to a sensory stimulus.

Dyskinesia. A movement disorder characterized by involuntary muscular movements, such as *dystonias* and *tremors*.

Dysmetria. Disturbed ability to judge range of motion. Dysmetria is demonstrated if there is "past pointing" when patients attempt to place a finger on an object held in front of them or touch their nose.

Dysphagia. Impaired ability to swallow.

Dysphasia. Term sometimes preferred in place of "aphasia" to denote a partial loss of language ability.

Dysthymia. Emotional or intellectual disorder, usually referring to depression. Dysthymia may also imply a condition caused by a dysfunctional thymus gland.

Eaton-Lambert myasthenia syndrome (LEMS). An autoimmune disorder sometimes found in association with small cell lung cancer; manifested by proximal leg or arm weakness and autonomic changes (e.g. dry mouth, impotence).

Echoic memory. Short-term auditory memory.

Edinger-Westphal nucleus. Nucleus innervating the ciliary and papillary sphincters of the eye. This nucleus is part of the parasympathetic innervation to the eye by the third cranial nerve (CN III).

Efferent. Going away from the neuronal cell body.

Empyema. Encapsulated collection of pus in a brain space, (e.g., subdural or epidural).

Encephalitis. Inflammation of the brain.

Endorphins. Natural body substances with properties similar to morphine.

Epicritic sense. Ability to perceive fine degrees of touch, pain, or temperature from the skin or mucosa.

Epidural. Above or outside of the dura mater covering of the brain.

Episodic memory. Memory processes related to temporal events (e.g., autobiographic information).

Evoked potentials. Electrical activity changes in the nervous system elicited by a sensory stimulus and detected by computerized averaging of responses to repeated sensory stimuli. Evoked potentials can be used to examine the visual, auditory, and somatosensory systems and the peripheral nerves.

Expressive aphasia. A term sometimes used to denote a type of aphasia (acquired language disorder) characterized by a notable difficulty with verbal expression. Expressive aphasia is generally synonymous with "Broca's aphasia," but may be applied indiscriminately in medical settings whenever verbal output is impaired.

Extension. Movement away from the body.

Extrapyramidal movement disorder, extrapyramidal cerebral palsy. Movement disorder resulting from disorders of the nervous system not involving the pyramidal cortico-spinal and cortico-bulbar pathways. Extrapyramidal disorders include the cerebellar and basal ganglia movement disorders.

Falx cerebri. Fold in the dura matter that *separates the cerebral hemispheres* in the midsagittal plane. The **falx cerebelli** is the dura fold separating the *cerebellar* hemispheres.

Fasciculation. Irregular contractions and relaxations of muscle unit, appearing as a twitch or ripple.

Febrile convulsion. Seizure in children associated with a high fever.

Fibrillation. Contraction of single muscle fibers, detectable by monitoring the electrical activity of the muscle.

Flaccid. Paralysis characterized by a loss of muscle tone.

Flexion. Pulling toward the body.

Focal. Limited to a designated area.

Fundus. Back of the eye.

Glabellar reflex. Reflex elicited by gently tapping the forehead causing momentary rhythmic eye blinks. This reflex normally extinguishes with repeated (2–3 taps) stimulation. Failure to extinguish this reflex is seen in parkinsonism.

Glia. Supportive tissues of the brain, includes astrocytes, microglia cells, and oligodendrocytes.

Global aphasia. Severe to profound loss of language ability in all modalities (speaking, listening, reading, writing).

Grand mal seizure. A generalized seizure characterized by loss of consciousness and tonic-clonic movements.

Graphesthesia. The ability to recognize shapes drawn on the palm.

Grasp reflex. One of the "frontal release" signs in which a reflexive grasp is elicited when the palm is stroked.

Hallucination. A perception or a sensation not founded on reality.

Halo brace. Ring and brace superstructure used to immobilize a patient with a high spinal cord injury. (See Appendix B for descriptions of other types of orthoses.)

Hemianopsia. Blindness for one-half of the visual field (see Figure 4–3 on page 144).

Hemiparesis. Weakness (partial paralysis) of one side of the body.

Hemiplegia. Paralysis of one side of the body.

Herniation. The abnormal protrusion of an organ or tissue through an opening or space. Brain herniations include *uncal herniation* through the tentorial notch, subfaucial *cingulate herniation, upward cerebellar herniation* through the tentorial notch, and *cerebellar tonsil herniation* through the *foramen magnum.*

Horner's syndrome. Neurologic syndrome characterized by unilateral ptosis (drooping of the eyelid), narrowing of the pupil, and diminished vasodilation and sweating present on the same side of the head as the brain lesion.

Hydrocephalus. An abnormal accumulation of fluid in the cranial vault. (See Disturbances in Cerebrospinal Fluid, Chapter 9, page 305)

Hyperesthesia. A heightened sensitivity to sensory stimulation.

Hypnagogic. State of rest coming just before sleep.

Hypotonia. An absence of muscle tone; floppy.

Iconic memory. Visual memory.

Illusion. False interpretation of sensory perception.

Insight. Ability to observe and evaluate oneself and to appreciate the relationship between events.

Intention tremor. Coarse, rhythmic movements elicited by intentional hand movements (e.g., reaching for objects).

Intractable pain. Constant, unrelenting pain.

Jaw jerk. A stretch reflex elicited by tapping the medial portion of the mandible.

Lennox-Gastaut seizures. Variant of petit mal seizure having other associated seizure patterns. (See Chapter 9, Seizure Disorders, pages 302–303 for in-depth descriptions of this and other types of seizures.)

Leptomeninges. The pia mater and arachnoid.

Lethargic. Awake, but drowsy, inactive and indifferent to external stimulation.

Lissencephaly. Unconvoluted cerebral hemispheres, associated with severe forms of retardation.

Logomania, logorrhea. Excessive, repetitious speech output.

Long-term memory. Secondary memory; memory processes allowing for a large capacity of long-term storage of information (acquired knowledge).

Lordosis. Anterior curve of the spinal column.

Lower motor neuron (LMN) lesion. Lesions involving the motor neurons of the bulbar (cranial) and spinal nerves and their peripheral roots. The LMNs refer to the final common output pathway of the central nervous system, consisting of the anterior horn cells and their axons which form the peripheral nerves that innervate the muscles. LMN lesions are characterized *acutely* by paralysis, hypotonia, and areflexia in the distribution of the involved peripheral nerve(s) or nerve root(s). Chronic states are characterized by fasciculations and atrophy of the muscles innervated by that nerve.

Medulla oblongata. Bulblike lower portion of the brain stem; an enlarged extension of the spinal cord where it enters the foramen magnum of the occipital bone.

Meninges. The three membranes covering the brain; the dura mater, pia mater, and arachnoid.

Meningitis. Inflammation of the membranes covering the brain.

Miosis. Constriction of the pupil resulting from decreased or increased parasympathomimetic tone.

Misoplegia. Condition sometimes observed in patients with right hemisphere cerebral damage in which the patient expresses anger or hatred toward an affected limb.

Moribund. Near death.

Myelitis. Inflammation of the spinal cord.

Myokymia. Persistent irregular twitching of muscles producing a "bag of worms" appearance.

Myotonia. Involuntary, painless delay in muscle relaxation after contraction.

Nasolabial fold. Crease running from the sides of the nose to the corners of the mouth. A "flattening" of the nasolabial fold noted during the neurologic examination may be an indication of weakness of that side of the face.

Near vision. Visual acuity tested at approximately 14 inches from the eye.

Neglect. A lack of awareness of or response to the environment or self on the side opposite to a parietal lobe lesion.

Neonatal seizures. Seizures in the newborn, usually caused by a metabolic abnormality or infection.

Neural tube defects/disease. The *neural tube* refers to the embryologic structure formed at approximately 23 days of gestation which closes to form the vestigial spinal cord and brain. Neural tube disorders arise from defects in this stage of human development (e.g., spina bifida).

Neuralgia. Pain in a particular nerve or its distribution.

Neurectomy. Surgical excision of a nerve.

Neuritis. Inflammation of a nerve.

Neuroleptic. Drugs producing favorable tranquilizing and antipsychotic effects.

Neuron. The fundamental unit of the nervous system, consisting usually of *dendrites* that receive messages, the *soma* (cell body), and the *axon* for transmitting messages.

Neurosis. A somewhat controversial term referring to a group of mental or emotional disorders (e.g., certain forms of compulsions, phobias, anxiety, obsessions) in which reality testing is intact. Patients with neuroses do not have the delusions or hallucinations characteristic of most forms of psychoses (see Chapter 9, Psychotic Disorders).

Neurotransmitter. Neurochemical substance, such as norepinephrine, dopamine, acetylcholine, that is released when the axon terminal of a presynaptic neuron is excited.

Nominal aphasia. Term sometimes used to denote a type of aphasia (acquired language disorder) characterized by a primary diffculty with naming. Patients with early to middle stage dementia are sometimes said to have "nominal aphasia," reflecting disintegrating lexico-semantic abilities.

Nuchal rigidity. Stiff neck.

Nystagmus. Abnormal, involuntary movement of eyes reflecting an imbalance in the complex neuronal network involving the visual pathways, the labyrinthine proprioceptive influences from neck muscles, the vestibular and cerebellar nuclei, the reticular formation of the pontine brain stem, and the oculomotor nuclei.

Obtunded, obtunderate. Dull, indifferent, with responsiveness limited to little more than fleeting wakefulness.

Occupational, or pendular, nystagmus. A type of pendular nystagmus (slow, coarse movements in both directions) resulting from prolonged work in poorly lit surroundings (e.g., mines) in which rods are required for vision. Since there are no rods in the macula, the nystagmus is a temporary condition caused by the eyes' attempts to compensate for poor light.

Ocular bobbing. Brisk, downward bilateral, conjugate eye movements followed by a slow return to a normal position, indicative of cerebellar hemorrhages or caudal pontine lesions.

Ocular flutter. Rapid, rhythmic eye movements of decreasing amplitude on fixation.

Oculoplethysmography. Auscultation of intracranial arteries by placing the diaphragm of the stethoscope on the eye.

Opsoclonus. Random, clonic, conjugate eye movements usually felt to represent cerebellar lesions.

Optic chiasm. The location where optic nerve fibers for the temporal visual field cross to the opposite side (see Figure 4–2).

Optic radiation. The white matter tract looping laterally and posteriorly from the lateral geniculate body to the sensory nuclei in the calcarine fissure of the occipital lobe. The temporal section of the optic radiation is called the *loop of Meyer.*

Optic tract. The white matter tract from the optic chiasm to the lateral geniculate body of the thalamus.

Optokinetic nystagmus. A normal visual response to the landscape or objects moving rapidly in a horizontal plane in front of the eyes. This response may be lacking in patients having parietal lobe lesions.

Palilalia. Compulsive verbal repetitions.

Papilledema. Swelling of the optic disk causing congestive changes in the optic nerve seen on fundoscopic examination.

Paralysis agitans. Parkinson's disease.

Paresthesia. Heightened response to sensory stimulation (touch, temperature, pain, etc.); "pins and needles" sensation.

Partial seizures. A seizure involving an abnormal electrical discharge in a focal brain area. This type of seizure may spread to become a generalized seizure (secondary generalization). Partial seizures may be *simple*, in which there is no impairment of consciousness, or *complex* (complex partial seizure), in which there is impaired consciousness. Complex partial seizures (or partial complex seizures) often arise in the temporal lobes.

Pattern-shift visual evoked response (PSVER). An evoked potential study widely adopted to examine for lesions in the visual system. It usually examines for any discrepancies between the left and right eyes, as might be found in patients with multiple sclerosis or retrobulbar neuritis.

Perception. Psychological awareness of a stimulus. Perception can occur without recognition.

Percussion hammer. Small, rubber tipped hammer used to elicit stretch reflexes during the neurologic examination.

Peripheral. Pertaining to the peripheral nervous system.

Persistent vegetative state. A state in which a person, although awake, shows no interaction with the environment. Such patients usually have suffered severe brain damage and are unable to speak or track objects visually and need to have all bodily functions cared for by others.

Petit mal seizure. A generalized seizure characterized by a momentary loss of consciousness; "absence spells."

Phantom limb pain. Pain felt after a body part has been amputated in which there is a sensation that pain is coming from the missing part.

Phobia. A persistent, irrational fear.

Photic stimulation, photic driving. The use of powerful stroboscopic light for evoked potential stimulation during EEGs.

Pons. Prominence on the ventral surface of the brain stem between the cerebral peduncles and the medulla. The pons, or "bridge," contains connections to and from the cerebrum and is the origin of the CN V Trigeminal), CN VI (Abducens), CN VII (Facial), and CN VIII (Vestibulocochlear) nuclei.

Pontine. Pertaining to the pons.

Postconcussion syndrome. Referring to a wide variety of symptoms following mild head injury, such as headache, complaints of impaired memory, difficulty sustaining concentration, dizziness, depression, apathy, and anxiety.

Post-traumatic amnesia (PTA). Referring to the time period following brain trauma during which the patient lacks continuous memory of the events of daily life.

Primitive reflexes. One of the chief signs of *static encephalopathy* (cerebral palsy) is the persistence of primitive reflexes beyond 6 to 12 months of age, when these reflexes normally disappear. Primitive reflexes may reappear in children or adults who have had head injuries or in association with acute encephalopathies or degenerative diseases of the central nervous system. Primitive reflexes include the **asymmetrical tonic neck reflex** (ATNR); the **tonic labyrinthine reflex** (TLR); the positive **support reflex**; and the **grasp, bite, rooting,** and **sucking reflexes**. In the developing child, primitive reflexes normally diminish with a corresponding emergence of **automatic movement reactions**, such as the *anterior protective response and lateral protective response*.

Pronation. Medial rotation of the forearm (palm backward) or foot.

Prosopagnosia. An impaired ability to recognize faces.

Psyche. Mind.

Psychogenic. Not related to a physical cause.

Psychomotor agitation. Motor unrest.

Psychomotor retardation. Lack of movement and/or motor initiation without paresis.

Psychosis. Pertaining to major psychiatric disorders which may require psychiatric hospitalization treatment and pharmacologic therapies. Patients with psychoses will have impaired reality testing. Delusions and hallucinations are features of the majority of psychoses (see Psychoses, Chapter 9, pages 332–333).

Ptosis. Weakness of the eyelids.

Pure word deafness, verbal agnosia. A type of agnosia in which there is a recognition impairment strictly limited to spoken words without an impairment in the ability to hear sounds or to recognize other sounds.

Quadriplegia, quadriparesis. Paralysis or paresis, respectively, of all four extremities.

Rachischisis. Disorders produced by a lack of fusion of the dorsal midline structures of the neural tube (e.g., spina bifida).

Receptive aphasia. Term sometimes used to describe an acquired language disorder in which there is a notable impairment of auditory comprehension; generally synonymous with "sensory aphasia" or "Wernicke's aphasia."

Resting tremor. Tremor present in a resting position. The "pill rolling" tremor characteristic of parkinsonism is a common example.

Retina. The location of receptors of visual stimuli in the back of the eye.

Retraction-conversion nystagmus. A nystagmus characterized by the eye adducting and jerking up into the orbit, associated with pretectal and tectal lesions of the midbrain.

Retrobulbar neuritis. Inflammation of the optic nerve.

Rigidity. Increased muscle tone that is present throughout the range of movement of a muscle.

Rinne test. Tuning fork test used by an examiner to compare air conduction (AC) versus bone conduction (BC) of sound. The vibrating tuning fork is first placed over the mastoid until the sound is no longer heard by the patient and then held near the external auditory meatus until the patient reports he or she can no longer hear the sound. Since sound conducted by air is normally heard longer than sound conducted by bone, air conduction is usually longer than bone conduction (AC > BC), unless there is conductive disease (BC > AC).

Romberg sign. Clinical sign to evaluate balance impairment due to proprioceptive loss. A positive Romberg sign is found when the patient, standing with feet together has a loss of balance after closing his or her eyes.

Rotary nystagmus. Nystagmus characterized by circular eye movements.

Rotation. Turning or circular motion.

Scoliosis. Abnormal curvature of the spine.

Scotomata. Blind spots in the visual field. Sparks or shimmering spots in the visual field are called *scintillating scotomata*.

Seizure. Abnormal discharge of electrical activity in the central nervous system.

Semantic memory. Memory process not tied to temporal or spatial factors or sequences in which a schema of information containing related concepts, propositions, and sensations are stored and retrieved.

Sensory ataxia. A condition characteristic of patients with proprioceptive deficits.

Short-latency somatosensory evoked potentials (SSEP). A computerized evoked potential examination used in neurophysiology laboratories to confirm lesions in the somatosensory system, including the peripheral nerves, posterior column of the spinal cord, brain stem, and cortex. This test is useful in the evaluation of conditions such as cervical spondylosis, Guillian-Barré syndrome, or multiple sclerosis.

Short-term memory. Primary memory; a stage of memory processing in which a relatively small amount of information can be briefly retained (e.g., remembering a phone number you have just heard long enough to place a call).

Simultagnosia. Inability to perceive more than one stiumlus at a time in a given modality.

Snout or rooting reflex. A normal response in infants, but in adults this reflex indicates bifrontal or diffuse cortical atrophy. The reflexive protrusion of the lips is elicited by tapping or touching the lips or corners of the mouth.

Soma. Body.

Somatic. Pertaining to the body.

Somatophrenia. Condition sometimes observed in patients with right hemisphere cerebral damage in which the patient denies ownership of a paretic limb, or attributes ownership of the limb to another person.

Somnolent. Sleepy, difficult to arouse from sleep, or difficult to sustain alertness.

Spasmus nutans. A benign condition of childhood which usually appears in infancy and lasts for months to a few years, characterized by bilateral or monocular horizontal or vertical nystagmus, with rhythmic head nodding.

Spastic. A velocity-dependent increase in muscle tone, with exaggerated tendon reflex jerks, following upper motor neuron and pyramidal tract lesions.

Static encephalopathy. Preferred term for **cerebral palsy** (see Chapter 9, Hereditary, Teratogenic, and Other Congenital Disorders, pages 313–318).

Strabismus. Improper alignment of the visual axes.

Stupor. State of responsiveness in which the patient can only be aroused by vigorous and persistent external stimulation.

Subdural. Beneath the dura mater.

Supination. Lateral rotation of the forearm (palm forward) or foot.

Support reflex. When an infant extends its legs to support weight when its feet are bounced against a surface.

Supratentorial. Above the sheath of dura mater (tentorium cerebelli) that extends between the cerebellum and cerebrum. The term supratentorial is also sometimes facetiously used, as with the comment that the patient's problem is "supratentorial," or "all in the head," not real.

Synapse. The junction between two neurons. Neurons communicate by passing chemicals (neurotransmitters) between each other. These chemicals may be *excitatory*, causing the receiving neuron to have an electrical discharge (impulse); or *inhibitory*, preventing the receiving neuron from having an electrical discharge; or *neuromodulatory*, altering the response of the receiving neuron.

Syncope. Fainting, "light headedness."

Synkinesia. Involuntary muscle contractions associated with movement.

Tentorium. The fold of the dura mater that forms a partition *between the cerebrum and the cerebellum*. The **falx cerebri** is the dura fold in the midsagittal separation of the two cerebral hemispheres.

Tic. A movement disorder characterized by a repetitive, involuntary, or compulsive movement. Complex compulsive movements are called *habit tics*.

Tonic labyrinthine reflex. In infants, the arms and legs are pulled in toward the body when the head is flexed, and they extend when the head is held back and up.

Transcortical motor aphasia. A type of aphasia (acquired language disorder) characterized by mild or moderate dysfluency of speech, which is improved during repetition tasks, with relatively good auditory comprehension.

Transcortical sensory aphasia. A type of aphasia (acquired language disorder) characterized by fluently articulated, paraphasic speech, with better auditory comprehension and repetition than typically found with Wernicke's aphasia.

Tremor. Rhythmic, alternating, oscillatory movements produced by repetitive patterns of muscle contraction and relaxation.

Trephination. Cutting a circular hole ("burr hole") into the brain; *craniotomy*.

Upper motor neuron (UMN) lesion. Lesions involving the motor cortex and/or corticobulbar or corticospinal tracts; lesions above the level of a lower motor nucleus. *Acute consequences* of upper motor neuron lesions can include paralysis or paresis, hypotonia, hyporeflexia, and the Babinski sign. Over time there is *hyperreflexia and hypertonicity of muscles (spasticity) contralateral to the lesion*, if the lesion is above the decussation of the cortico-spinal (pyramidal) tract.

Vertigo. A sensation of movement that is often, but not always, a sensation of rotating or spinning.

Vestibular nystagmus. Nystagmus, usually rotary nystagmus, resulting from diseases in the semicircular canals and their central connections.

Vestibulo-cephalic reflex. See doll's eye phenomenon, occulocephalic reflex, above.

Visceral. Pertaining to the large internal organs of the three truncal cavities of the body.

Visual allesthesia. Phenomenon in which patients with hemi-inattention replace an image from the non-attended visual field to the attended visual field.

Wasting. Loss of muscle mass.

Weber test. Tuning fork test used by an examiner to test for a differential impairment in air versus bone conduction of sound. With this test, the tuning fork stem, when placed on the midline of the forehead, will be heard louder on the side with conductive disease. When disease of the cochlea is present, the sound vibration will be reported to lateralize to the better, or nondiseased, ear.

Wernicke's aphasia. A form of aphasia (acquired language disorder) characterized by relatively poor auditory comprehension and fluently articulated verbal expression marked by paraphasic distortions ranging from occasional phonologic errors to jargon.

B. Abbreviations Used in the Neurologic and Mental Status Examination

ACA. Anterior cerebral artery

ACh. Acetylcholine

AC < BC; AC > BC. Air less than bone air greater than bone

AD. Alzheimer's disease

ADD-H. Attention deficit disorder with hyperactivity

AKM. Akinetic mutism

ALS. Amyotrophic lateral sclerosis

AOS. Anterior operculum syndrome; apraxia of speech

ANS. Autonomic nervous system

BAD. Bipolar affective disorder

BAER (p). Brain stem auditory evoked response (potential)

C1, C2, etc. Cervical (vertebrae) number

CBS. Chronic brain syndrome

CN. Cranial nerve

CNS. Central nervous system

CPA. Cerebellar pontine angle

CPS. Complex partial seizure

CSF. Cerebrospinal fluid

CT, CAT, C CT. Computerized tomography, computerized axial tomography, contrast CT

CT CVA. Cerebrovascular accident

DAT. Dementia of the Alzheimer's type

DCS. Dorsal cord stimulation

DSM-IV. *Diagnostic and Statistical Manual of Mental Disorders IV,* (American Psychiatric Association) .

EEG. Electroencephalography

EMG. Electromyography

ENG. Electronystagmography

EOM. Extra ocular movements

EST, ECT. Electroshock therapy, electroconvulsion therapy

FOI. Flight of ideas

GII. General intellectual impairment

HDS. Herniated disk syndrome

HNP. Herniated nucleus pulposus

ICP. Intracranial pressure

L1, L2, etc. Lumbar (vertebrae) number

LOA. "Looseness" of associations

LOC. Loss of consciousness

LP. Lumbar puncture

MANSCAN. Mental Activity Network Scanner (method of computerized EEG analysis)

MCA. Middle cerebral artery

MG. Myasthenia gravis

MRI. Magnetic resonance imaging

MS. Multiple sclerosis

ncCT. Noncontrast CT

NCV. Nerve conduction velocity

NDT. Neurodevelopmental therapy

OPCD. Olivopontocerebellar degeneration

PCA. Posterior cerebral artery

PCS. Postconcussion syndrome

PDD. Primary degenerative dementia

PERLA. Pupils are equal and (equally) reactive to light and accommodation

PET. Positron emission tomography

PICA. Posterior inferior cerebellar artery

PNS. Peripheral nervous system

P Sz. Paranoid schizophrenia

PTA. Posttraumatic amnesia

S1, S2, etc. Sacral (vertebrae) number

SDAT. Senile dementia— Alzheimer's type

SIADH. Syndrome of Inadequate Antidiuretic Hormone

SPECT. Single photon emission tomography

SzDis. Seizure disorder

T1, T2 etc. Thoracic (vertebrae) number

TBI. Traumatic brain injury

TC. Tonic-clonic

TENS. Transcutaneous electrical nerve stimulator

VA shunt. Ventriculo-atrial shunt

VP shunt. Ventriculo-peritoneal shunt

V-B A. Vertebro-basilar artery

V-B D. Vertebro-basilar disease

VBI. Vertebro-basilar insufficiency; vertebro-basilar ischemia

VER (p). Visual evoked response (potential)

II. MENTAL STATUS ASSESSMENT

The neurologic examination begins with a brief mental status assessment, followed by examination of the cranial nerves, the motor system, coordination, reflexes, the sensory system, and gait and stability. While conducting the neurologic interview, subjective indicators of cognitive or psychiatric disturbances are noted. Psychiatric disturbances are identified from relatively subjective behavioral observations, whereas cognitive functions are more objectively examined with a series of tasks that compose a mental status screening. Patients with notable problems with cognition or with psychiatric disorders are referred for further evaluation.

A. Subjective Psychiatric Observations

Part of the mental status examination includes observations of the patient's appearance and behaviors during the interview. **When making subjective remarks about the patient's mood, affect, thinking processes, or content of thoughts in notes or reports, it is best to be as descriptive as possible and to include verbatim examples of the patient's statements.** For example, it is better to report, "Pt. said, 'I don't know what the point of all of this is, I'm no good to anyone,'" than to say, "Patient seemed depressed."

1. **Appearance.** Describes the patient's general habitus (grooming, hygiene, clothes, jewelry, etc.), use of gestures, any odd mannerisms, posture, or body language.

2. **Motor activity.** Describes the patient's rate of initiation of movement, any excessive activity or notable inactivity, pacing, agitation, repetitive movements, or tremors.

3. **Speech.** Describes the rate of speech, any evidence of a flight of ideas, lack of coherence, any inappropriate content, and the characteristics of articulation and language.

4. **Thought content.** Describes any indicators of delusions, paranoia, hallucinations, low self-esteem, denial, worry, hypochondriasis, suspiciousness, panic, or irritability. *Thought content refers to the ideas and preoccupations evident in the patient's language content.*

5. **Thought processes.** Describes any indicators of distractibility, evasiveness, displays of lapses or blocks, delayed or slow mental processing, impulsivity, or uncooperativeness. *Thought processes refer to the progression of the patient's thinking patterns.*

6. **Insight.** Describes any indicators of the patient's lack of appreciation of his or her condition or situation. *Insight refers to the patient's ability to interpret his or her condition or situation in a manner consistent with the perceptions of others.*

7. **Judgment.** Describes any indicators of an inability to form appropriate responses to everyday social situations. *Judgment refers to the ability to understand consequences and to form appropriate responses to everyday situations.*

8. **Mood.** Describes any indicators of anger, sadness, euphoria, apathy, fear, or depression. *Mood refers to the prevailing, general emotional state of the patient.*

9. **Affect.** Describes any notable affective displays, such as tearfulness, smiling, frowning, emotional lability, giddiness, or angry outbursts. *Affect refers to the fluctuating physical displays of emotions in facial expression, body movements, and voice.* Affect usually reflects a person's mood, but mood and affect can also be out of synchrony, as in parkinsonism, where a flat, masked affect may fail to reveal the patient's underlying emotion.

B. Bedside Assessment of Mental Status and Higher Cortical Functions

The standard bedside mental status interview includes tasks related to **language functions** (assessing naming, repeating, reading, writing, and comprehension of verbal directions); **orientation** (determining if they know where they are, who they are, and the date and time); **memory** (assessing short-term memory and recall of information after a brief delay); **attention** and **calculation** (asking the patient to subtract by 7s from 100); **drawing**; and **abstract reasoning** (assessing proverb interpretation). Some of the published, brief tests of mental status are described in the next section. These instruments vary in the extent to which their reliability and validity have been documented. Since they are screening tests, they may not be sensitive enough to identify subtle problems and, therefore, yield false negatives. Also, because mental status screening tests require language facility to perform nearly all of the tasks, patients with subtle aphasia could be inappropriately diagnosed to have generalized intellectual impairment (a false positive finding).

C. Standardized Cognitive Screening Examinations

1. **Mini-Mental State Examination (MMSE) (Folstein, Folstein, & McHugh, 1975).** The MMSE is a brief questionnaire with items related to orientation, registration (short-term memory), attention, calculation, language (naming, repeating, reading, writing), and drawing. This test requires approximately 15 to 20 minutes to administer. It is probably the most frequently used "standardized" mental status examination by physicians. The MMSE is used to screen for patients requiring further testing or as a means for longitudinal probes when progressive, dementing illness is suspected (see Table 4–1).

2. **Short Portable Mental Status Questionnaire (SPMSQ) (Pfieffer, 1975).** This assessment format is also popular in medical settings because it is brief and simple to administer. The patient is asked:

What is the date today?

What day of the week is it?

What is the name of this place?

What is your telephone number?

How old are you?

TABLE 4–1. Mini-Mental State Examination (Folstein, Folstein, & McHugh, 1975)

Score		
	I.	**Orientation**

____/5   What is today's date? Can you tell me the *season? year? day? month?*

____/5   Where are we? *state, county, town, hospital, floor*

II. Registration

____/3   I'm going to test your memory now. I'm going to say the names of three things and I want you to repeat them and remember them. OK? Here they are, say "Ball, flag, tree." (If the patient repeats the names completely and accurately the first time the maximum score is given. Keep saying them until all three are repeated, if cannot repeat all three after six trials, **Recall**, see below, cannot be tested.)

____/5   **III. Attention and Calculation**

        Ask the patient to subtract serial 7s from 100 or to spell the word "world" backward.

____/3   **IV. Recall**

        Ask the patient to recall the three words you previously asked to be repeated (ball, flag, tree).

____/9   **V. Language**

        Ask the patient to name the objects *pencil* and *watch.*

        Ask the patient to repeat, "No ifs, ands, or buts."

        Ask the patient to follow a three-stepped command: "Take the paper in your right hand, fold it in half, and put it on the floor."

        Write the sentence: "Close your eyes" in large letters and ask the patient to do what it says.

        Ask the patient to write a sentence (must contain a subject and a verb and be grammatical).

        On a clean piece of plain, white paper draw a design of two intersecting pentagons and ask the patient to copy it. The copy should be accurate, though any tremor or rotation of the drawing is permissible.

Total Score:____/30

     VI. Check level of Consciousness:

        ____Coma ____Drowsy ____Stupor ____Alert

Interpretation:

     28–30 Normal; 20–27 Mild Dementia; 12–19 Moderate Dementia; and

     0–11   Severe Dementia

When were you born?

Who is the President of the United States?

Who was the President just before him?

What was your mother's maiden name?

Subtract 3 from 20 and keep subtracting 3 from each new number, all the way down.

The total number of errors is interpreted to indicate the degree of cognitive impairment; extra points are allowed for educational and racial factors.

3. **The Neurobehavioral Cognitive Status Examination (NCSE) (Schwamm, Van Dyke, & Kierman, 1983).** The screening items from this mental status examination can be administered in a brief time, but if the "metric" items (additional items of graded difficulty in each subtest) are administered, testing time is about 30 minutes. This test is seldom used in routine mental status screening, as it requires pictures and other materials, (i.e., block design blocks) in its administration. However, this test enjoys some popularity in medical research as a quick cognitive assessment with populations having, or at risk for, central nervous system damage.

4. **Cognitive Capacity Screening Examination (CCSE) (Jacobs, Bernard, & Delgado, 1977).** This cognitive screening instrument contains 30 items and requires about 10 to 20 minutes to administer. It can be administered by any health care professional and tests orientation, concentration, attention, mental control, language (including concept formation), and short-term memory.

5. **Galveston Orientation and Amnesia Test (GOAT) (Levin, O'Donnell, & Grossman, 1979).** This evaluation protocol is used mainly with patients who have had traumatic brain injuries. It evaluates the major spheres of orientation (time, place, and person) and memory functions.

III. NEUROLOGIC EXAMINATION

A. Neurologic Review

The purpose of the neurologic examination is first to localize the site(s) of neurologic damage and then to determine what is causing the problem. The examination begins with a neurologic review (neurologic "review of systems"). The neurologist's examination usually presumes a neurologic problem exists; thus, during the neurologic review, the patient will be asked to describe any problems with *headache, vision, hearing, tinnitus, vertigo, movement, numbness, bowel and bladder control, memory, and speech* and *language.* This interview usually precedes the mental status examination and the rest of the neurologic examination.

B. Neurologic Physical Examination

The neurologic physical examination is organized by systems, generally in the following manner:

Cranial nerves examination

Motor and muscle strength assessment

Coordination examination

Station and gait examination

Sensation assessment

Reflex testing

1. Muscle strength testing in the neurologic examination is graded on a 0 to 5 rating scale:

0 = total paralysis

1 = inability to contract against gravity

2 = able to contract against gravity

3 = active movement against gravity, no resistance

4– = active movement against slight resistance

4 = active movement against moderate resistance

4+ = active movement against strong resistance

5 = normal strength

2. Reflexes are numerically graded on a 0–4 rating scale, as follows:

0 = absent

1+ = diminished

2+ = normal

3+ = increased

4+ = clonic

Both muscle strength and reflexes will be illustrated in the medical record by using a stick figure to represent the patient.

3. **Graded scales for specific muscle groups** are sometimes used in specialized assessments (See Facial Grading System, Figure 4–1).

C. Examining the Cranial Nerves (CN)

Table 4–2 lists the cranial nerves, their functions, and disorders associated with damage to particular cranial nerves. Figure 4–2 illustrates the anatomical location of cranial nerves.

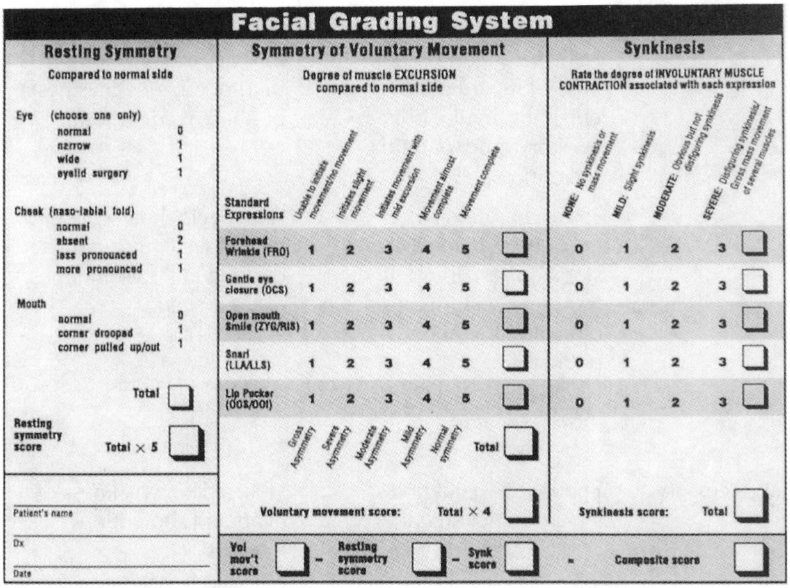

Facial Grading System

Resting Symmetry

Compared to normal side

Eye (choose one only)		
	normal	0
	narrow	1
	wide	1
	eyelid surgery	1
Cheek (naso-labial fold)		
	normal	0
	absent	2
	less pronounced	1
	more pronounced	1
Mouth		
	normal	0
	corner drooped	1
	corner pulled up/out	1

Total ☐

Resting symmetry score — Total × 5 ☐

Patient's name

Dx

Date

Symmetry of Voluntary Movement

Degree of muscle EXCURSION compared to normal side

Synkinesis

Rate the degree of INVOLUNTARY MUSCLE CONTRACTION associated with each expression

Standard Expressions	Unable to initiate movement/no movement	Initiates slight movement	Initiates movement with mild excursion	Movement almost complete	Movement complete		NONE: No synkinesis or mass movement	MILD: Slight synkinesis	MODERATE: Obvious but not disfiguring synkinesis	SEVERE: Disfiguring synkinesis/ Gross mass movement of several muscles	
Forehead Wrinkle (FRO)	1	2	3	4	5	☐	0	1	2	3	☐
Gentle eye closure (OCS)	1	2	3	4	5	☐	0	1	2	3	☐
Open mouth Smile (ZYG/RIS)	1	2	3	4	5	☐	0	1	2	3	☐
Snarl (LLA/LLS)	1	2	3	4	5	☐	0	1	2	3	☐
Lip Pucker (OOS/OOI)	1	2	3	4	5	☐	0	1	2	3	☐
	Gross Asymmetry	Severe Asymmetry	Moderate Asymmetry	Mild Asymmetry	Normal symmetry	Total ☐					

Voluntary movement score: Total × 4 ☐

Synkinesis score: Total ☐

Vol mov't score ☐ – Resting symmetry score ☐ – Synk score ☐ = Composite score ☐

Figure 4–1. Facial Grading System (from Ross, B. G., Fradet, G., & Nedzelski, J. M. Development of a sensitive facial grading system. *Otolaryngology—Head and Neck Surgery, 114*(3), p. 382, 1996, with permission.)

Table 4–2. Cranial nerves and their functions, and problems associated with their dysfunction

Cranial Nerve	Function	Disorders Associated with Lesions
I Olfactory	Smell	Anosmia
II Optic	Vision	Vision loss
III Oculomotor	Eye movements, pupillary constriction, and accommodation	Ptosis, diplopia, loss of accommodation
IV Trochlear	Eye movement	Diplopia
V Trigeminal	Facial sensation, mastication, and proprioception	Facial numbness and weakness
VI Abducens	Eye movement	Diplopia
VII Facial	Facial expression; taste; sensation of tonsils, soft palate, external and middle ear; salivation	Upper and lower facial weakness, loss of taste for anterior two-thirds of tongue, dry mouth, dysarthria
VIII Vestibulocochlear	Equilibrium and hearing	Vertigo, nystagmus, disequilibrium, deafness
IX Glossopharyngeal	Pharyngeal elevation; taste; sensation of the base of the tongue, epiglottis, uvula, pharynx, auditory tube; parotid secretion	Dysphagia; dysarthria; loss of taste, posterior one-third of tongue; anesthesia of pharynx; dry mouth
X Vagus	Taste; sensation of epiglottis, larynx, trachea, stomach, small intestine, transverse colon; muscles of deglutition and phonation; cardiac suppression; visceral movement and secretions	Dysphagia, hoarseness, palatal weakness, cardiac dysfunction, dysfunctions of the viscera
XI Spinal Accessory	Phonation, head and shoulder movement	Hoarseness, weakness of head and shoulder muscles
XII Hypoglossal	Tongue movements	Dysarthria, weakness or wasting of tongue muscles

Source: Adapted from Gilroy, J. (1990). *Basic neurology.* New York: Pergamon.

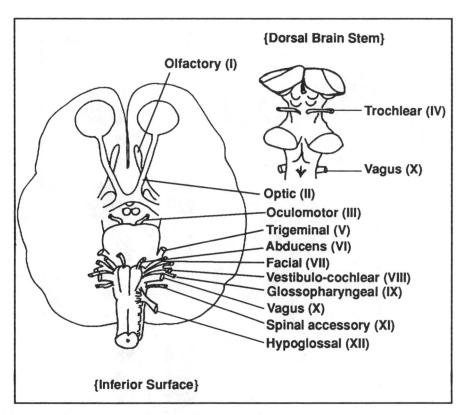

Figure 4–2. Location of the cranial nerves

CN I (Olfactory). To test the olfactory nerve the neurologist may present substances with odors (not noxious), such as coffee, lemon oil, and cloves, for the patient to smell.

CN II (Optic). Visual acuity will be examined with a Snellen chart or equivalent. In addition, an ophthalmoscopic examination of eyes is done to examine the fundus. Vision testing can locate sites of lesion along the visual pathway from the retina to the visual cortex (see Figure 4–3). Visual field testing may be done grossly, by asking the patient if he or she can see fingers wiggling in the upper, middle, and lower thirds of his or her left and right visual fields; or a precise mapping of the patient's area of vision can be made by an opthalmologist using visual stimuli adjustments on a projection screen (Goldman fields). Neurologists may use a "Maddox rod," an instrument used to detect subtle evidence of double vision, in vision testing.

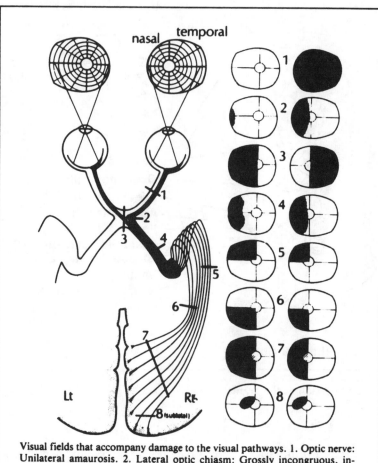

Visual fields that accompany damage to the visual pathways. 1. Optic nerve: Unilateral amaurosis. 2. Lateral optic chiasm: Grossly incongruous, incomplete (contralateral) homonymous hemianopia. 3. Central optic chiasm: Bitemporal hemianopia. 4. Optic tract: Incongruous, incomplete homonymous hemianopia. 5. Temporal (Meyer's) loop of optic radiation: Congruous partial or complete (contralateral) homonymous superior quadrantanopia. 6. Parietal (superior) projection of the optic radiation: Congruous partial or complete homonymous inferior quadrantanopia. 7. Complete parieto-occipital interruption of optic radiation. Complete congruous homonymous hemianopia with psychophysical shift of foveal point often sparing central vision, giving "macular sparing." 8. Incomplete damage to visual cortex: Congruous homonymous scotomas, usually encroaching at least acutely on central vision.

Figure 4–3. Visual system lesions and visual field deficits (From Plum, F. [1985]. Neuro-opthalmology. In J. B. Wyngaarden & L. H. Smith [Eds.], *Cecil textbook of medicine* [17th ed.]. Philadelphia: W. B. Saunders, p. 2032, with permission.)

CN III (Oculomotor), IV (Trochlear), VI (Abducens). Pupillary responses are mediated by CN II (afferent arc) and CN III (efferent arc). The neurologist stimulates pupillary responses (to test size, shape, and equality) with light and accommodation to objects near the eye. If pupils respond equally to contralateral light and accommodation stimulation, this finding is recorded as **PERLA** (**p**upils are **e**qual and **r**esponsive to **l**ight and **a**ccommodation) or equivalently PERRLA and PEERLA. When pupils are dilated (widely open), as one sometimes sees in association with drug effects, the condition is referred to as *mydriasis.*

Figure 4–4 illustrates pupillary reactions in association with different lesions and disorders. This area of cranial nerve testing also examines volitional and pursuit eye movements or extra-ocular movements (EOMs). Cranial nerve III elevates the upper eyelid and CN VII (Facial nerve) closes the eyelid. CN IV provides some downward and outward movement, and CN VI provides lateral movement.

CN V (Trigeminal). CN V is tested by assessing facial sensation, eliciting a corneal reflex (eye blink with light touch or air puff), checking for opening and closing the jaw against resistance; and examining for the jaw jerk reflex. (Afferent aspects are a part of CN V, and efferent aspects are a part of CN VII.)

CN VII (Facial). To test CN VII, the neurologist will see if patient can do such things as close the eyes, wrinkle the brow, show the teeth, smile, or whistle. A lower quadrant, facial weakness occurs with a contralateral upper motor neuron disease, and an upper and lower facial weakness will be found ipsilateral to disease involving the lower motor neuron.

CN VIII (Vestibulocochlear). To test CN VIII, the neurologist will have the patient listen to a watch tick, will conduct tuning fork tests, or request an audiologic evaluation. Vestibular testing might include a *Barany test, caloric test,* or *posturography.*

CN IX (Glossopharyngeal), X (Vagus). These functionally integrated cranial nerves are tested mainly by listening to the patient speak. The neurologist will ask the patient to phonate and will examine the symmetry of palate with "ah," elicit a gag reflex, and ask the patient to swallow. Figure 4–5 illustrates the innervation for the head and neck muscles.

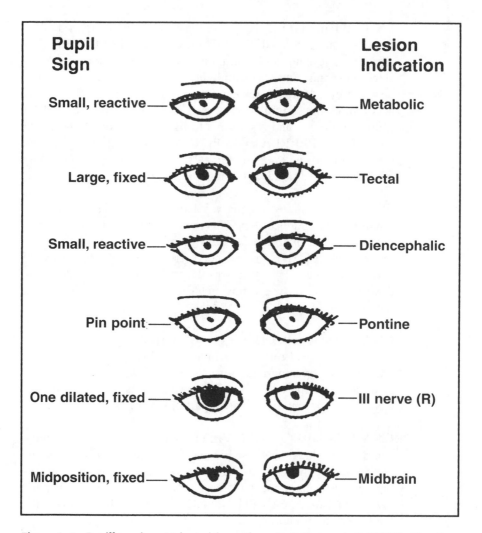

Figure 4–4. Pupillary signs (Adapted from Plum, F., & Posner, J. B. [1980]. *The diagnosis of stupor and coma* (3rd ed.). Philadelphia: F. A. Davis.)

CN XI (Spinal Accessory). To test CN XI, the patient will be asked to shrug the shoulders and push the head left and right against resistance.

CN XII (Hypoglossal). To test CN XII, the patient is asked to stick the tongue in and out of the mouth and to push against a tongue depressor to the left and right.

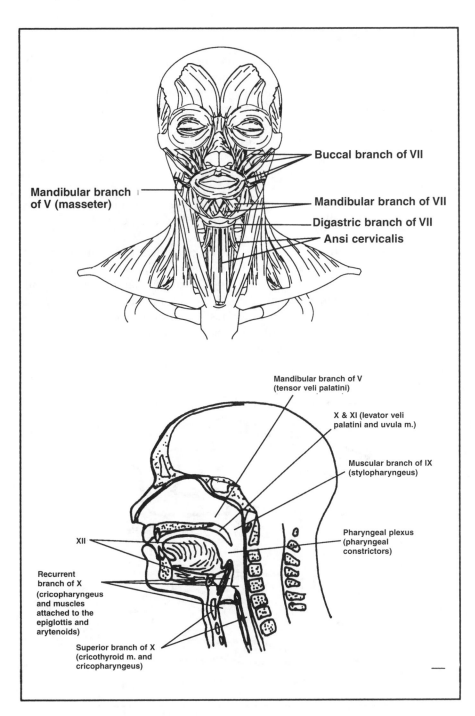

Figure 4–5. Efferent innervation for head and neck muscles

147

D. Motor Examination

1. **Motor.** Motor testing may begin with an inspection of the patient's posture in bed (see Figure 4–6) and determining if the patient is able to sit. The patient's muscle tone, range of movement, and strength in all extremities is then tested.

2. **Coordination and balance.** Coordination is tested with rapid alternating movements, finger-to-nose test, heel-to-shin test, and standing with eyes closed.

3. **Gait.** Gait is examined by watching the patient walk and by asking the patient to walk on the toes and heels.

4. **Sensation.** Sensation testing examines responses to *touch, pain, temperature, vibration, proprioception* (position sense), *stereognosis* (ability to recognize objects), *graphesthesia* (ability to recognize numbers drawn on the palm), *and two-point discrimination.* Sensation testing will reveal patterns of sensory loss within the distributions of segmental nerve roots, or *dermatomes* (see Figure 4–7).

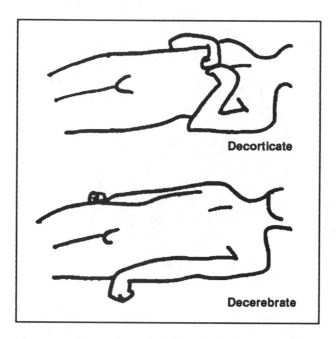

Figure 4–6. Decorticate and decerebrate arm postures

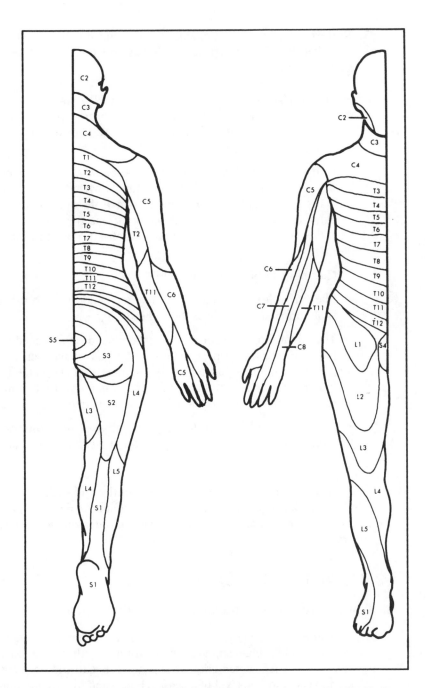

Figure 4–7. Dermatomes (From Budassi, S. A., & Barber, J. M. [1981]. *Emergency nursing: Principles and practice.* St. Louis: C. V. Mosby, p. 225, with permission.)

5. **Reflexes.** Reflex testing examines for reduced, heightened, or so-called pathologic reflexes. **Reflexes the neurologist tests generally include:**

- **Tendon/stretch reflexes.** *Jaw jerk*, CN V and CN VII; *biceps,* C5 and C6; *triceps,* C7 and C8; *brachioradialis,* C5 and C6; *quadriceps,* L3 and L4; *ankle* (Achilles tendon), S1 and S2; and *patellar*, L2, L3, and L4.

- **Uritogenital reflexes.** Including the *bulbo-cavernosal reflex*, in which the anal sphincter contracts when the tip of the penis is grasped; the *anal wink* in which the anal sphincter contracts with stroking of the buttocks; and the *cremasteric reflex* (retraction of the testicles when stroking the inner thigh).

- **Cutaneous abdominal reflexes.**

- **Plantar reflex.** Flexion of the great toe is normal, extension is abnormal and known as the *Babinski sign.*

- **Thumb adduction reflex.** Wartenberg hand sign, elicited by hooking your fingertips with those of the patient and then asking the patient to pull against your fingers; if the patient's thumb adducts across the palm into a simian grasp, then the abnormal thumb adduction reflex is demonstrated.

- **Other pathologic reflexes, or release phenomena.** Including the *snout*, or rooting, *reflex*; *glabellar reflex*; and *bite reflex.*

In neonates, demonstrations of the Moro (startle) and suck reflexes are normal. During the first year of life the infant's *primitive reflexes* diminish corresponding to an emergence of *automatic movement reactions.*

IV. COMA, DELIRIUM, AND DEMENTIA

A. Coma and Post-Coma Cognitive Status

1. **Examination.** The physical examination of the comatose patient involves a neurologic appraisal to determine whether the disease is supratentorial, subtentorial, or metabolic. **Breathing patterns** are indicators of the level of disease. Hyper- and hypoventilation occur most often with metabolic disorders. Cheyne-Stokes respi-

rations (see Chapter 7, Terminology, page 238) are usually associated with hemispheric or pontomedullary disease. A **fundoscopic** examination of the eye will be made, looking principally for **papilledema** or **subhyaloid hemorraging**, the classic sign for a subarchnoid hemorrhage. **Oculocephalic responses** will be examined using the *doll's eyes maneuver* (see Terminology, page 120), unless there is reason to suspect a neck injury. **Pupillary reflexes** and **gaze** positioning will be examined. The extent and symmetry of stretch reflexes and motor responses will be examined and the limb, neck, and jaw posturing of the patient will be noted. Decorticate posturing, decerebrate posturing, mixed posturing, or flaccid quadriplegia indicate different sites of lesions. The examination of a comatose patient and the patient emerging from coma will also include a rating of the level of **consciousness** and **responsiveness**.

2. **Ratings.** Coma is a state of unresponsiveness brought on by *intracranial causes* (supratentorial and subtentorial), *diffuse lesions,* and *metabolic disturbances.* States of stupor and coma may be described with terms such as *lethargic, obtundurate, stuporous,* and *comatose,* but are best described by using a standardized rating scale. One of the most commonly used methods for rating coma levels is the **Glasgow Coma Scale** (GCS), or Glasgow Rating Scale, shown in Table 4–3. The **Rancho Los Amigos Scale** is often applied when rating levels of *cognitive responses following coma during stages of recovery* (see Table 4–4).

B. Eye Movements in Pursuit and Gaze

Eye positions and movements can indicate sites of lesion in the poorly responsive patient. Coma can be caused by diffuse lesions in both cerebral hemispheres or by focal lesions of the midbrain and upper pons. Most comatose patients have **roving dysconjugate gaze** (unable to fix their vision on objects). This type of movement indicates the brain stem is, to some extent, intact. Patients displaying a **forced downward gaze** may have had *thalamic hemorrhages,* lesions in the *region of the pineal gland or metabolic encephalopathies.* A **forced upward gaze** occurs when the *frontal eye fields* (area 8 in the frontal cortex) exert a tonic effect on horizontal eye movements. With destructive lesions, the tonic control from the intact hemisphere forces the gaze *toward the damaged hemisphere.* **Forced horizontal gaze** can occur with brain stem lesions. Patients with progressive supranuclear palsy often have difficulty with vertical and, later, horizontal gaze movements.

Table 4–3. Glasgow Coma Scale

Response	Score
Eye opening	
None	1
To pain	2
To speech	3
Spontaneous	4
Verbal response	
None	1
Incomprehensible sounds	2
Inappropriate words	3
Confused conversation	4
Oriented conversation	5
Motor response	
None	1
Abnormal extension (decerebrate rigidity)	2
Abnormal flexion (decorticate rigidity)	3
Withdrawal	4
Localizes pain	5
Obeys commands	6
Total GCS:	_____

Source: Adapted from Teasdale, M. J., & Jennett, B. (1974). Assessment of command impaired consciousness: A practical scale. *Lancet, 11,* 81–84.

C. Delirium, Depression, and Dementias

1. **Delirium.** Delirium is caused by *systemic factors* (cardiovascular disease, infections, medications, neoplasm, metabolic disturbances, post-operative status, trauma, and substance abuse) or *central nervous system factors* (infection, neoplasm, trauma, vascular disorders, stroke, subdural hematoma, postictal status, subarachnoid hemorrhage, vasculitis, and arteriosclerosis). Delirium is often in evidence in the presence of a life threatening condition; after medical correction, cognitive faculties may return to baseline.

2. **Depression.** In any patient, but particularly in the elderly, the diagnosis of depression is an essential feature of the differential examination of mental status. Depression can be associated with dementia, or its presence can cause the patient to display cogni-

Table 4–4. Rancho Los Amigos Cognitive Scale for Head Injury

Level	Indicators
I	*No response* to pain, touch, sound, or sight.
II	*Generalized reflex response* to pain.
III	*Localized response.* Blinks to strong light, turns toward/away from sound, responds to physical discomfort, inconsistent response to commands.
IV	*Confused, inappropriate, and agitated.* Alert, very active, aggressive or bizarre behaviors, performs motor activities but behavior is nonpurposeful, extremely short attention span.
V	*Confused, inappropriate, and nonagitated.* Gross attention to environment, highly distractible, requires continual redirection, difficulty learning new tasks, agitated by too much stimulation. May engage in social conversations but with inappropriate verbalizations.
VI	*Confused, appropriate.* Inconsistent orientation to time and place, retention span/recent memory impaired, begins to recall past, consistently follows simple directions, goal-directed behavior with assistance.
VII	*Automatic, appropriate.* Performs daily routine in highly familiar environment in a nonconfused but automatic manner. Skills noticeably deteriorate in unfamiliar environment. Lacks realistic planning for own future.
VIII	*Purposeful, appropriate.*

Source: From Hagen, C., & Malkmus, D. (1979, November). *Intervention strategies for language disorders secondary to head injuries.* Paper presented at the American Speech-Language-Hearing Association Annual Convention, Atlanta, GA, with permission.

tive deficits. In such cases, treatment for depression can reverse the cognitive deficits. Formal assessment of depression is not normally a part of the routine neurologic examination.

3. **Reversible dementias.** Dementia is potentially reversible when the cognitive declines are related to *depression, drug toxicity, normal pressure hydrocephalus, infection, nutritional deficiencies, cardiopulmonary disorders,* and *resectable brain lesions.*

4. **Irreversible dementias.** Causes for dementia that are not reversible include *AIDS, Creutzfeldt-Jacob disease, Alzheimer's disease, Pick's disease, alcoholic dementia syndromes, cerebro-cerebellar degenerations, Huntington's chorea,* and *multi-infarction* (see Chapter 9 for more elaboration). Alzheimer's disease (AD), multi-infarct dementia (MID), mixed AD and MID, and alcoholic dementia make up the majority of chronic dementing illnesses.

Multi-infarct dementia (MID) can be found in conditions such as *multiple lacunar infarctions* in the central nervous system as seen with *Binswanger's disease* (hypertensive atherosclerotic disease leading to multiple subcortical lesions), *large vessel atheromas, vasculitis, systemic hypoprofusion* (due to occlusion of a major body vessel, such as the aorta, or heart attacks), and *anoxic episodes.*

Alzheimer's disease (AD) is, at present, an irreversible, progressive disease resulting in profound dementia in its latter stages. The neuropathology includes degeneration and loss of nerve cells, particularly in those regions essential for memory and cognitive associations. It is characterized by neuritic plaques and neurofibrillary tangles. In addition, aggregates of amyloid protein can be found adjacent to and within blood vessels of patients with AD.

Alcoholic dementia refers to a multifactorial disorder associated with long-term metabolic disruption, blows to the head following falls, poor nutrition, and other factors. **Wernicke-Korsakoff syndrome** is a form of dementia known to be associated with *alcoholism, severe vitamin-impoverished diets*, and anoxic or hemorrhagic cerebral *ischemia*, producing a selective, bilateral loss of neurons in the medial diencephalon and hypothalamus. Wernicke-Korsakoff syndrome usually reflects chronic thiamine depletion. Wernicke's *encephalopathy* is usually the acute manifestation, characterized by global confusion, ocular disturbances, apathy, and ataxia. *Korsakoff 's amnestic syndrome* (Korsakoff's disease, Korsakoff's psychosis, Korsakoff's dementia) is viewed as a chronic state, or later stage, of this syndrome. Korsakoff amnesics have a profound memory loss for **recent events**, with spared language functions and relatively spared **retrograde** memory (memory for past events), a severe **anterograde** amnesia (impaired ability to acquire new information), and often, but not always, a related **confabulation**. Confabulation refers to the tendency to claim falsely to have seen, experienced, or done something.

V. COMMONLY ORDERED NEUROLOGIC STUDIES

For a discussion of specific neurologic imaging studies, refer to Chapter 8, Radiologic Studies and Therapies.

A. Muscle and Nerve Conduction Studies

1. **Edrophonium (tensilon) testing.** Test done to differentially diagnose an acetylcholine deficiency in myoneural junction disease (myasthenia gravis). This test requires introducing timed intravenous injections of edrophonium chloride (tensilon) and conducting tests of muscle strength improvements as an effect of this drug.

2. **Electromyography (EMG).** EMG is an examination of the electrical impulses produced by a muscle. A needle electrode is inserted into a muscle and the electrical wave pattern (frequency and amplitude of the electrical impulse) is read from an oscilloscope. The graphic copy is called the *electromyograph*. An EMG study can detect abnormalities in the muscle itself or the consequences of damage to the nerve innervating the muscle.

3. **Nerve conduction studies (NCS) or nerve conduction velocity (NCV) testing.** This test measures the velocity of electrical impulses along nerves. One electrode is placed along the course of the nerve to provide electrical stimuli, and a measurement is taken of the time required for the electrical stimuli to reach either a second electrode (for sensory nerves) or the time necessary to reach the muscle innervated by that nerve (for motor nerves). In NCS, *F-responses* refer to measures of conduction in the proximal portions of a motor nerve and ventral root. The *H-reflex* provides the equivalent of a stretch reflex in which sensory fibers of the posterior tibial nerve in the popliteal fossa are stimulated electrically and the efferent evoked action potential from the soleus muscle is recorded.

B. Nystagmus and Eye Movements

1. **Barany test.** A labyrinthine nystagmus test in which nystagmus is induced by rotating the patient in a specially designed chair.

2. **Caloric test.** A test used to examine the connections between the vestibular nuclei of the eighth cranial nerve and the oculomotor nerves. This test is performed by irrigating the external ear canal with water at a controlled temperature with the head at a 30° angle. In testing comatose patients, ice water is used. In the awake subject, temperatures of 30 to 40° F are typical. Ice water in both ears simultaneously can be used to test vertical eye movement.

3. **Electronystagmography (ENG).** Evoked potential test used as an alternative to or to substantiate the caloric testing for nystagmus. This test is performed with the patient in a supine position with electrodes affixed with paste to the skin under the eyes. With the eyes closed, positional or caloric stimuli are introduced to elicit nystagmus. Eye movement recordings are made on an *electronystagmograph*. ENGs help to differentiate vestibular from nonvestibular balance disorders.

C. X-Ray and Other Imaging Studies

Additional studies are described in Chapter 8.

1. **Cerebral angiography/arteriography.** An x-ray study of the brain done following the injection of a contrast dye into the major arteries.

2. **Computerized tomography (CT) scans.** This computerized x-ray study of the brain requires that the patient lie inside a large, donut-shaped scanner while x-ray beams make a complete circle through segments of the brain. As the beams pass through tissues, the scanner detects density differences, and the aggregate data are analyzed by the computer to construct a "picture" of the scanned segments. An intravenous infusion of an **iodinated contrast agent** (radiopaque dye containing iodine) is often injected into a vein prior to the study. This allows identification of vascular structures and disruption of the brood-brain barrier, providing *enhancement*; thus, when a contrast agent is used the study will be called an "enhanced CT." Disruption of the blood-brain barrier is abnormal. Therefore, *enhanced studies can delineate blood vessels, vascular malformations, vascular tumors, and regions in which the blood-brain barrier is lacking.* Additional discussion of the CT scan is found in Chapter 8, and Figure 8–1 represents the anatomical areas demonstrated by CT scans. Figure 4–8 demonstrates the structures examined in a CT scan taken through the middle of the third ventricle.

3. **Myelography.** An x-ray study made of the subarachnoid space of the spinal cord with an injection of a contrast dye for the purpose of examining for impingement of nerve exits, intervertebral disc protrusions and herniations, or abnormal bony pressures on the cord or nerves.

4. **Magnetic resonance imaging (MRI).** Like the CT scan, the MRI produces a computerized picture of the brain, or other body

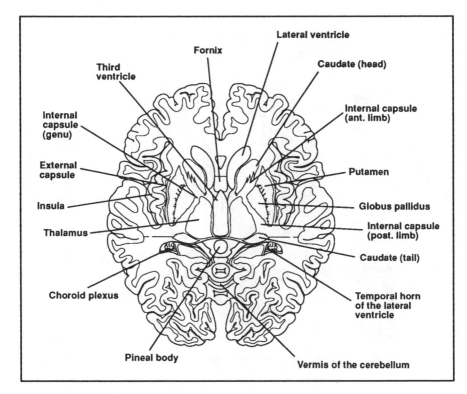

Figure 4–8. Anatomical structures revealed in a CT scan through the middle of the third ventricle

structures, but uses radio waves and magnetism instead of X rays and does not require ionizing radiation. The MRI is based on the principle that all atoms have magnetic properties. This energy, when subjected to a radio wave, can be detected; and (like the CT scan) the detectors feed data to a computer to construct remarkably clear images which are then interpreted by a neurologist or radiologist. Figure 4–9 provides an anatomical illustration corresponding to a midsagittal plane of the MRI. Additional discussion of the MRI is found in Chapter 8.

5. **Functional Magnetic Resonance Imaging (fMRI).** Functional magnetic resonance imaging (fMRI) technology uses the principles and techniques of static nuclear magnetic resonance (NMR) imaging and earlier developed methods of imaging brain metabolic activity, PET scanning, SPECT scanning and rCBF studies. fMRI is a safer, cheaper procedure than these

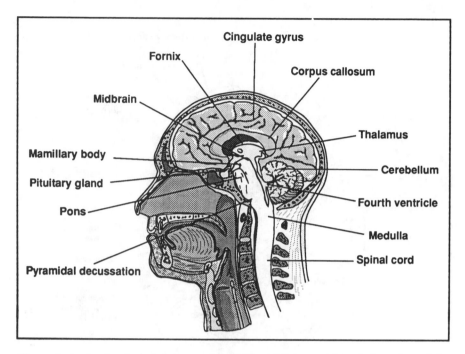

Figure 4–9. Anatomical structures revealed by MRI in a midsaggital section of the brain

nuclide scanning methods and the spatial and temporal resolution with fMRI and visualization of the brain when engaged in a mental activity are equivalent or better. fMRIs have been used experimentally to examine for areas of brain activity and networks of brain regions and structures involved in motor functions, sensory perceptions, and memory. The principles of fMRI involve the link between increases in regional metabolic functions during certain brain activities as shown by tracking oxygen consumption. The Blood Oxygen Level Dependent (BOLD) mechanism, in which the blood in an active region or the brain becomes more oxygenated, influences the brain's nuclear properties, and these changes are detected by NMR and analyzed by a computer to generate images of brain activity.

6. **Pneumoencephalography (PEG).** This x-ray study involves the injection of air or gas into the subarachnoid space for the purpose of delineating the cisterns and the ventricular system. The PEG is especially useful for the evaluation of posterior fossa, suprasellar, and ventricular tumors.

7. **Skull series.** Plain film radiograms taken in four views used to examine for bony and soft tissue abnormalities of the cranium.

D. Cortical Electrical Activity

1. **Electroencephalography (EEG).** The EEG is a recording of electrical impulses in the brain made while the patient is awake, asleep, or receiving stimulation while staring at a pattern board or a flashing light (photic stimulation). The majority of EEG machines have 8, 12, 16, or 20 channels. Depending on the technique used, approximately 16 to 30 small chlorided silver electrodes are attached to the patient's scalp with a special paste, allowing a graphic recording of electrical impulses. The EEG tracings are *voltage versus time graphs* and record slow waveform (0.5–30 Hz) activity across specific areas of the brain. Studies require from 45 to 90 minutes. Findings can be analyzed *on line*, during actual examination, or *off line*, from recordings of the examination. The EEG is useful in studying seizure activity, to determine brain death, and to evaluate focal versus diffuse conditions (refer to Table 4–5 and Figure 4–10).

2. **Mental Activity Network (MAN) Scanning.** This is an example of a computerized analysis of EEG signals taken from 124 sites (instead of the usual 8 to 20). This technology is being used experimentally to examine patterns of electrochemical activity in the brain during various mental activities.

E. Other Studies

1. **Intracranial pressure (ICP) monitoring.** Intracranial monitors may be placed when there is suspicion of cerebral edema, hemorrhage or hematoma, obstruction hydrocephalus, brain herniation, or clinical signs of a space-occupying or expanding lesion. The devices used for ICP include *intraventricular catheters, subarachnoid screws*, and *epidural fiber-optic sensors*. These devices measure pressure within the cranium, displayed on a monitor as pressure (mm Hg) over time (minutes). ICP waves within normal parameters are referred to as "C-Waves."

2. **Neuropsychiatric and neuropsychologic testing.** Whenever appropriate, patients with emotional or cognitive deficits will be referred for neuropsychiatric or neuropsychologic evaluation. This testing may be an important part of the overall neurodiagnostic evaluation to examine for secondary emotional and cognitive deficits.

Table 4–5. EEG patterns

Pattern	Description
Alpha	Frequencies of 8–13 Hz, but may be slower in children. An alpha frequency is often found as the posteriorly dominant rhythm present in the awake, alert individual with his or her eyes closed that disappears when the eyes are opened.
Beta	Symmetrical frequencies of 14–35 Hz of lower amplitude than alpha rhythms. Beta rhythms are normally found in the frontal areas and will be depressed over focal lesions.
Theta	Mild slowing with frequencies of 3–7 Hz. Slow waves are normal during sleep and are commonly seen in association with metabolic disorders and destructive lesions.
Delta	Severe slowing with frequencies less than 3 Hz.
Sharp	Waves showing a brief high voltage electrical discharge from a focal area of the brain, often indicative of epilepsy, also called "spike and dome" waves.
Negative	EEG pattern felt to represent a sudden burst of electrical activity from the brain surface, suggestive of epilepsy.
Asymmetric	EEG patterns corresponding to large areas of the left and right hemispheres are graphically displayed. The waves correspond to patterns of connections between the electrodes and the recording channels, known as *montages*. Location schematics of the montage reference sites and linkages are illustrated on the electroencephalogram tracing, as if you were looking at the top of the head. *Asymmetric* patterns reflect destructive lesions to one of the hemispheres.
Mu	Frequencies of 7 to 11 Hz located centrally or centro-parietal that attenuate with movement.
Lambda	Transient waves from the occipital area occurring during visual scanning.

3. **Cerebral spinal fluid (CSF) analysis.** Laboratory analysis of CSF is done to determine if there are **changes in the normal constituents** (water, glucose, sodium chloride, and protein), which indicate brain disease, or if **blood**, which indicates hemorrhage, **bacteria**, or increased **leukocytes** (which indicate infection) are present. Appendix C contains a list of normal values in CSF analysis.

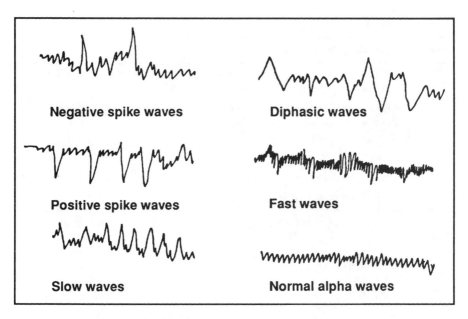

Figure 4–10. Illustration of EEG patterns

VI. DSM–IV CLASSIFICATIONS

The American Psychiatric Association publishes a standardized classification system for psychiatric disorders currently called the *Diagnostic and Statistical Manual of Mental Disorders–IV*, referring to the fourth edition of these published categories. DSM–IV classifications provide descriptive guidelines for psychiatric diagnoses. All DSM–IV codes are included in the International Classification of Disease codes, (ICD–9, CM). The DSM–IV classification system relies on what the patient says and does as indicators for how the patient thinks and feels. This system is *multiaxial*. The first three axes relate to the diagnostic assessment. Axis I codes clinical syndromes. Axis II codes personality disorders and developmental disorders. Axis III identifies relevant medical disorders and conditions. Axis IV codes the severity of the psychosocial stressors, and Axis V designates the Global Assessment of Function (GAF), based on a 100-point scale (see Table 4–6). Classifications also include conditions not attributable to the disorders that are the focus of treatment (see further discussion in Chapter 9).

Table 4–6. DSM IV classifications

Axis	Area Described
I	Clinical disorders and other disorders that may be the focus of clinical attention (e.g., major depression or paranoia)
II	Personality disorders and mental retardation (e.g., anti-social, schizoid, passive-aggressive personalities)
III	General medical conditions (e.g., chronic medical conditions such as stroke)
IV	Psychosocial and environmental problems (e.g., loss of job or bereavement)
V	Global assessment of functioning

Source: *Quick Reference to the Diagnostic Criteria from DSM-IV.* American Psychiatric Association, Washington, DC (1994).

VII. PAIN AND SLEEP

A. Pain

Complaints related to pain are reported in the neurologic examination. Pain is described relative to its *quality* (pulsing, sharp, tingling, dull, etc.), *intensity* (slight, mild, moderate, severe), *location, and duration* (acute, chronic, intermittent, and intractable).

B. Sleep

It is sometimes necessary to examine the patient's sleep pattern or to conduct EEG studies during sleep. In these cases, sleep patterns will be described in terms of "stages." Sleep has five stages: *Substage I* (relaxed, hypnagogic pre-sleep stage), *Sub-stage II* (asleep but easily aroused), *Sub-stage III* (aroused from sleep with difficulty), *Deep* (Delta) *Sleep* (when brain waves are slow and metabolism slows), and *REM* (rapid eye movement) stage sleep (when dreaming is present and respiration is irregular; there may be apnea during this stage and arousal is difficult).

VIII. NOTES

_____

_____

_____

IX. REFERENCES

American Psychiatric Association. (1987). *Diagnostic and statistical manual of mental disorders* (3rd ed., rev.). Washington, DC: American Psychiatric Association.

American Psychiatric Association. (1994). *Quick reference to the Diagnostic Criteria from DSM-IV™.* Washington, DC: American Psychiatric Association.

Chenitz, W. C., Stone, J. T., & Salisbury, S. A. (1991). *Clinical gerontological nursing.* Philadelphia: W. B. Saunders.

Folstein, M., Folstein, S. E., & McHugh, P. (1975). Minimental state, a practical method for grading the cognitive status of patients for the clinician. *Journal of Psychiatric Research, 12,* 189–198.

Gilroy, J. (1990). *Basic neurology.* New York: Pergamon.

Hagen, C., & Malkmus, D. (1977, November). *Rancho Los Amigos scale for head injury.* Paper presented at the American Speech-Language-Hearing Association Annual Convention, Atlanta, GA.

Heilman, K. M., Watson, R. T., & Greer, M. (1977). *Handbook of neurologic signs and symptoms.* New York: Appleton-Century-Crofts.

Jacobs, J. W., Bernard, M. R., & Delgado, A. (1977). Screening for organic mental syndromes in the medically ill. *Annals of Internal Medicine, 86,* 40–46.

Levin, H. S., O'Donnell, V. M., & Grossman, R. G. (1979). The Galveston Orientation and Amnesia Test: A practical scale to assess cognition after head injury. *Journal of Nervous System and Mental Disorders, 167,* 675–684.

Pfeiffer, E. (1975). A short portable mental status questionnaire for the assessment of organic brain deficits in elderly patients. *Journal of the American Geriatric Society, 23,* 433–441.

Plum, F. (1985). Neuro-opthalmology. In J. B. Wyngaarden & L. H. Smith (Eds.), *Cecil textbook of medicine* (17th ed.). Philadelphia: W. B. Saunders.

Plum, F., & Posner, J. B. (1980). *The diagnosis of stupor and coma* (3rd ed.). Philadelphia: F. A. Davis.

Ross, B. G., Fradet, G., & Nedzelski, J. M. (1996). Development of a sensitive facial grading system. *Otolaryngology—Head and Neck Surgery, 114*(3), 382.

Samuels, M. A. (Ed.). (1978). *Manual of neurologic therapeutics.* Boston: Little, Brown.

Schwamm, L. H., Van Dyke, C., & Kierman, R. J. (1987). The neurobehavioral cognitive status examination: Comparison of the Cognitive Capacity Screening and MMSE in neurologic populations. *Annals of Internal Medicine. 107,* 486–491.

Teasdale, M. J., & Jennett, B. (1974). Assessment of coma and impaired consciousness: A practical scale. *Lancet, 11,* 81–84.

Weisberg, L. A., Strub, R. L., & Garcia, C. A. (1983). *Essentials of clinical neurology.* Baltimore: University Park Press.

CHAPTER

5

Nutrition, Hydration, and Swallowing

Speech-language pathologists usually are consulted when patients have **dysphagia**. They may be asked to determine if any behavioral therapy, oral exercises or stimulation, dietary adjustment, feeding assistance or technique, postural change, oral prosthesis, or adaptive equipment would benefit oral intake. They may be asked to participate in determining if a risk for aspiration prevents consideration of oral intake. Medical staff generally understand that dysphagic and malnourished patients have delayed recoveries and more frequent complications leading to increased hospitalization lengths and costs for care. **Any involvement with nutritionally compromised or fluid-deficient patients necessitates a basic understanding of normal nutrition and hydration requirements, the medical management of nutrition, and fluid and electrolyte balances.**

This chapter reviews medical terminology commonly used to discuss disorders of nutrition and hydration and describes procedures for the medical management of nutrition, hydration, and deglutition disorders.

I. TERMINOLOGY RELATED TO NUTRITION, HYDRATION, AND SWALLOWING

A. Anatomic Terminology in Nutrition, Hydration, and Swallowing

Bile duct. Duct formed by the union of the common hepatic duct and the cystic duct; carries bile into the duodenum.

Cardia. Small area of the stomach near the esophagastric junction.

Cardiac valve, cardiac orifice, cardiac sphincter. Opening into the stomach at the junction of the esophagus.

Cecum. First part of the large intestine.

Celiac. Pertaining to the abdomen.

Cervical esophagus. Upper portion of the esophagus.

Chief salivary glands. Three pairs of glands with ducts opening into the oral cavity, including the **parotid glands** (with *Stensen's duct*) located below the ear; **sublingual glands** with 10 to 30 ducts located on the floor of the mouth; and the **submandibular glands** *(Wharton's duct)* located below the mandible.

Colon. Large intestine from the cecum to the rectum including the *ascending colon*; *transverse colon*; *descending colon*; and *sigmoid*, or pelvic, *colon*.

Common hepatic duct. Duct formed by the union of the right and left hepatic ducts which receive bile from the liver.

Duodenum. First part of the small intestine extending from the *pyloric valve* to the *jejunum*.

Enteric. Pertaining to the intestine.

Epigastric. Pertaining to the region above the stomach.

Fundus. Enlarged upper portion of the stomach extending to the left of the *cardiac valve* (stomach orifice).

Gallbladder. A small, pear-shaped organ located next to the liver; stores and concentrates bile for release in digestion.

Jejunum. Second part of the small intestine extending from the *duodenum* to the *ileum*.

Kidneys. Two bean-shaped organs located behind the abdominal cavity on either side of the spinal cord in the lumbar region. The kidneys filter wastes (urea, creatinine, and uric acid) from the blood and reabsorb materials the body needs to retain in the bloodstream before producing urine. The kidneys produce a substance called *renin* which controls blood pressure.

Ileum. Third part of the small intestine extending from the *jejunum* to the *cecum*.

Liver. This organ manufactures a thick greenish or yellowish-brown fluid called **bile**. Bile contains a fatty substance *(cholesterol)*, bile acids, and pigments. One of the pigments manufactured by the liver is called *bilirubin*, produced when red cells are destroyed in the liver. The liver helps to keep the amount of sugar (glucose) in the blood in a normal balance through a process called **glycogenesis**. It can also convert glycogen into glucose when blood sugar levels are low. The liver manufactures blood proteins, removes old erythrocytes, releases bilirubin, and removes poisons from the bloodstream. Bile released by the liver travels down the *hepatic duct* into the *cystic duct* and into the *gallbladder* where it is concentrated and then mixed with pancreatic juices for digestion. The term **portal system** refers to the blood vessels passing to and from the liver.

Mesentery. Peritoneal fold which carries the blood supply and attaches the jejunum and ileum to the posterior abdominal wall.

Mesocolon. Mesentery attaching the colon to the posterior abdominal wall.

Omenta. Peritoneal sheets connecting the stomach with other visceral organs (liver, spleen, and transverse colon).

Pancreas. Organ located next to the duodenum leading out of the stomach. The pancreas is both an **exocrine gland** (excreting amylase and lipase outward into the duodenum through the pancreatic duct to aid in digestion) and an **endocrine gland** (secreting insulin and glucagon into the blood stream). Insulin is essential for the metabolism of blood sugar and for maintenance of the proper blood sugar level.

Peritoneum. A serous membrane sac composed of the *parietal peritoneum* lining the abdominal wall and *visceral peritoneum* containing the viscera in position.

Pylorus, pyloric sphincter, pyloric valve. Valved opening between the stomach and the duodenum.

Small intestine. Proximal portion of the intestine from the *pylorus* to the *ileocecal junction*.

Small salivary glands. Salivary glands distributed throughout the tongue, cheeks, and lips.

Stomach. Organ that prepares food both chemically and mechanically for transport into the small intestine for further digestion.

Thoracic esophagus, distal esophagus. Lower esophagus which passes through the thorax.

B. Illustration of the Digestive and Urinary Tracts

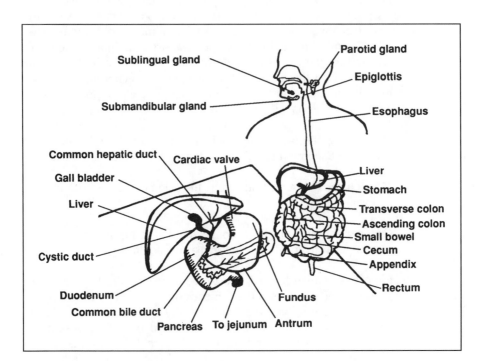

Figure 5–1. Anatomy of the digestive tract

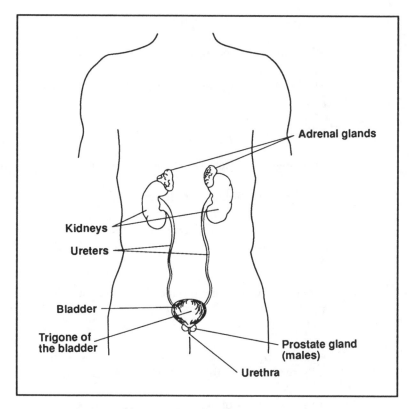

Figure 5–2. Anatomy of the urinary tract

C. Descriptive and Diagnostic Terminology in Nutrition, Hydration, and Swallowing

Achalasia. A common disorder characterized by dilation of the esophagus caused by failure of the cardiac sphincter to relax. This condition can produce aspiration tendencies when the patient is supine (lying on the back). Patients with achalasia typically complain of chest pain, regurgitation, or nocturnal cough. An **epiphrenic diverticulum** occurring just above the diaphragm can be associated with achalasia and other esophageal motility disorders.

Achlorohydria. Lack of hydrochloric acid in the stomach juices.

Acidosis. A condition in which the pH level of the blood falls *below* 7.35.

Acoria. A lack of satisfaction after eating, not due to hunger.

Ageusia. A loss of taste sensation.

Albumin. A plasma protein.

Alkalosis. A condition in which the pH level of the blood is *above* 7.45.

Alliaceous. Tasting like onions or garlic.

Allotriogeusia. Referring to a perverted appetite or sense of taste.

Amblygeusia. Reduced taste sense.

Amino acids. Small substances which are the chief structure of proteins and are produced when proteins are digested and broken down.

Amylase. An enzyme produced by the pancreas that breaks down starch. **Lipase**, also produced by the pancreas, breaks down triglycerides and lipids.

Anabolism. *Constructive phase* of metabolism in which the body cells synthesize protoplasm for growth and repair.

Anorexia. Loss of appetite or desire for food.

Anthropometric assessment. Measures of body size, weight, and proportion as a part of the nutritional assessment.

Ankyloglossia. Tongue tied.

Aphagia. A complete inability to swallow.

Aphthous stomatitis. Small ulceration of the mucous membrane of the mouth.

Aposia. Lack of thirst.

Aptyalism. Lack of saliva secretion.

Ascites. An accumulation of fluid in the peritoneal cavity.

Aspiration. The entry of secretions, fluids, food, or any foreign substance into the airway.

Asterixis. A motor condition usually associated with hepatic coma and other conditions in which there are intermittent lapses in sustained contractions of muscle postures of the extremities; "liver flap."

Atresia of the esophagus. A congenital absence of the esophageal opening or a congenital esophageal stricture.

Azotemia. Excessive urea or other nitrogenous substances in the blood. *Prerenal azotemia* refers to decreased renal profusion secondary to congestive heart failure (CHF), shock, or volume depletion.

Barrett's esophagus, Barrett's metaplasia. Referring to a condition characterized by metaplastic epithelium occurring in the lower esophagus following chronic peptic esophagitis.

Basal energy expenditure (BEE). An individual's energy needs for basic tissue metabolism can be calculated by a mathematical equation that determines caloric requirements depending on *age, sex, weight*, and *height* of the patient. The *BEE equation* is sometimes referred to as the **Harris-Benedict equation** or formula (see Dietitian's Nutritional Assessment, Table 5–9, on page 200).

Bile. Digestive substances produced in the liver and stored in the gallbladder.

Biliary. Carrying or containing bile.

Bilirubin. Pigment produced from the destruction of hemoglobin in the liver and released into bile.

Borborygmi. Rumbling or splashing bowel sounds.

Bougie. Tapered, flexible, sausage-shaped tubes of varying diameters used to dilate an orifice.

Buccal. Pertaining to the cheek.

Bulimia. A voracious appetite.

Cachexia. A general wasting away of body tissue; state of malnutrition, emaciation, debilitation, and anemia.

Cacogeusia. Referring to a bad taste.

Calorie. The amount of heat necessary to raise the temperature of 1 gram of water 1° C.

Candidiasis (moniliasis, thrush). Curdlike creamy patches of fungal growth. *Candida albicans* in the mouth or upper gastrointestinal tract may be found in association with antibiotic therapy, diabetes, immune suppression therapy, or immunodeficiency diseases.

Catabolism. *Destructive* phase of metabolism in which body stores are broken down to maintain basal energy requirements.

Cathartics. Drugs that induce opening of the bowels (laxatives).

Cheilosis. An abnormal condition of the lip characterized by reddening and fissures at the corners, seen in riboflavin and other B-complex vitamin deficiencies.

Cholecystitis. Inflammation of the gallbladder.

Chyle. The milkylike fluid secreted during intestinal digestion made up of lymph and emulsified fats.

Cirrhosis. A degenerative liver disease characterized by changes in the lobes of the liver and in fat infiltration of the liver's cells.

Colostrum. The first milk secreted by mothers after delivery.

Congenital intestinal obstruction. Disorders in neonates which can include *atresia* and *stenosis of the bowel, meconium ileus, meconium plug syndrome, small left colon syndrome* (SLCS), and *hypertrophic pyloric stenosis.*

Continence. The ability to control bowel or bladder elimination.

Creatinine. One of the nonprotein constituents of blood and a component of renal products (urine) formed as the end product of creatine metabolism.

Creatinine height index (CHI). A urine test used to determine lean body mass and degrees of protein depletion.

Deglutition. Swallowing.

Deglutition therapist. An individual trained to provide therapy specifically for swallowing disorders. Deglutition therapy may be a subspecialty of nursing, speech-language pathology, or other health professions.

Dehydration. A condition that results from a low volume of body water.

Dentalgia. Pain in a tooth.

Dermatomyositis. A collagen disease characterized by edema; muscular weakness; skin rash; and, in some cases, mucosal lesions.

Diabetes insipidus. A rare form of diabetes characterized by excessive thirst and the passage of large volumes of dilute urine caused by the inability of the kidney tubules to reabsorb water, also called *nephrogenic diabetes. Diabetes insipidus* is associated with hypothalamic damage affecting mechanisms that cause an *antidiuretic hormone (ADH) deficiency.*

Diabetes mellitus. The most common form of diabetes, in which there is a disorder in the metabolism of insulin (hormone produced by the pancreas) and of carbohydrate, protein, and fat, with associated disorders of the structures or functions of the blood vessels. **Type I insulin-dependent diabetes mellitus (IDDM)**, formally referred to as *juvenile diabetes*, is characterized by little or no endogenous insulin secretion. **Type II noninsulin-dependent diabetes mellitus (NIDDM)**, the more common form of diabetes mellitus, is characterized by abnormalities in insulin secretion and resistance to the action of insulin, contributing to *hyperglycemia. Secondary diabetes* can be drug-induced or occur as a consequence of other conditions, such as pancreatic disease, hormonal dysfunction, pregnancy, and genetic defects. The term *brittle diabetes* refers to diabetes that is difficult to control with medication and/or diet.

Diarrhea. The passage of watery, unformed stools accompanied by abdominal cramping.

Diverticula. Abnormal pouches in the walls of a hollow structure, such as the esophagus or the intestines.

Diverticulitis. Inflammation of diverticula.

Duodenal atresia. Total obstruction of the intestinal lumen (duodenum); often seen in conjunction with Down syndrome.

Dumping syndrome. Condition, frequently occurring after a gastrectomy, in which the patient experiences sweating faintness, flushing, and diarrhea.

Dysphagia. An impaired ability to chew or swallow solid and/or liquid substances, often associated with discomfort and aspiration.

Dysphagia Management Team. A group of health care professionals who collaborate on the evaluation and management of dysphagic persons. At a minimum, these teams usually include: a dietitian, speech-language pathologist or occupational therapist, nurse, and physician.

Edema. An excess of water in the interstitial space within body tissues.

Edentulous. Lacking teeth.

Electrolytes. Chemical compounds that dissolve and separate molecules carrying either a positive or negative electrical charge.

Emesis. Vomited stomach contents.

Enteritis. Inflammation of the intestine.

Enterostomal therapist. A nurse who has been certified or trained in the care of patients' ostomies.

Eructation. The discharge of gas from the stomach through the mouth (belching).

Fick Equation. Formula to determine directly the amount of oxygen consumed, in which cardiac output = oxygen consumed (mL/minute $\times$ 100) divided by arterial oxygen content minus venous oxygen content. A *reverse Fick equation* refers to an indirect oxygen consumption computation in which resting energy expenditure (REE) = VO_2 1/minute $\times$ 5 kcal $\times$ 60 minutes $\times$ 24 hours.

Flatus. Intestinal gas released from the rectum.

Fluid balance. The state in which water remains in normal amounts and percentages in the body's tissues.

Fluid intake. All sources of fluid consumed or introduced into the body.

Fluid output. All fluid eliminated from the body (through drainage tubes, catheters, wounds, sweating, exhalation, vomiting, defecation, or urination).

Free water. Fluid contained in solid foods, enteral feedings, and humidified air.

Gastralgia. Pertaining to pain in the stomach.

Gastric paresis, gastroplegia. Paralysis of part or all of the stomach, sometimes associated with diabetes.

Gastric ulcers, peptic ulcers. Erosions of gastric mucosa. *Acute gastric ulcer* can be caused by trauma, major surgery, alcohol abuse, or increased steroid secretions. *Chronic gastric ulcer* can be caused by *chronic peptic disease* usually involving the nonacid secreting antral area of the stomach (antrum). *Chronic peptic disease* can also produce *peptic strictures* of the esophagus.

Gastrocele. A hernia of the stomach.

Gastrodynia. Pain in the stomach.

Gastromegaly. Abnormally large stomach.

Gastroschisis. Antenatal herniation of the abdominal contents through a paraumbilical (around the umbilicus) defect in the abdominal wall.

Glossodynia. Painful tongue due to a chronic inflammatory process or nutritional deficiency.

Halitosis. Offensive mouth odor.

Hematemesis. Vomiting blood.

Hemoptysis. Expectoration of blood.

Hiatus hernia, hiatal hernia. A protrusion of part of the stomach through the esophageal opening of the diaphragm.

Hirshsprung's disease. A congenital aganglionosis with disruption of the normal colonic transport.

Hypercalcemia. An *excessive* amount of calcium in the blood. *Hypo*calcemia is a *deficit* of calcium in the blood.

Hyperchloremia. An *excessive* amount of chloride in the blood. *Hypo*chloremia is a *deficit* of chloride in the blood.

Hyperemesis. Excessive vomiting.

Hyperkalemia. An *excessive* amount of potassium in the blood. *Hypo*kalemia is a *deficit* of potassium in the blood.

Hypermagnesemia. An *excessive* amount of magnesium in the blood. *Hypo*magnesemia is a *deficit* of magnesium in the blood.

Hypernatremia. An *excessive* amount of sodium in the blood. *Hypo*natremia is a *deficit* of sodium in the blood.

Hyperphosphatemia. An *excessive* amount of phosphate in the blood. *Hypo*phosphatemia is a *deficit* of phosphate in the blood.

Hypertonic solution. A mixture of water with a higher amount of dissolved substances than normally found in the blood.

Hypervolemia. Excessive amount of fluid (water) in the blood.

Hypovolemia. Below average amount of fluid (water) in the blood.

Iatrogenic malnutrition. Malnutrition inadvertently produced by medical treatment.

Icterus. Jaundice; yellowish discoloration of the skin, sclera membranes (whites of the eyes), and secretions due to high levels of bilirubin in the blood.

Ileus. Obstruction of the small intestine.

Imperforate anus. A group of congenital anorectal anomalies often associated with infants who have **tracheo-esophageal fistulae (TEF)** or VATER (vertebral, anal, tracheal, esophageal, and renal congenital abnormalities) syndromes. In most cases of imperforate anus, the rectum terminates with a fistula into either the urethra in the male or into the vagina in the female.

Kwashiorkor syndrome. A malnutrition syndrome associated with a severe protein deficiency.

Malabsorption syndromes. Syndromes resulting in impaired absorption of nutrients by the small bowel.

Mallory-Weiss syndrome. Laceration of the distal esophagus and proximal stomach caused by retching, vomiting, or hiccups. This disorder is seen frequently in chronic alcoholism, but may be found in association with other conditions affecting the upper gastrointestinal tract.

Malnutrition. A condition resulting from a lack of proper or adequate nutrients in the diet or from malabsorption.

Marasmus. Malnutrition associated with chronic illness, especially when patients have been maintained on inadequate diets.

Megadose. Ingesting more of a substance than the amount recommended to sustain health (e.g., a megadose of some vitamins can be harmful).

Melena. Black stool or black vomit due to the presence of blood in the gastrointestinal tract.

Metabolic rate, basal metabolic rate (BMR). The rate at which the body burns calories.

Micturition. Urination, the act of voiding.

Mild alkali syndrome. A disorder that, if unrecognized, can cause irreversible kidney disease; brought on by excessive use of antiacids.

Milliequivalent. The unit of measure used to measure electrolytes (mEq/liter).

Nausea. The feeling of sickness with a desire to vomit.

Necrotizing enterocolitis. A severe, often fatal, disease occurring most frequently in premature infants, characterized by temperature instability, abdominal distention, residual aspirates, bloody stools, bilious vomiting, acidosis, disseminated intravascular coagulation, and *pneumotosis intestinalis*. Necrotizing enterocolitis is associated with conditions such as asphyxia, hyaline membrane disease, patent ductus arteriosus, sepsis, and polycythemia.

Nitrogen balance. The state of the body relative to ingestion and excretion of protein. A *positive nitrogen balance* indicates adequate protein ingestion. A *negative nitrogen balance* indicates protein depletion and malnutrition.

Obesity. A condition in which there is an excessive amount of body fat.

Occlusal. In dentistry, pertaining to the contacting (biting) surfaces of the teeth; referring generally to closure.

Odynophagia. Pain associated with swallowing.

Omphalocele. A congenital defect that can vary from a small bulge at the base of the umbilicus to a sac containing the intestines.

Patent. A tube or vessel that is open and unobstructed.

Periodontal disease. Disease of the gums leading to tooth decay and tooth loss, related to inadequate oral hygiene or conditions producing poor oral hygiene, such as deficient salivation.

Peristalsis. The rhythmic muscular contractions that move contents through the alimentary (gastrointestinal) tract.

Pica. A craving to eat unusual or nonnutritive substances.

Piecemeal swallow. An inability to clear the entire bolus with one swallow.

pH. The expression of hydrogen ion concentration in fluids.

Pitting edema. A condition in which a "pit" or impression is left after pressure is applied to edematous skin tissue.

Plasma. The fluid component of blood (synonymous with *serum*).

Polydipsia. Excessive thirst.

Polyphagia. Excessive eating.

Polyuria. Excessive urination.

Presbyphagia, presbyesophagus. Swallowing and esophageal dysmotility problems related to normal physiologic changes in aging and associated pathologic conditions.

Proctalgia. Pertaining to pain in or around the rectum.

Projectile vomiting. Vomiting with great force.

Pseudodiverticula. Esophageal glands which have become dilated, appearing to be diverticula.

Ptyalism. Excessive secretion of saliva.

Pyloric stenosis. A congenital condition seen in newborns characterized by an overgrowth of muscle fibers diminishing the lumen of the pylorus.

Pyrosis. Heartburn.

Recommended daily (dietary) allowance (RDA). The daily amount of nutrients the body needs (varies by age, weight, and activity level).

Reflux. The explusion of stomach material into the esophagus or hypopharynx.

Renin. A substance produced by the kidney which controls the narrowing of blood vessels all over the body, thus controlling blood pressure.

Retropulsion, reverse peristalsis. Esophageal or intestinal dysmotility causing contents to be pushed upward through the esophagus or gastrointestinal tract.

Rhabdomyolysis. Disintegration or breakdown of muscle characterized by myoglobin in the urine.

Riley-Day syndrome. Familial dysautonomia in which there is a delay in the cricopharyngeal sphincter relaxation resulting in aspiration tendencies.

Rokitansky's diverticulum. A traction diverticulum in the esophagus.

Rumination. Rechewing food regurgitated from the stomach; more often seen in infants.

Saliva. The secretions which contain amylase and serve to moisten, dissolve, and transport food for digestion.

Schatski's ring. Lower esophageal stricture in the region of the squamocolumnar junction.

Scleroderma, progressive systemic sclerosis. A systemic disease characterized by skin tightening and fibrosis of smooth muscles, with which there may be an associated dysphagia.

Serum albumin and transferrin. A measure of visceral protein stores and malnutrition.

Short bowel syndrome. State of malabsorption caused by resection of a large part of the small intestine (to correct colitis, atresia, volvulus, etc.).

Sialoadenitis, sialadentitis. Inflammation of a salivary gland, usually characterized by painful swelling of the gland.

Sjögren's syndrome. Inflammation of the lacrimal glands and salivary glands sometimes affecting swallowing.

Skin turgor. The fullness of the skin in relationship to the underlying tissue; an indicator of fluid balances in the body.

Stasis. Not moving.

Stomatitis. Inflammation of the mucosa of the mouth.

Strangury. Painful urination due to spasmodic muscle contraction.

Swallow center. An area of the medulla oblongata on the *floor of the fourth ventricle* where the central nervous system nuclei that control swallowing are located.

Third spacing. A condition in which body fluids become trapped in interstitial areas due to a loss of plasma proteins. Third spacing can occur suddenly when a patient is *burned*, suffers a *crushing injury*, or has an *allergic reaction*; or it can occur slowly in certain types of liver or kidney diseases.

Trench mouth (Vincent's infection). An inflammatory condition of the gums associated with pain, ulcerations, fever, bleeding, and lymphadenopathy.

Trismus. An inability to open the mouth fully; can occur in patients who have undergone surgery or radiation treatment to the mouth.

Turgor. The fullness of the skin relative to the underlying tissue.

Tympanites. A condition that results when intestinal gas accumulates and is not expelled (intestinal distention); meteorism.

Urgency. A sensation of needing to urinate immediately.

Volvulus. A twisting of the bowel (or other organ) on itself causing an obstruction.

Waterbrash. Stomach contents that are regurgitated into the mouth.

Xerostomia. Insufficient secretion of saliva; dry mouth.

Zenker's diverticulum. A posterior diverticulum of the esophagus, usually in the cervical esophagus.

Zollinger-Ellison syndrome. A syndrome of extreme gastritis marked by hypergastrinemia, gastric hypersecretion, and peptic ulceration.

II. PROCEDURES, TESTS, AND THERAPIES FOR NUTRITION, HYDRATION, AND SWALLOWING MANAGEMENT

Also see section on Commonly Ordered Laboratory Tests in Chapter 3; Chapter 8 for elaborated descriptions of radiologic studies; Chapter 4 for descriptions of neurologic studies; and the list of Gastrointestinal and Abdominal surgeries, Chapter 12.

Acid perfusion test. A test comparing subjective responses to saline versus decinormal hydrochloric acid perfused into the esophagus through a nasogastric tube; used to differentiate cardiovascular midchest pain from painful esophageal reflux.

Artificial saliva. Oral wetting agent prepared with properties similar to saliva and used to diminish "dry mouth," or *xerostomia*, and to assist with digestion of foods.

Auscultation of swallowing. Listening by means of a stethoscope to swallowing sounds *(cervical auscultation)* to determine the presence of aspiration; or listening to stomach sounds *(stomach auscultation*, or *left upper quadrant* [LUQ] *auscultation)* to determine if a nasogastric tube is properly placed. In the latter procedure, an air bolus is injected through the nasogastric tube after placement, and LUQ auscultation is used to listen for the air released ("whoosh" sound) into the stomach.

Balloon tamponade. An emergency procedure using a balloon catheter to control bleeding from esophageal varices.

Barium fluoroscopy; upper G.I. study; upper esophageal series; barium fluorogram; cinesophagram. Radiologic studies of oral, pharyngeal, hypopharyngeal, and esophageal structures and dynamic functions through the use of x-ray with barium (or barium with air). Depending on its purpose, the study may utilize fluoroscopy, rapid series films, videofluoroscopy (videotapes), or cinefluoroscopy (motion picture flms).

Barium swallow (BaS); modified barium swallow (MBS). Radiologic study using thin and thick liquid barium, paste barium, barium pills, barium-coated cookies, or barium mixed with soft solid food substances (e.g., pudding, marshmallows, applesauce) for the purpose of examining swallowing structures and dynamic swallowing functions with particular attention to the oral and pharyngeal phases of swallow and aspiration risks.

Cholecystography. X-ray examination of the gall bladder using radiopaque dye.

Colonoscopy. Examination of the *upper* portion of the colon. A **sigmoidoscopy** refers to an examination of the rectosigmoid, or *lower* part, of the large bowel.

Dialysis. A procedure that removes water and toxic chemicals from the body when the kidneys can no longer perform that function. *Hemodialysis* is a procedure using an artificial kidney machine to filter wastes from the bloodstream. *Peritoneal dialysis* is a procedure in which fluid is introduced through a peritoneal catheter into the abdominal cavity causing highly concentrated wastes circulating in the peritoneum to diffuse out of the bloodstream and into the fluid for removal. *Continuous arterio-venous hemofiltration* (CAVH) is a method similar to dialysis in which blood is removed from the body and waste is filtered out. This procedure is amenable for use in intensive care units with critically ill patients.

Dilation, dilatation. Expansion of an organ, orifice, or stricture in a tube, such as the esophagus, usually with an instrument such as specially gauged dilators, or "bougies," referred to as *bouginage dilation*.

Electroglottography (EGG). Technique used to examine laryngeal displacement and glottal motions during speech and swallowing through the use of a two-channel oscilloscope, a pressure transducer (with electrodes placed on each side of the thyroid cartilage), and an amplifier.

Enteral hyperalimentation. Nutrition and hydration support through feeding tubes introduced into the gastrointestinal tract.

Enterostomy. The creation of an opening into the intestine.

Esophageal gastric tube airway, esophageal obturator airway. Tube with an inflatable balloon cuff obturator inserted into the esophagus to occlude the esophagus and prevent aspiration of stomach contents during endotracheal intubation and ventilation (see Figure 5–3).

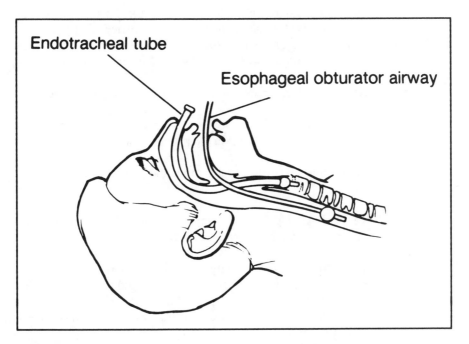

Endotracheal tube

Esophageal obturator airway

Figure 5–3. Illustration of esophageal obturator airway [From Parsons, C. B. (1987). *Critical care procedures and protocols.* Philadelphia: J. B. Lippincott, Co., p. 245, with permission.]

Extracorporeal hemoperfusion. A procedure used to remove potential toxins, such as the removal of ammonia, and other products from the patient in hepatic coma.

Fiberoptic endoscopic examination of swallowing safety (FEESS). Endoscopic examination of oropharyngeal functions during swallowing. FEESS studies may be videotaped.

Fiberoptic endoscopy. Visualization and, in some cases biopsy tissue sampling through the use of a fiberoptic, flexible endoscope inserted into a hollow organ (*nasendoscopy, colonoscopy, duodenoscopy, gastroduodenoscopy, esophagastroscopy, gastroscopy, peritoneoscopy, laryngoscopy, proctosigmoidoscopy,* etc.).

Gamma-glutamyl transferase (GGT). A test performed on blood serum to determine the level of an enzyme found in the liver, kidney, prostate, heart, and spleen. Increased levels of GGT can indicate a number of conditions, including cirrhosis, liver necrosis, hepatitis, alcoholism, neoplasm, acute pancreatitis, acute myocardial infarction, nephrosis, and acute cholecystitis.

Gastraview, Gastragrafin study. Trademarked names for contrast preparations used in radiologic studies. Gastraview studies are usually ordered to examine for fistulae in the gastrointestinal tract prior to abdominal surgeries *when barium residues are not wanted.*

Gavage. Feeding directly into the stomach by way of a tube.

Heme Quant test. A quantitative assay to detect a heme-positive reaction (presence of blood) in the patient's stool (feces).

Hepatic antigen. A test to determine the presence of the hepatitis B virus.

Intraesophageal pH monitoring. Procedure for monitoring gastric reflux across a 24-hour sampling period.

Lavage. To wash out a cavity. *Gastric lavage* is used to remove stomach contents by aspiration and flushing out contents with a stomach tube ("stomach pump"). *Diagnostic peritoneal lavage* (DPL) is a procedure used to examine for a ruptured bowel or bleeding into the peritoneum.

Manometry. An intraluminal measure of pressures used to determine the force and velocity of peristalsis of the upper and lower esophageal sphincters. *Manofluoroscopy* combines computerized manography with barium fluoroscopy to examine for pressure gradients relative to bolus flow actions.

Mecholyl test. A test using a cholinergic drug, mecholyl, to evaluate esophageal achalasia.

Murphy drip. Continuous bladder irrigation through a triple-lumen urinary catheter (Foley catheter).

Nasendoscopy, nasopharyngoscopy. Procedures for directly visualizing the nasal, palatal, pharyngeal, laryngeal, and esophageal entry structures, usually with a fiberoptic endoscope.

Nasogastric feedings. Enteral nutrition and hydration support through the use of a tube passed into the nasal passages through the pharynx and esophagus into the upper gastrointestinal tract.

Nasojejunal feedings. Feedings by way of a tube inserted through the nose and into the stomach for passage through the pyloric sphincter and duodenum into the jejunum.

Oral glucose tolerance test (OGTT). Test for levels in the blood following the oral administration of a volume of glucose.

Orogastric feedings. Enteral feedings preferred for infants in which oral tubes rather than nasogastric tubes are used. Newborns are "nose breathers" and the nasogastric tube may partially occlude the airway and compromise the infant's respiration.

Panorex. Trademarked name of a radiologic procedure using two axes of rotation to obtain a panoramic radiograph of the dentition and the dental arches.

Parenteral hyperalimentation. A method to supply the necessary nutrients directly into the bloodstream usually by means of a catheter inserted through a **central venous catheter placement**, or cannulation, referred to as a **"central line."** The subclavian vein or a right atrial catheter placement is most often used for parenteral hyperalimentation. (See Figure 5–5 on page 191). The term **total parenteral nutrition** (TPN) is a synonym (see definition on the next page).

Percutaneous endoscopic gastrostomy (PEG). An endoscopic procedure performed for insertion of a gastrostomy tube. This endoscopic procedure is preferred in cases where a patient cannot tolerate a general anesthetic, and, thus, may be performed by a gastroenterologist with only local anesthesia and mild sedation. (See Chapter 12, Gastrointestinal and Abdominal Surgeries, pages 396–399, for additional discussion.)

Pharyngotomy. Creation of an opening into the pharynx, usually for the purpose of providing a feeding method.

Prealbumin (PAB) assessment. A blood test used to determine the adequacy of nutritional support. A PAB level of ≤15 mg/dL indicates *protein caloric malnutrition*.

Renal biopsy. A percutaneous technique used to examine kidney tissue.

Scintigraphy. A radionuclide study used to detect gastroesophageal reflux, esophageal motility, and aspiration.

Small bowel biopsy and duodenal aspiration. To achieve this small bowel study, a lubricated mercury-filled Rubin-Quinton tube or Carey capsule is placed in the oropharynx and swallowed by the patient allowing the tube to enter the stomach. It is then manipulated under fluoroscopic guidance through the pylorus into the duodenum. With negative pressure (suction), contents and mucosa can be aspirated from the tip of the tube.

Small bowel studies, lower G.I. studies, large bowel studies, barium enemas. Radiologic examinations of the small and large intestines.

Stool culture. A test performed on feces to determine the presence of organisms.

Total parenteral nutrition (TPN). *Parenteral hyperalimentation* is synonymous. Long-term intravenous nutrition, or total parenteral nutrition (TPN), is a nutritional support method in which an **amino acid-glucose-lipid infusate** is introduced directly into a central vein (usually the subclavian vein) by means of disposable tubing and an *infusion pump* to maintain a constant infusion rate through a large intravenous catheter. TPN is used with patients who have severe digestive abnormalities and is prescribed to provide an amount of nitrogen that meets or exceeds the amount required to maintain nutritional equilibrium to allow protein synthesis and weight maintenance or gain. Patients likely to receive TPN include: those who are in a *mild catabolic state* following surgery or are severely malnourished and require nutritional therapy prior to surgery; those in a *hypermetabolic state* (as found after trauma, severe burns, head injury, cancer, and sepsis); those with *pancreatitis*; those *without a functioning gut*; and those with a *gastrointestinal obstruction*, or *short bowel syndrome*.

Tube feedings. Introducing nourishment through an enteral tube. The term *gastric gavage* is synonymous.

Ultrasonographic examinations of dysphagia. Use of ultrasound for detecting soft tissue movements during swallow and determining any aspiration tendencies. This technique is felt to be useful with infants or other patients who are not easily studied with fluoroscopy.

Urinary catheter. A small bore tube usually placed into the bladder to drain urine. *Indwelling catheters*, such as the triple-lumen Foley catheters, have small inflatable balloons to secure the tube for an extended period of time. Condoms attached to tubing ("condom catheters") and external urinary devices with adhesive bags may be used for the collection of urine from males and infants.

III. NUTRITION AND HYDRATION ABBREVIATIONS

a.c. Before meals (*ante cibum*)

ACBE. Air contrast barium enema

ADH. Antidiuretic hormone

A/G. Albumin globulin (ratio)

Alb. Albumin

ALP. Alkaline phosphatase

AODM. Adult onset diabetes mellitis

Aq. Water (*aqua*)

ATC. Around the clock

ATP. Adenosine triphosphate

Ba. Barium

BaE. Barium enema

BAO. Basal acid output

BEE. Basal Energy Expenditure

b.i.d. Two times a day (*bis in die*)

BM. Bowel movement

BRP. Bathroom privileges

B.S. Blood sugar

BUN. Blood urea nitrogen

BW. Body weight

Ca. Calcium

CCK-PZ. Cholecystokinin-pancreotzymin

C & DB. Cough and deep breaths

CDCA. Chenodeoxycholic acid

CHO. Carbohydrate

Cho. Cholesterol

cib. Food (*cibus*)

Cl. Chloride

CRF. Chronic renal failure

CUC. Chronic ulcerative colitis

DAT. Diet as tolerated

D5W. 5% dextrose in water

D5RL. 5% dextrose in Ringer's lactate

D5S. 5% dextrose in saline

DHFT. Dobbhoff (enteric) feeding tube

E. coli. *Escherichia coli*

EGD. Endoscopic gastroduodenoscopy

EIP. Esophageal intraluminal pseudodiverticulosis

ERCP. Endoscopic retrograde cholangiopancreatography

ESRD. End stage renal disease

FB. Foreign body

FBS. Fasting blood sugar

Fe. Iron

F/F. Removable full denture

FN. Fully nourished

FOS, FOF. Full of stool, full of feces

GB. Gall bladder

GEJ. Gastroesophageal juncture

GER. Gastroesophageal reflux

GERD. Gastroesophageal reflux disease

GGT. Gamma-glutamyl transferase

GI. Gastrointestinal, gastroenterology

GIP. Gastric inhibitory peptide

GNB. Gram-negative bacillus

GTT. Glucose tolerance test

G.U. Genitourinary

HAA. Hepatitis-associated antigen

HAV. Hepatitis A virus

HBIG. Hepatitis B immune globulin

HBV. Hepatitis B virus

HCl. Hydrochloric acid

HCV. Hepatitis C virus

Hyper al. Hyperalimentation

I & O. Intake and output

IBS. Irritable bowel syndrome

IBW. Ideal body weight

ICG. Indocyanine green

IDDM. Insulin-dependent diabetes mellitus

INF. Intravenous nutritional fluid

IRDM. Insulin resistant diabetes mellitus

IV. Intravenous

IVC. Intravenous cholangiography

IVP. Intravenous pyelogram

JJT/JT. Jejunostomy tube

K. Potassium

KUB. Kidney, ureter, and bladder

LB. Large bowel

LDH. Lactic dehydrogenase

L.E.S. Lower esophageal sphincter

LFT. Liver function test

LGI. Lower gastrointestinal (tract)

LS scan. Liver spleen scan

MN. Midnight

MOM. Milk of magnesia

M & R. Measure and record

MVit. Multivitamin

Na. Sodium

NCS. No concentrated sweets

NG. Nasogastric tube

NH3, NH4. Ammonia, ammonium

NIDDM. Noninsulin-dependent diabetes mellitus

NIT. Nasointestinal tube

NN. Negative for sugar and acetone

NPO. Nothing by mouth (*non per os*)

NPO **p MN.** Nothing by mouth after midnight

N&V. Nausea and vomiting

Nx. Nourishment

OCG. Oral cholecystography

O&P. Ova and parasites

P. Phosphorus

PAB. Prealbumin

p.c. After meals (*post cibum*)

PCM. Protein caloric malnutrition

PEG. Percutaneous endoscopic gastrostomy

PEJ. Percutaneous endoscopic jejunostomy

PKU. Phenylketonuria

p.o. By mouth (*per os*)

PP. After meals (*post parandial*)

PTC. Percutaneous transhaptic cholangiography

PUD. Peptic ulcer disease

q. Every (*quaque*)

q. **a.m.** Every morning

q.d. Every day (*quaque die*)

q.h. Every hour (*quaque hora*)

q. s. Every shift

q. 2 h. Every two hours

q.i.d. Four times a day (*quarter in die*)

RDA. Recommended daily allowance

SB. Small bowel

SBS. Short bowel syndrome

S-G. Swan-Ganz (catheter)

TEF. Tracheo-esophageal fistula

t.i.d. Three times a day (*ter in die*)

TPN. Total parenteral nutrition

U/A. Urinalysis

UDCA. Ursodeoxycholic acid

U.E.S. Upper esophageal sphincter

UTI. Urinary tract infection

VCU. Voiding cystourethrogram

IV. ENTERAL AND PARENTERAL NUTRITION

When oral intake is not possible, safe, nor sufficient to meet a patient's nutritional needs, then **enteral hyperalimentation** (*nutrition by way of tubes placed in the gastrointestinal tract*) or **total parenteral nutrition (TPN)** (*nutrition by way of solutions infused directly into the blood stream*) is necessary (see Figures 5–4 and 5–5). Enteral hyperalimentation is usually achieved through a lubricated, small-bore, weighted feeding tube (such as a Dobbhoff feeding tube) that is passed through a nostril into the nasopharynx and esophagus into the stomach or directed through the stomach for transpyloric passage into the duodenum or jejunum. Enteral feeding may be temporary, through the use of nasogas-

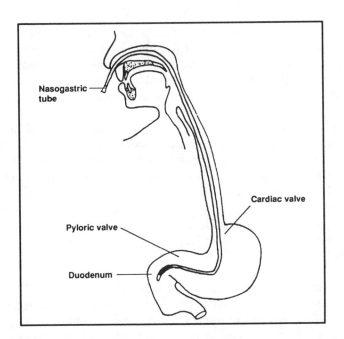

Figure 5–4. Illustration of nasogastric tube placement

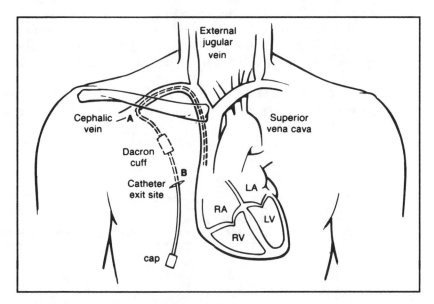

Figure 5–5. Illustration of Total Parenteral Nutrition (TPN). A. Vascular access site. B. Cutaneous exit site of catheter. [From Persons, C. B. (1987). *Critical care procedures and protocols.* Philadelphia: J. B. Lippincott Co., p. 225, with permission.)

tric, nasoduodenal, or nasojejunal tubes, or long-term, through the use of **gastrointestinal tubes (G-tubes)** which are placed *percutaneously* directly into the stomach, duodenum, or **jejunum (JJTs)**. Percutaneous feeding tubes can be removed or "taken down," once the patient achieves the ability to maintain nutrition and hydration needs safely by oral intake.

When enteral feeding tubes are inserted, placement is confirmed through left upper quadrant auscultation and/or x-ray. The hospital's dietitians select the formulas and rates for the enteric feeding solutions. Feedings may be *intermittent* or *continuous*, depending on the type of solution required and patient's status.

Volume and feeding rates will be calculated according to the individual factors for adults and children. Table 5–1 lists suggested feeding rates for infants.

Gravity infusion or an *infusion pump* specifically designed for prescribed infusion rates with enteral feeding may be selected, depending on the patient's needs and tolerances. Enteral feeding products commonly used include *Dobbhoff feeding tubes* with Dobbhoff enteric feeding bags and pump (Biosearch Medical Products, Inc.); *Corpak feeding tubes*; *Flexiflo Flexitainer feeding bag* and enteral feeding formula (Ross Laboratories); *Kangaroo tube-feeding set* with a Kangaroo 220 enteral feeding pump (Chesebrough-Ponds, Inc.); *Life Care Pump* (Abbott Laboratories); *IVAC Enteral feeding pump* (IVAC Corporation); and *Moss compression feeding catheters* designed for surgical patients.

TPN, or *total parenteral nutrition*, is used with nutritionally depleted patients for whom enteral hyperalimentation is not an option (see definition of TPN). TPN solutions consist of a *nitrogen source* (protein), *hypertonic dextrose* and *lipids*, and *supplementary vitamins* and *minerals*

Table 5–1. Suggested initial feeding rates for infants

Birth Weight (gm)	Initial Volumes (per mL)	Average Increment Increase
1000	2–3	1–2
1001–1250	3–4	2–5
1251–1500	6–10	3–5
1501–2000	10–15	5–10

Source: Adapted from Willett, M. J., et al. 1986. *Manual of Neonatal intensive care nursing.* Boston: Little, Brown.

which are infused into a central vein, typically the subclavian vein. *Right atrial catheters* are placed for long-term TPN, and the most commonly used catheters are *Hickman, Broviac*, and *Centracil* catheters (see Figure 5–5). Other intravenous solutions are not recommended to be "piggy backed" onto a TPN line; however, a Hickman catheter has a double lumen which allows for continuous TPN infusion and intermittent infusion of medications and additional therapies. TPN can be infused through a **peripherally inserted central venous catheter** (PICC) line. These lines are preferred in the home setting, because they have a low infection rate. Peripheral parenteral support utilizes a moderate osmolality formula and lipids.

V. INFANT NUTRITION, HYDRATION, AND SWALLOWING

The gastrointestinal tract of the *premature* infant often does not tolerate adequate fluid volumes to meet the infant's fluid or caloric demands. Additionally, prior to reaching a gestational age of approximately 32 to 34 weeks, the infant lacks a coordinated suck and swallow pattern and, thus, is not adequately developed to allow intake from a breast or bottle. Consequently, enteral feeding is used until the infant reaches a gestational age of 32–34 weeks and has no evidence of respiratory distress. Table 5–1 provides a reference for infant feeding volumes.

VI. ADULT NUTRITION AND HYDRATION

Nutrition is the process by which the body uses foods and fluids to reach and maintain health. To maintain proper nutrition the body needs *calories, water, carbohydrates, proteins, fats, vitamins*, and *minerals*. Vitamins are the chemical substances necessary for normal tissue growth and maintenance of health. Except for vitamin K and biotin, vitamins cannot be manufactured by the body. The functions of various vitamins are outlined in Table 5–2.

Severe nutritional deficiencies can accompany debilitating diseases, such as *metastatic cancer, infections, thyrotoxicosis, impaired intestinal absorption disorders, connective tissue diseases, chronic behavioral disorders*, and conditions associated with ***alcoholism***. Nutritional deficiencies can result from the lack of a single vitamin or deficiencies in multiple nutrients. The lack of the vitamin **thiamine** is commonly associated with *neurologic nutritional deficiencies*, especially alcoholic neuropathies. **Alcoholic-nutritional peripheral neuropathies** are found in advanced stages of alcoholism. This disorder is characterized by axonal degeneration mainly involving the small pain and temperature-mediating fibers in the lower distal extremities.

Table 5-2. Vitamins and their functions

Vitamin	Function
A (Retinol)	Growth of cells; promotion of skin, hair, and epithelial cells
B_1 (Thiamine)	Normal digestion, carbohydrate metabolism, nervous system functions
B_2 (Riboflavin)	Normal growth, light accommodation, formation of certain enzymes
B_3 (Niacin)	Carbohydrate, fat, and protein metabolism; prevents loss of appetite
B_6 (Pyridoxine)	Healthy gums and teeth; red cell formation; carbohydrate, fat, and protein metabolism
B_9 (Folic acid)	Red cell formation, protein metabolism, normal intestinal tract functioning
B_{12} (Cyancobalamin)	Protein metabolism, red cell formation, healthy nerve cells
C (Ascorbic acid)	Healthy bones, teeth, and gums; formation of blood vessels and capillary walls; proper healing; facilitation of iron and folic acid absorption
D (Calciferol)	Absorption of calcium and phosphorus
E (Alpha-tocoperal)	Red cell formation, protection of essential fatty acids
Pantothenic acid	Metabolism
H (Biotin)	Enzyme activity; metabolism of carbohydrates, fats, and proteins
K (Menadione)	Production of prothrombin (for blood clotting)

Source: Adapted from Lewis, L. W., & Trimby, B. K. (1988). *Fundamental skills and concepts in patient care* (4th ed.). Philadelphia, PA: J. B. Lippincott.

The signs of nutritional deficiencies include:

- Apathy and listlessness;
- Darkening of the skin;
- Red, sore mouth with fissuring at the corners;
- Sore, red tongue;
- Burning feet;

- Anemia; and

- Weight loss.

Caloric needs vary by body size, level of activity, and other factors, but most active adults require between 2000 and 3000 calories per day. To achieve, or maintain, ideal body weight (IBW), dietitians generally recommend a daily intake of 25 calories per kilogram of body weight. Plant and animal sources provide the amino acids the body refashions into the protein it requires. The term "protein complementation" refers to a process by which two or more *plant sources* are ingested together at the same meal to provide the same total protein found in a single animal source.

Carbohydrates provide an easily metabolized source of energy, and many carbohydrate sources (grains, cereals, fruits, vegetables) have undigestible fiber, which promotes elimination. Fats have a higher energy value than carbohydrates and protein sources (2½ times the amount of either). Alcohol is also high in calories, providing 7 calories per gram.

Water is an essential part of wellness, and fluid intake must be maintained at a fairly constant level (see Tables 5–3 and 5–4). Minerals, such as potassium, calcium, phosphorus, and so on, are the substances which, when dissolved in the body, help to regulate the body's processes—such as conduction of nerve impulses. The healthy body maintains regulatory processes to ensure that fluid reserves and electrolytes are in proper balance. Following neurologic damage to the **hypothalamus**, water balance disorders can arise from disturbances in the neuromechanisms affecting the release of the **antidiuretic hormone (ADH)**, causing conditions such as *diabetes insipidus* and *hypo-*and *hypernatremia*. Hypothalamic damage can also lead to temperature regulation disorders. Tables 5–4 and 5–5 summarize the conditions indicative of fluid or electrolyte imbalances. (For further discussion of specific disorders, see Chapter 10.)

Table 5–3. Average water balances (70 kg male)

Intake	2,500 mL/day (about 35 mL/kg/day baseline)
Oral Liquids	1,500 mL
Oral Solids	700 mL
Metabolic	250 mL (through internal metabolic resources)
Output	1,400–2,300 mL/day
Urine	800–1,200 mL
Stool	250 mL
Insensible losses	600–900 mL (through lungs and skin)

Source: Adapted from Gomella, L. G. (Ed.). (1989). *Clinician's pocket handbook* (6th ed.). Norwalk, CN: Appleton & Lange.

Table 5-4. Indicators of fluid imbalance

Changes in weight
Changes in blood pressure
Elevated body temperature (fluid deficit)
Weak, rapid, thready pulse (fluid deficit)
Full, bounding pulse (fluid excess)
Shallow respiration (fluid deficit)
Moist and labored respiration (fluid excess)

Table 5-5. Indicators of electrolyte imbalances

Condition	Indicators
Hypernatremia	Confusion, stupor, coma, muscle tremors, seizures, pulmonary, and peripheral edema.
Hyponatremia	Lethargy, confusion, coma, muscle twitches, irritability, seizures, nausea, vomiting, ileus.
Hyperkalemia	Weakness, flaccid paralysis, hyperactivity, deep tendon reflexes, confusion, EKG changes.
Hypokalemia	Weakness, flaccid paralysis, hyperactivity, deep tendon reflexes, confusion, EKG changes.
Hypercalemia	Anorexia, nausea, vomiting, polyuria, polydipsia, abdominal pain, kidney stones, fatigue, hypotonia, lethargy, coma.
Hypocalcemia	Peripheral and perioral paresthesia, hyperactive deep tendon reflexes, carpopedal spasm, abdominal cramps, Chvosteks' sign (facial twitches), lethargy and irritability (in infants), EKG changes, generalized seizures, tetany, laryngospasm.
Hypermagnesemia	Nausea, vomiting, hypotension, hyporeflexia, weakness, drowsiness, coma, bradyrhythmias, respiratory failure.
Hypomagnesemia	Weakness, muscle twitches, asterixis, tremors, vertigo, convulsions, tachycardia.
Hyperphosphatemia	Renal failure.
Hypophosphatemia	Weakness, rhabdomyolysis, cardiac and respiratory failure, impaired leukocyte and platelet function, paresthesia, hemolysis.

Source: Adapted from Gomella, L. G. (Ed.). *Clinician's pocket handbook* (6th ed.). Norwalk, CT: Appleton & Lange, and from Lewis, L. W., & Timby, B. K. (1988). *Fundamental skills and concepts in patient care* (4th ed.). Philadelphia: J. B. Lippincott.

VII. IATROGENIC MALNUTRITION IN THE ELDERLY

Malnutrition and dehydration caused by improper or inadvertent errors in nutrition and hydration care are serious problems with the elderly. Malnutrition and dehydration can be caused by **polypharmacy**, *using combinations of drugs that affect the body's management of fluid stores, metabolism, or appetite.* Diuretic drugs need to be monitored to ensure that proper fluid balance is maintained.

Other factors potentially leading to malnutrition include:

- Pain, affecting appetite;

- Poor oral hygiene;

- Improper dietary restrictions;

- Poorly fitting dentures;

- Improperly packaged food items; and

- Decreased mobility (inability to obtain food or water on their own when needed).

Environmental factors, including unpleasant surroundings or odors, the lack of sensory aids (hearing aids, glasses) during meals, and neurogenic deficits (e.g., as visuospatial disturbances, or neglect of one side of the food tray) can also affect the patient's appetite, ability to eat independently, and, consequently, nutritional status.

VIII. PRESCRIBED DIETS

In hospitals, diet orders are written by the physician, and the nurse or ward clerk is responsible for communicating the orders to the dietary service or department. Hospitals vary somewhat as to the diet styles that can be ordered for the patient, and the characteristics of a particular diet style (e.g., "mechanical soft" diet) may differ among institutions. Table 5–6 provides a volume equivalent reference for metric measurements of dietary intake. Table 5–7 lists diet styles commonly found in medical facilities. Determination of dietary orders will usually require a **nutritional assessment** by a dietitian, as described in Table 5–8.

IX. READING AND WRITING NUTRITION NOTES

A. Fluid and Electrolyte Management

The "Doctor's Orders" section of the patient's medical chart will contain the stated **dietary orders**, any **I.V. fluid orders**, and orders

Table 5-6. Volume equivalents

1 Teaspoon	=	5 mL*
1 Tablespoon	=	15 mL
1 Ounce	=	30 mL
Juice glass	=	120 mL (4 oz.)
Average drinking glass	=	240 mL (8 oz.)
Coffee cup	=	210 mL
Milk carton	=	240 mL
1 Quart	=	946 mL

* 1 mL equals 1 cc; however, it has become more acceptable in medicine to use **mL** as the preferred volume measurement.

Table 5-7. Prescribed diet styles

Diet Style	Description
Prescribed therapeutic diets	Diets for special needs such as sodium restricted, protein restricted, low residue, or diabetic diet therapies
Clear liquid diet	A diet consisting of water, clear fruit juice, clear broth, gelatin, tea, or coffee.
Full liquid diet	A diet of liquid and strained fruit juices, soups, vegetable juice, milk, ice cream, gelatin, tea, and coffee.
Pureed diet	A diet similar to a full liquid diet but including pureed fruits, vegetables, and meats.
Mechanical soft diet	A diet style that includes ground meats and in which fruits and vegetables are well-cooked and soft enough to be easily chewed by edentulous persons.
Light or convalescent diet	A diet in which fried, rich, or raw foods are eliminated; and foods are generally prepared by steaming or boiling for easier digestion.
Dysphagia diet	Diet style usually ordered for patients with dysphagia related to oropharyngeal weakness and/or dycoordination who have some risk of aspiration or other swallowing difficulties.
Regular diet	Standard diet served from the kitchen for patients who do not require any dietary therapies.

Table 5-8. Dietitian's nutritional assessment

Assessment	Purpose
Nutrition History	Examines the patient's food habits, preferences, weight, and any weight changes.
Somatic Protein	Includes a height-to-weight ratio and mid-arm circumference measure to indicate skeletal muscle stores.
Triceps Skinfold	Indicates fat stores.
Visceral Proteins	Examines serum albumin, serum transferrin or total iron binding capacity (TIBC) and total lymphocyte count.
Nitrogen Balance	Indicates the adequacy of nutritional support.
Basal Energy Expenditure (BEE) Requirement	Requirements for energy and protein will vary depending upon the nutritional status of the patient, stresses, and activity factors. The Harris-Benedict formula for computing BEE is:

$$\text{Male} = 66 + (13.7 \times \text{weight, in kg}) + (5 \times \text{height, in cm}) - (6.8 \times \text{age, in years})$$

$$\text{Female} = 665 + (9.6 \times \text{weight, in kg}) + (1.8 \times \text{height, in cm}) - (4.7 \times \text{age, in years}).$$

for **replacement fluids or electrolyte imbalance therapies**. These orders are based on findings from the admitting physical examinations, daily vital signs, laboratory findings, I & O records, the nutritional assessment, and related studies, such as those pertaining to dysphagia. Certain prescribed diets, such as those restricting *potassium* (**K**) and *sodium* (**Na**), are intended to correct electrolyte and fluid imbalances.

B. Bedside Charting

Usually, at the end of the bed or in a rack near the patient's bed, there will be a chart for daily recording of vital signs and, when ordered, all **intake and output** (I & O). Nurses are responsible for recording all measurable daily food and liquid ingestion and excretion. Certain medical conditions, such as dehydration, necessitate more frequent monitoring. Infants require especially careful monitoring of nutrition/hydration intake during illness to ensure they take recommended volume (see Table 5–9).

Table 5–9. Infant formula guidelines

Age	Formula Volume Per Feeding	Feedings Per Day
1 month	126 ml (4.1 oz)	6
2 months	142 ml (4.6 oz)	5
3 months	161 ml (5.2 oz)	5
4 months	168 ml (5.4 oz)	5
5 months	191 ml (6.2 oz)	4
6 months	179 ml (5.8 oz)	5
7–9 months	131 ml (4.2 oz)	5
10 months	136 ml (4.4 oz)	5
11 months	125 ml (4.0 oz)	5
12 months	141 ml (4.5 oz)	4

Source: From Kenner, C. A. (1992). *Nurse's clinical guide: Neonatal care*, p. 133. Springhouse, PA: Springhouse Corporation. Reprinted with permission.

C. Special Dietary Orders

The speech-language pathologist's findings regarding indications for special dietary orders, feeding precautions, and feeding guidelines should be clearly and concisely written in the *consultation report* or *progress notes* **and** in place where the information is *readily accessible to nurses or others who are feeding the patient*. Warning "stickers," armbands, and posters are commercially available to alert nurses to special feeding precautions; and feeding guidelines can be posted above the patient's bed or on the bedstand (as long as the patient's confidentiality is protected). When special dietary adjustments, such as a dysphagia diet style, are recommended by the speech-language pathologist's assessment, it may be best to communicate these recommendations directly to the physician and the dietitian or in a conference with the **Dysphagia Management Team**.

Typically, dysphagia diet styles for aspirating patients restrict thin liquids and solid foods and are prepared for easier movement through the oral and pharyngeal phases of swallow. Thickening agents are usually added to liquids.

Dysphagia diet style consistencies can range from solids, prepared similarly to the mechanical soft diet, to thickened paste/pureed solid foods. Patients with an esophageal stricture or obstruction, who are not at risk of thin liquid aspiration, may benefit from a pureed or full liquid diet style. Dysphagia diets need to be tailored to the individual needs and problems of the patient.

X. NOTES

XI. REFERENCES

Arvedson, J. C., & Brodsky, L. (Eds.) (1993). *Pediatric swallowing and feeding: Assessment and management.* San Diego: Singular Publishing Group, Inc.

Ayres, S. M., Schlichdrig, R., & Sterling M. J. (1988). *Care of the critically ill* (3rd ed.). Chicago: Yearbook Medical Publishers.

Bender, A. (1982). *Dictionary of nutrition and food technology* (5th ed.). London: Butterworth.

Chenitz, W. C., Stone, J. T., & Salisbury, S. A (1991). *Clinical gerontological nursing.* Philadelphia: W. B. Saunders.

Gomella, L. G. (Ed.). (1989). *Clinician's pocket handbook* (6th ed.). East Norwalk, CT: Appleton & Lange.

Gomella, L. G. (Ed.) (1993). *Clinician's pocket reference* (7th ed.). Norwalk, CT: Appleton & Lange.

Groher, M. E. (Ed.). (1984). *Dysphagia: Diagnosis and management.* Stoneham, MA: Butterworth.

Karnell, M. P. (1994). *Videoendoscopy: From velopharynx to larynx.* San Diego: Singular Publishing Group, Inc.

Kenner, C. A. (1992). *Nurse's clinical guide: Neonatal care.* Springhouse, PA: Springhouse Corporation.

Langmore, S., Schatz, K., & Olsen, N. (1988). Fiberoptic endoscopic examination of swallowing safety: A new procedure. *Dysphagia, 2,* 216–219.

Lewis, C. M. (1986). *Nutrition and nutritional therapy.* East Norwalk CT: Appleton-Century-Crofts.

Lewis, L. W., & Timby, B. K. (1988). *Fundamental skills and concepts in patient care* (4th ed.). Philadelphia: J. B. Lippincott.

Logemann, J. A. (1983). *Evaluation and treatment of swallowing disorders.* San Diego, CA: College-Hill Press.

Perlman, A L. (1991). Neurology of swallowing. *Seminars in Speech and Language, 12,* 171–184.

Persons, C. G. (1987). *Critical care procedures and protocols.* Philadelphia: J. B. Lippincott.

Robinson, C. H., Lawler, M. R., Chenoweth, W. L., & Garwick A E. (1986). *Normal and therapeutic nutrition* (17th ed.). New York: Macmillan.

Rosenthal, S. R., Sheppard, J. J., & Lotze, M. (1995). *Dysphagia and the child with developmental disabilities.* San Diego: Singular Publishing Group, Inc.

Willett, M. J., Patterson, M., & Steinbock B. (1986). *Manual of neonatal intensive care nursing.* Boston: Little, Brown and Company.

CHAPTER

6

Infectious Diseases and Infection Controls

All health care personnel must be cognizant of infection precautions when they have contact with patients. Patients should not be exposed to unnecessary risks for infection, and employees should avoid exposure to contagious diseases. Certain populations, such as transplant patients taking immunosuppression therapies, burn patients, critically ill patients, elderly patients, and neonates, are especially susceptible to infection. Precautions also apply in cases where the patient has a suspected or diagnosed infectious disease. The need for the speech-language pathologist to understand and apply techniques that promote **asepsis** cannot be overemphasized.

Clinicians who have contagious diseases or exudative lesions on the skin should avoid physical contact with patients. Clinicians must be especially careful to ensure that equipment used in the mouth (such as equipment used during oral examinations, tracheo-esophageal puncture prosthesis fittings, laryngeal stroboscopies, fiberoptic nasendoscopies, etc.) has been properly cleaned and then sterilized. Any equipment used in or near the mouth that has been loaned to a patient needs to be sterilized before it is distributed and again after it is returned. Speech-language pathology ward rounds, where the clinician moves from patient to patient, mandate the use of **Universal Precautions** (see Section III). Any contact with patients in intensive care units, patients with uncovered tracheostomies, patients receiving enteric therapies, patients referred shortly after head and neck surgeries, or any time there is probable contact with blood or body secretions, requires the use of appropriate **barrier practices**.

This chapter reviews terminology related to infection control, describes methods for infection prevention, and discusses common infectious diseases.

I. TERMINOLOGY USED IN INFECTION CONTROL AND INFECTIOUS DISEASES

Also see Hematologic Terminology in Chapter 7.

Acid fast bacilli (AFB) isolation. Infection control practice to prevent the spread of the organism causing tuberculosis.

Acquired immunodeficiency syndrome (AIDS). See *human immunodeficiency virus* and HIV Positive Patients on page 218.

Aerobic. With oxygen.

AIDS-related complex (ARC). A term previously used to refer to symptoms of night sweats, diarrhea, and wasting in association with HIV infection.

Air borne transmission. Air route for the spread of pathogens.

Anaerobic. Without oxygen.

Antibiotic. Drug used to treat infection.

Antimicrobial agent. Chemical used to kill or inhibit the growth of microorganisms.

Antiseptic. Chemical used to kill or inhibit the growth of microorganisms, usually safe to apply on living tissue.

Asepsis. Lack of infection.

Autoclave. An apparatus for pressurized steam sterilization.

Autoclave film. A continuous roll of transparent plastic tubing or bags for packaging items exposed to autoclave *sterilization.*

Autoclave tape. A tape with ink that is sensitive to heat or chemical agents and visible only after exposure to sterilization. The ink changes to a dark color during the sterilization process.

Bacteremia. When bacteria are present in the blood.

Bacteria. Single-celled organisms that reproduce asexually and multiply rapidly. Bacteria are classified by their shape: *cocci* are spherical, *bacilli* are rodlike, and *flagella* have whiplike extensions. Bacteria requiring oxygen to multiply are called aerobic, and those not requiring oxygen to function and reproduce are called *anaerobic.* Some types of bacteria are essential to normal body functions, such as the bacteria lining the intestinal tract.

Bacteriostatic. Chemical used to prevent or inhibit the growth of microorganisms and safe to use on living tissues.

Barrier. Technique, instrument, or garment used to block the transfer of pathogens.

Blood and body fluid precautions. Method of infection control that prevents contact with blood or body fluids; for example, used with patients who have HIV infection or the hepatitis B virus.

Centers for Disease Control (CDC). Referring to the government agency located in Atlanta, Georgia, which conducts and collates research data related to infectious diseases.

Colonization. Growth of microbial agents; a stage of infection.

Communicable. Contagious.

Contact isolation. Procedures applied to eliminate physical contact with infected individuals and any articles they have touched.

Contact route. Contact with infection can come directly through touching an infected person, indirectly through contaminated surfaces or objects, and by droplets when in close proximity to the patient's breath or expectorate.

Contaminate. To unsterilize, or to expose to pathogens.

Cultures. Examinations of bacteria in body fluids, cells, and samples, including throat sputum, cerebrospinal fluid, urine, pus, wounds, drains, genital secretions, and stool.

Deinfestation. Elimination of parasitic insects.

Direct fluoroscent antibody (DFA) test. Test for syphilis.

Disease-specific isolation. Special treatment and isolation procedures for designated infectious diseases.

Disinfectant. Chemical that will *kill microorganisms* but not necessarily their spores.

Double-bagging technique. Procedure used with patients having infectious diseases which involves placing a bag holding contaminated items into a clean bag that has not been in contact with the isolation (contaminated) room.

Drainage and secretion precautions. Procedures applied to eliminate contact with infected wounds and body secretions; used primarily with burn patients and patients with conjunctivitis.

Empyema. Collection of pus within a body cavity.

Encephalitis. Acute viral, or other infectious causes, producing inflammation of the central nervous system characterized by fever, headache, and stiff neck.

Endocarditis. Referring to infection involving the lining of the membrane of the cardiac chambers.

Enteric precautions. Procedures applied to eliminate contact with infected feces; used primarily with patients who have Hepatitis A virus.

Epiglottitis. Usually referring to an aggressive disease occurring in young children in which there is sore throat, copious oral secretions, severe pain of the pharyngeal area without reddening, and respiratory difficulty.

Fever. Condition in which the body temperature is above a normal range, usually in excess of 37.8° C or 100.2° F. Causes of fever can include *infections* (viral, bacterial, or fungal); *tissue injury, drugs, malignancy, immune-mediated disorders, endocrine disorders,* and *other inflammatory disorders.*

Flora. Bacteria normally present in a given location.

Hepatomegaly. Enlargement of the liver and spleen; indicative of infection.

Host. Person (or animal) carrying an organism.

Human immunodeficiency viruses (HIV-1, HIV-2). Referring to the viral agents of acquired immunodeficiency syndrome (AIDS), formerly called *human T-lymphotropic virus type III* (HTLV-III) or *lymphadenopathy-associated virus* (LAV). HIV is transmitted through the exchange of body fluids, such as between a mother and fetus, within breast milk, sharing contaminated needles, receiving contaminated blood products, and sexual intercourse. HIV causes the individual to be susceptible to *opportunistic infections* due to several immunological changes that occur. Lymphopenia with a decreased helper lymphocyte to suppressor lymphocyte (T 4 to T 8 ratio) is characteristic of HIV infections. Many patients acquire cytomegalovirus (CMV), Epstein-Barr virus (EBV), and herpes simplex virus (HSV). See HIV Positive Patients on page 218.

Humidifier. A method for saturating gas with vapor.

Iatrogenic infection. Infection inadvertently resulting from a medical or surgical procedure.

Infectious period. Time when pathogens can be transmitted from a host.

Interferons. A family of proteins produced by lymphocytes, fibroblasts, epithelial cells, and macrophages which provide a major host defense against viruses.

Ludwig's angina. A condition characterized by cellulitis of the floor of the mouth usually due to an odontogenic infection. The tongue may be pushed upward with induration (firm hardening) of the submandibular space.

Meningitis. An inflammation of the leptomeninges (pia and arachnoid) caused by infectious or noninfectious processes (e.g., cancer, hemorrhage). The types of infectious meningitis include *bacterial meningitis, aseptic meningitis, herpes simplex, viral meningitis,* and *tuberculosis meningitis.* See Neurologic Infections, Section VII, and Chapter 9, Neurologic and Psychiatric Disorders.

Microorganisms. Minute forms of life capable of causing diseases.

Mononuclear phagocyte. Macrophages degrade and kill bacteria directly and in antibody-dependent reactions.

Myelitis. Inflammation of the spinal cord; several viruses, such as varicella-zoster, are associated with myelitis.

Natural killer (NK) cells. Lymphocytes that are defined by their ability to break down (lyse) certain tumors.

Nebulizer. Device producing an aerosol.

Neutropenic. Having a low white (neutrophil) cell count and at risk for infection.

Neutrophils. Cells that ingest bacteria and kill them.

Nonpathogenic organism. Harmless microorganism.

Nosocomial infection. Infection occurring within a health facility. Nosocomial infections can result from indwelling catheters, decubitus ulcers (pressure sores), intravenous catheterization, drugs, surgical wound infections, pulmonary emboli, and pneumonia.

Otitis externa, otitis media. Referring to infections of the external auditory canal and the middle ear, respectively.

Pathogenic organism. Microorganism that is contagious or can cause an infection.

Pediculosis. Lice infection.

Pharyngitis. Referring to inflammation of the pharyngeal mucosa. The causes of pharyngitis include *viruses* (respiratory viruses, herpes simplex, Epstein-Barr virus, coxsackie virus A); *bacteria* (Group A streptococcus, Vincent's fusospirochetes, *corynebacterium diphtheriae, corynebacterium hemolyticum),* and *gonorrhea.*

Pneumonia. Referring generally to an inflammation of the lungs caused by bacteria, viruses, or chemical and physical agents. *Acute* *pneumonia* is synonymous with "lobar pneumonia," or *pneumococcal pneumonia*, usually brought on by pneumococcus bacteria. *Aspiration pneumonia* results from inhalation of secretions. Aspiration of normal oropharyngeal flora may lead to *necrotizing pneumonia*. Some degree of aspiration is fairly common, especially during sleep. The effects of minimal amounts of aspiration depend on the individual's mechanical defenses, including cough and mucociliary clearance. A condition called *hypostatic pneumonia* can result in poorly ventilated areas of the lungs in people who lie in the same positions for long periods of time. A condition called *mycoplasmal pneumonia* is caused by the *mycoplasma pneumoniae organism* causing a chronic, severe cough. Milder forms are sometimes called "walking pneumonia." *Pneumocystis carinii pneumonia* is an often fatal lung disease occurring most frequently in premature infants, neonates, individuals receiving immunosuppressant drugs, and individuals with human immunodeficiency virus disease. (See Nosocomial Infections, Section VIII.)

Portal of entry. Site of infection entry.

Quinsy. A unilateral peritonsillar abscess. This condition may require surgical drainage to prevent glottal edema and respiratory distress.

Reservoir. Site where microorganisms reproduce.

Resistant organisms. Infectious organisms that do not respond to antibiotics.

Respiratory isolation. Procedures applied to prevent the spread of contagious diseases through airborne means; used with patients having rubeola (measles), rubella (German measles), pertussis (whooping cough), mumps, and tuberculosis.

Retropharyngeal space abscess, lateral pharyngeal space abscess. Referring to soft tissue infections in the back and sides of the pharyngeal walls, respectively. A lateral pharyngeal space abscess can be life-threatening if erosion of the carotid artery occurs resulting in *carotid exsanguination*.

Reverse isolation. Procedure applied to prevent the spread of infection to a noncontagious but highly susceptible patient; used with certain cases of leukemia, burn patients, transplant patients, and other immunosuppressed patients.

Rhinitis. Watery nasal discharge.

Rickettsiae. A group of organisms that are larger than viruses but smaller than bacteria. Some rickettsiae cause human disease (e.g., typhus and Rocky Mountain spotted fever).

Secondary infection. Infection resulting from another condition.

Sepsis, septicemia. Infectious state; patient will be said to be "septic."

Seroconversion. A conversion from a negative status in blood analysis for a given antibody to positive status, indicating infection is present.

Seropositive. An indicator in blood analysis of exposure to a virus.

Spore. A microbial state that allows survival until a growth environment is provided.

Sterile field. Area where all surfaces are sterile and kept free of microorganisms and their spores.

Sterile technique. Application of procedures to keep instruments and surfaces **free of microorganisms and their spores**.

Sterilization. A process for destroying microorganisms and their spores; *decontamination* is not the same as sterilization.

Stomatitis. Inflammation of the mouth. *Aphthous stomatitis* refers to shallow, painful ulcers on the labial or buccal mucosa. *Vincent's stomatitis* is an ulcerative infection of the gingival mucosa due to an anaerobic fusobacteria and spirochetes. This condition is characterized by foul breath and purulent gray ulcerations. Other conditions associated with oral ulcers and vesicles include *herpangina* (a childhood disease that causes tiny ulcerations of the soft palate due to infection with the coxsackie virus A), *fungal diseases*, and *systemic illnesses*.

Strict isolation. Procedure used to limit contact with patients having highly contagious diseases; used with patients having small pox, chicken pox, or diphtheria, and with burn patients.

T-cells. T-lymphocytes that are present in the immune system to combat infections; the HIV attacks T-lymphocytes.

Thrush. Infection of the oral mucosa by *candida*.

TORCH. Acronym for *T*oxoplasma, *O*ther infections, *R*ubella, *C*ytomegalo, and *H*erpes virus, type 2.

Vaccine. Derivative given to promote the body's immune defenses against a contagious disease.

Vector. Person or animal (or insect) that spreads pathogenic micro-organisms.

Vehicle of transmission. Transmission media of pathogens can occur through **airborne** means (by exposure to air particles containing pathogens), **vector borne** means (by exposure to animals or insects carrying pathogenic microorganisms), and **contaminated substances** (e.g., blood, food, water, or drugs).

Viruses. Viruses are not living organisms. They are large nucleoprotein particles which are capable of entering specific types of cells. Viruses are nearly as small as a single molecule of protein. Many of the infections caused by viruses can create a lasting immunity; thus, *inoculation* (vaccination) with weakened forms of a virus can help to prevent infection.

II. ABBREVIATIONS RELATED TO INFECTIOUS DISEASES

Ab. Antibody

AFB. Acid fast bacilli

AIDS. Acquired immune deficiency syndrome

AIHA. Autoimmune hemolytic anemia

ARC. Aids-related complex

AZT. Azidothimidine

CDC. Centers for Disease Control

EBV. Epstein-Barr virus

E. coli. Escherichia coli

ELISA. Enzyme-linked immunosorbent assay

FUO. Fever of unknown/undetermined origin

GC. *Gonococcus* (gonorrhea)

GNB. Gram-negative bacillus

GNID. Gram-negative intracellular diplococci

GP. Gram-positive

GVHD. Graft versus host disease

HAA. Hepatitis-associated antigen

HAV. Hepatitis A virus

HBc. Hepatitis B core antigen

HBeAg. Hepatitis B e antigen

HBsAg. Hepatitis B surface antigen

HBIG. Hepatitis B immune globulin

HBV. Hepatitis B virus

HCV. Hepatitis C virus (non-A, non-B hepatitis)

HIV, HIV-1, HIV-2. Human immunodeficiency virus, type 1, type 2

HIVD. Human immunodeficiency virus disease

HSV. Herpes simplex virus

ID. Infectious disease

Inf. Infected, infectious

MBC. Minimum bacterial concentration

MMR. Measles, mumps, rubella

MO. Multiple organisms

MRSA. Methicillin resistant *Staphylococcus aureus*

O & P. Ova and parasites

OPV. Oral polio vaccine

PAIDS. Pediatric AIDS

PCP. *Pneumocystis carinii* pneumonia

PML. Progressive (cranial nerve) multifocal lymphencephalopathy

PPD. Purified protein derivative

RT. Rubella titer

STD. Sexually transmitted disease

Syph. Syphilis

TB. Tuberculosis

TBC. Tuberculin calibrated (syringe)

TDT. Tetanus-diphtheria toxoid

TOPV. Trivalent oral polio vaccine

TORCH. Toxoplasma, other (syphilis), rubella, cytomegalovirus, and herpes virus

URI. Upper respiratory infection

UTI. Urinary tract infection

VD. Venereal disease

VDRL. Venereal Disease Research Laboratory (test)

III. UNIVERSAL PRECAUTIONS

Health care facilities currently apply what are called **Universal Precautions** (UP), meaning **everyone** (patients and staff is considered an infectious risk. **This approach to infection control is based on the presumptions that:**

- Infectious agents are present before symptoms are present;

- Multiply resistant organisms may be present before they are detected; and

- Air and blood borne infections are always potential hazards to staff and patients.

Special precautions for infection controls will be required for conditions such as tuberculosis, multiresistant bacterial infection or colonization, herpes simplex, varicella zoster, scabies (pediculosis), measles, and mumps.

When Universal Precautions are part of the infection control policies, **all patient contact requires:**

- Handwashing before and after contact;
- Gloves be worn if there is any contact with body fluids, mucous membranes, or broken skin;
- Gowns be worn if clothing is likely to become soiled;
- Eye and mouth protection be worn if any expectorant, blood, or body fluid splashes are likely; and
- All disposable intact needle/syringes and sharp instruments be placed in the "sharps disposal" container.

IV. PROTECTION METHODS

A. Handwashing

When Universal Precautions are applied, hands must be washed with soap and water before and after contact with any patient and immediately after contact with blood or body fluids. A suggested handwashing technique for routine protection is described below.

Routine Handwashing

- Remove or push up the wristwatch and sleeves and remove jewelry.
- Turn water on and off using a clean paper towel.
- Wet hands and apply a liquid disinfecting soap.
- Rub hands and forearms vigorously in a circular motion for 1 minute (or longer if directly exposed to contamination).
- Rinse and dry with clean paper towels.
- Use a paper towel to push open the door, or turn the doorknob, when entering or leaving the room.

B. Gloves

Gloves should be worn any time there is to be contact with a person who has a known infectious disease, especially when contact with blood or body secretions is likely. Gloves need to be put on in such a way as to avoid touching the outside of the glove with your bare skin. Although the sterile technique is not routinely required, the techniques for donning and removing sterile gloves are described below.

Putting on Sterile Gloves

- Open the glove package without touching the gloves.

- Touching only the folded cuff of the glove, lift the right hand glove and place it on your hand avoiding touching outside surface of the glove.

- With the gloved right hand, insert your fingers under the outside edge of the cuff of the left glove to lift it.

- Place it on the left hand avoiding any contact between the outside surface of the clean glove and the bare skin of the left hand.

- Carefully fold back the glove cuffs without touching bare skin or the inside of the gloves.

Removing Contaminated Gloves

- With your gloved right hand, grasp the wrist fold of your left glove and remove the glove.

- With your now-bare left hand, reach into the inside of the right glove and remove the glove without touching the outside of the glove; dispose of the contaminated glove.

C. Masks

Masks are worn with any patient likely to transmit pathogens through airborne means or splashing. Use of masks with clear plastic eye protectors is encouraged, as the eye can provide a portal of entry for infection.

D. Sterile Gowns and Hair and Shoe Coverings

Sterile gowns are worn in surgery or when required by **isolation precautions**, which are usually *posted at the patient's door*. Sterile gowns may be made of cloth or disposable paper and usually will be provided just outside of the patient's room. Sterile masks, gloves, and hair and shoe coverings will be used to protect a susceptible patient (such as a burn patient) from exposure to pathogens or in cases where the patient has a highly contagious disease.

Applying a Sterile Gown

- After applying a mask and hair and shoe coverings, pick up the sterile gown by the neck area.

- Allow it to unfold and insert your arms without touching the outside surfaces and do not extend your hands out from the sleeves.

- Ask an assistant who is wearing sterile gloves to secure the neck and to pull up on the sleeves to allow you to extend your hands.

- Apply sterile gloves in the manner just described.

E. Obtaining Signatures

Patients susceptible to or having an infectious disease can sign documents by placing a clean paper towel beneath the document paper and another clean paper towel on top of the paper, exposing the surface as necessary to be read. The patient can then rest his or her hand on the paper towel and sign without touching the document.

F. Disinfecting, Sterilizing, and Disposing of Contaminated Equipment

1. **Decontamination.** Medical treatment areas are kept *decontaminated* with various cleaning agents. Some areas require at least low to medium level decontamination; other areas, such as surgical suites, require a sterile environment, or high level decontamination.

2. **Disinfecting.** *Disinfecting* refers to a process that will destroy most microorganisms but may not destroy their spores; thus, cleaning with disinfecting agents does not necessarily eliminate a risk for infection. *Quaternary ammonium compounds*, or "Quats," are commonly used as *low level disinfectants. Chlorine* (household bleach) and *iodine* are halogens and are considered *medium level disinfectants.* Soaking in isopropyl alcohol solution, wiping surfaces with alcohol wipes, or wiping surfaces with hydrogen peroxide offers little more than low level disinfection. Your facility's infection control policies will state the appropriate agents and cleaning procedures to use for various surfaces.

3. **Sterilization.** High level decontamination, or *sterilization*, is directed toward destroying both the pathogenic microbes and their spores. Sterilization requires special methods which usually include heat, ethylene oxide gas, or chemical immersion agents. *Dry heat* is used to sterilize sharp instruments and

reusable syringes. Pressurized steam, or an *autoclave*, is considered a dependable method for destroying microorganisms and their spores but cannot be used with sharp instruments or devices affected by moisture.

Hospital infection control practices include *washer-sterilizers* which provide medium to high level disinfection. *Ultrasound* washers are used to agitate and loosen tiny particles from instruments, a process called "cavitation."

Chemical gas sterilization is useful when instruments or equipment would be damaged by other methods. *Ethylene oxide gas* can penetrate outer coverings well and is advantageous when equipment would be damaged by heat or liquid. Instruments that have been contaminated require heat or gas sterilization or a prolonged chemical cleaning before they can be reused. Chemical agents, such as hexachlorophene ("Cidex"), phenolic compounds, and glutaraldehyde solutions, are not considered as effective as gas or heat sterilization; thus, prolonged emersion (several hours) is advised. Some instruments, such as the end piece of a stroboscope, may be damaged by prolonged immersion in compounds like Cidex. The facility's Infection Control Officer or I.D. Nurse Practitioner should be consulted for advice on an adequate immersion cleaning time. Contaminated disposable items and contaminated linens need to be placed in the designated receptacles for disposal.

V. INFECTION CONTROL PRACTITIONER

Every medical facility will have an Infection Control Committee which usually is chaired by an Infection Control Practitioner (I.C.P.). The I.C.P. may be an Infectious Disease (I.D.) physician or an I.D. Nurse Practitioner. The Infection Control Committee is responsible for ensuring that the hospital environment minimizes the exposure of both the patient and staff to infectious complications. It monitors infections and identifies sources of contamination risks. It develops stated policies and procedures for infection prevention and reporting infections and infectious complications. The Infection Control Committee's policies and procedures typically cover: visiting policies, isolation policies and standard cleaning procedures in your area, insertion and maintenance procedures for intravascular devices and their dressing changes, serologic testing, care and maintenance of dialysis equipment, timing of equipment changes, preparation and delivery of enteral feeding solutions, orientation, and staff education, guidelines for the patient or staff immunization program, and oversight of nosocomial infections. These policies should be available from the infection Control Practitioner.

VI. COMMON INFECTIOUS PROBLEMS AND DISEASES

A. Bacterial Infections

Bacterial infections are classified clinically based on the result of the **gram stain**. This test consists of exposing specimens to a series of staining chemicals and examining for color changes or decolorization. **Gram-positive** organisms include: **Staphylococcus** (*S. aureus* and *S. epidermidis*); **streptococcus** *(S. pneumoniae, S. viridans*, and *enterococci)*; and some **bacilli** *(bacillus, listeria, corynebacterium)*.

Gram-negative organisms include: *Pseudomonadaceae* (*P. aeuruginosa* and *P. mallei*); *hemophilus*; Legionella; and various bacilli (including shigella, salmonella, proteus, and others).

B. Viral Infections

Viral infections frequently found among critically ill patients include: herpes simplex; varicella-zoster; cytomegalovirus; Epstein-Barr virus; hepatitis A and hepatitis B virus, hepatitis C; and retro viruses (human immunodeficiency viruses, HIV). Hospital workers who routinely come in contact with body fluids should undergo hepatitis B vaccination.

C. Fungal Infections

Fungal conditions often found among clinically ill patients include: *candida, aspergillus, cryptococcus neoformans*, and histoplasmosis.

VII. NEUROLOGIC INFECTIONS

Meningitis can result from **bacterial causes** (hemophilus influenza; gram-negative bacilli; gram-positive bacilli, including tetanus; *S. aureus, S. epidermidis*; nocardia; syphilis; and meningitides); **viral causes** (HIV; cytomegalovirus; enterovirus, such as coxsackie virus; measles; mumps; herpes simplex virus; and varicella-zoster virus); **fungal causes** (histoplasma, *candida, aspergillus, mucoraceae, coccidioides, cryptococcus*); **tuberculosis**; or **parasitic causes** (toxoplasmosis). The clinical manifestations will vary depending on the type of organism responsible for causing the infection. Cerebrospinal fluid (CSF) findings, blood cultures, and CT scans are usually ordered for the diagnosis. The CSF findings are examined for their **appearance**, the amount of **protein** and **glucose** present, the number of **lymphocytes** and other cells per cubic mm, and any increase in **CSF pressure**.

Another neurologic manifestation of infection is **septic shock**. *Septic shock* is the systemic response to an infectious process and results in fever, hypothermia, metabolic abnormalities, hypotension, impaired organ perfusion, and multiple organ systems failure (MOSF).

Tuberculosis and poliomyelitis (polio) are infectious diseases known to attack cranial nerves. Recurrent symptoms have been found in some patients who were treated for poliomyelitis decades earlier.

VIII. NOSOCOMIAL INFECTIONS

Infections acquired during hospitalization are called *nosocomial infections*. These infections typically include wound infections from surgeries or decubitus ulcers, urinary tract infections (UTIs), upper respiratory infections (URIs), pneumonia, contamination of enteral formula, or intravascular (I.V.) infections. **Aspiration pneumonia** is a complication common to patients receiving tube feedings or having tracheostomies and translaryngeal intubation. The risk for aspiration pneumonia increases with depressed consciousness. **Enteric gram-negative aerobic bacterium** (EGNAB), the flora from the gastrointestinal tract, are the organisms of nosocomial pneumonia which tend to colonize in the elderly and chronically ill patient. The patient's immobility, coupled with respiratory disease, are the main contributors.

Patients vary in their susceptibility to pneumonia following aspiration of the bacteria-laden secretions in the oropharynx. The clinical manifestations of aspiration pneumonia include increased production of purulent sputum, fever, and progressing pulmonary infiltrates. Some patients have **"silent,"** or *small volume,* **aspiration** that can be identified through a modified barium swallow (MBS) or similar study if the patient is alert enough.

Frequently, silent aspiration is surmised after the development of fever and a chest x-ray has revealed a new infiltrate. Aspiration consequences depend on the size of the food particles, pathogenic organisms, and pH of the material aspirated.

IX. HIV POSITIVE PATIENTS

The term *immunodeficient* means that a patient's immune defenses are less effective than normal. Patients found to have antibodies to the Human Immunodeficiency Viruses (HIV) are at known risk for opportunistic infections. The natural history for infections associated with the HIV (type I or type 2) is not yet known. The etiology is a retrovirus which selectively enters OK T4 ("helper") lymphocytes and becomes integrated into the genome of the host. A severe deficit in cellular immunity is ultimately manifested. Serologic testing for HIV is done with an Enzyme-Linked Immunosorbent Assay, or ELISA, followed by a Western Blot test (see Chapter 3).

Patients seropositive for HIV ultimately develop what was previously called "Aids Related Complex" (ARC), manifested by unexplained fevers, weight loss, fatigue, diarrhea, viral leukoplakia and/or oral candidiasis, and lymphadenopathy. Most patients with AlDs will ultimately develop *pneumocystis carinii* pneumonia and Kaposi's sarcoma, as well as other opportunistic infections and lymphomas. The neurologic complications associated with AIDS include: progressive dementia with disorientation, cognitive problems, and, sometimes, focal neurologic signs; encephalitis; meningitis; space-occupying lesions, including metastatic Karposi's sarcoma and primary and systemic lymphoma; and peripheral neuropathies, including inflammatory polyneuropathy, transverse myelitis, and cranial nerve involvement. The acquisition and progression of opportunistic infections in association with HIV differ between children and adults.

X. INFECTIONS IN NEWBORNS

Infections in newborns are classified as either **transplacental** (occurring during birth) or **acquired** (occurring after birth). Transplacental infections tend to be viral and usually include: toxoplasmosis, cytomegalo virus, rubella, and syphilis. Although the source of infection is the mother, she may be asymptomatic. Herpes virus can be transmitted during passage through the birth canal.

Most acquired infections are bacterial. The mode of infection in the neonatal intensive care unit is the same as that in adult intensive care units, transmission by the *hands of the caregivers*; thus, the Universal Precautions discussed in this chapter apply to infants as well as other patients.

XI. NOTES

_____

_____

_____

NOTES *(continued)*

XII. REFERENCES

Avery, M., & Imdieke, B. (1984). *Medical records in ambulatory care.* Rockville, MD: Aspen.

Ayres, S. M., Schlichtig, R., & Sterling, M. J. (1988). *Care of the critically ill* (3rd ed.). Chicago: Yearbook Medical Publishers.

Fein, I. A., & Strasberg, M. A. (1987). *Managing the critical care unit.* Rockville, MD: Aspen.

Gray, B. H., & Field, M. J. (Eds.). (1989). *Controlling costs and changing patient care?* Washington, DC: National Academy Press.

Haller, R. M., & Sheldon, N. (1976). *Speech pathology and audiology in medical settings.* New York: Stratten International Medical Book.

Lewis, L. W., & Timby, B. K. (1988). *Fundamental skills and concepts in patient care* (4th ed.). Philadelphia: J. B. Lippincott.

Miller, R. M., & Groher, M. E. (1990). *Medical speech pathology.* Rockville, MD: Aspen.

Nicolosi, L., Harryman, E., & Kresheck, J. (1983). *Terminology in communication disorders* (2nd ed.). Baltimore: Williams & Wilkins.

Persons, C. G. (1987). *Critical care procedures and protocols.* Philadelphia: J. B. Lippincott.

Sande, M. A., & Voldering, P. A. *The medical management of AIDS.* Philadelphia: W. B. Saunders.

Wolper, L. F., & Pena, J. J. (Eds.). (1987). *Health care administration.* Rockville, MD: Aspen.

CHAPTER

7

Cardiac, Pulmonary, and Hematologic Functions

Patients with hematologic, circulatory, cardiac, and pulmonary diseases make up a substantial proportion of the speech-language pathologist's caseload in a medical setting. This chapter expands the areas discussed in Chapter 3 (Vital Signs and Physical Examination) and contains additional review of cardiac, pulmonary, and hematologic diagnostic procedures. Related information is found in subsequent chapters. Chapter 8 (Imaging Studies and Radiologic Therapies) discusses specific radiologic and imaging techniques used to examine ventilation and circulatory functions in greater detail. Chapter 9 (Neurologic and Psychiatric Disorders) provides descriptions of cerebrovascular diseases; Chapter 10 (Acute and Critical Illnesses) provides descriptions of acute and critical illnesses, including cardiac, pulmonary, and hematologic conditions; and Chapter 12 (Surgeries and Other Procedures) includes a list of some thoracic and vascular surgeries potentially encountered in medical histories.

I. CARDIAC FUNCTIONS AND DISEASES

A. Cardiac and Circulatory Terminology

Aneurysm. A widening or ballooning-out of a weakened blood vessel wall.

Angina. Organ pain during ischemia. Some people will have a sensation of choking during *cardiac angina* attacks due to ventricular dysfunction. Angina is usually clinically described by **levels of pain**, using the following scale: **1+** = *light or barely noticeable*; **2+** = *moderate, bothersome*; **3+** = *severe and very uncomfortable*; and **4+** = *most severe pain ever experienced.*

Angiocarditis. Inflammation of the heart and/or its vessels.

Aorta. Largest artery of the body, receives blood pumped from the left ventricle as the initial point of circulation to the rest of the body.

Artery. Blood vessels that carry blood away from the heart to various parts of the body.

Arrhythmia. A lack of rhythmic heartbeats resulting from ischemia, metabolic dysfunction, drug toxicity, or atrial distention. Various forms of arrhythmia include: *atrial fibrillation, atrial flutter, paroxysmal atrial tachycardia, atrioventricular nodal arrhythmias, ventricular arrhythmias,* and *conduction disturbances.*

Arteriosclerosis. Induration or hardening, of the arteries.

Atria. Smaller, upper heart chambers.

Atrial septal defect. Congenital abnormality in which there is a communicating opening between the atria.

Atrioventricular bundle (Bundle of His). Part of the conducting system of the heart with fibers extending from the atrioventricular (AV) node into the intraventricular septum causing ventricular heart contractions.

Atrioventricular node (AV node). Point between the upper and lower chambers of the heart where electrical excitatory impulses from the sinoatrial (SA) node are promulgated on to the ventricular heart muscle.

Bicuspid valve. Heart valve located between the left atrium and ventricle; mitral valve.

Bradycardia. Slow heartbeat.

Capillary. Tiny networks of blood vessels that connect the venules and arterioles.

Cardiac arrest. Cessation of heart action.

Cardiac arrhythmias. Irregularities of heart rate and rhythm action due to disturbances in conduction. Arrhythmias include: **atrial arrhythmias** (*atrial fibriliation; atrial flutter;* and *paroxysmal atrial tachycardia,* or PAT); **atrioventricular nodal arrhythmias;** and **ventricular arrhythmias** (*ventricular fibrillation; premature ventricular contractions,* or PVCs; and *ventricular tachycardia,* or "V tach").

Cardiac tamponade. Compression on the heart by hemorrhage or effusion in the pericardium.

Cardiomegaly. Enlarged heart.

Cardioplegia. Paralysis of the heart muscle.

Cardiopulmonary arrest. Sudden cessation of respiration and circulation.

Carditis. Inflammation of heart tissues.

Claudication. An impaired ability to walk due to pain from inadequate blood supply to the muscles of the legs.

Coarctation of the aorta. Narrowing of the aorta.

Conduction disturbances. Heart abnormalities resulting from disturbances in myocardial neural impulses including: **atrioventricular block** (first, second, or third degree heart block); **bundle branch block** (BBB); **hemiblock; Stokes-Adams syndrome** (cardiac stasis); and **Wolff-Parkinson-White syndrome** (a congenital conduction disorder).

Congestive heart failure. Condition in which the heart is unable to pump adequately to supply the body's tissues. **Left sided fail-**

ure with left ventricular dilatation leads to pulmonary congestion, edema, cerebral hypoxia, and coma. **Right sided failure** involving the right ventricle leads to *portal system* involvement causing *ascites* and enlargement of the liver and spleen.

Cor triatriatum. Congenital condition in which the heart has three atrial chambers.

Cor triloculare. Congenital condition in which the heart has three chambers due to a lack of interatrial or interventricular septa.

Coronary arteries. Arteries supplying the heart muscle; includes the left main coronary artery (LMCA), *left anterior descending artery* (LADA), *circumflex artery,* and *right coronary artery* (RCA). It should be noted that **coronary artery bypass grafts (CABGs)** are grafting anastomoses surgeries most often performed on these four heart arteries.

Coronary atherosclerotic disease. Condition in which fibrous fatty plaques have accumulated on the walls of the arteries supplying the heart muscle, potentially causing ischemic heart disease.

Cyanosis. Having a blue appearance to the skin due to a lack of oxygenation.

Dextrocardia. Having the heart on the right side of the body.

Diastole. Relaxation of the ventricular heart muscle.

Embolus. A particle, air bubble, or clot carried in the bloodstream.

Endocardium. The inner lining of the heart.

Extracorporeal. Circulation of blood outside of the body, as in hemodialysis.

Extrastole. Heart contraction not initiated by the sinoatrial node.

Hypertension. High blood pressure; **essential hypertension** is idiopathic (of unknown cause) whereas secondary hypertension is a condition resulting from an associated disease, such as *glomerulonephritis, pyelonephritis,* or *adenoma* of the adrenal cortex.

Hypotension. Low blood pressure.

Infarction. Tissue death caused by lack of adequate oxygenation due to impaired blood supply.

Ischemia. Inadequate blood supply to tissues.

Isolated pulmonary stenosis. A congenital stenotic defect characterized by narrowing of the pulmonary valve.

Murmur. A rasping heart sound heard during auscultation of cardiac blood flow.

Myocardial infarction (MI). A condition usually caused by atherosclerotic disease of the vessels supplying the heart muscle, characterized by intense, constrictive chest pain with *diaphoresis* (profuse sweating), *pallor, hypotension, dyspnea, nausea, vomiting,* and *fainting*.

Myocardium. The heart muscle (middle layer of the heart).

Occlusion. Blockage.

Patent. Open.

Patent ductus arteriosus (PDA). A congenital condition in which the communicating duct between the pulmonary artery and aorta fails to close following birth. PDA is sometimes associated with **Infant Respiratory Distress Syndrome (IRDS)**.

Pericardium. Pertaining to the sac covering the heart.

Petechiae. Small, pinpoint hemorrhages on the skin.

Phlebitis. Inflammation of a vein.

Pulmonary artery. The artery that carries (deoxygenated) blood from the heart to the lungs to be oxygenated.

Pulmonary vein. The vein that carries oxygenated blood from the lungs to the heart.

Pulse sites, peripheral pulse sites. Body locations providing good access to arterial pulses for checking heart rate and rhythms; includes *radial pulse* (thumb side of wrist), *brachial pulse* (in the antecubital space of the elbow), *high brachial pulse* (inside the upper arm), *carotid pulse* (on the sides of the neck), *temporal pulse* (at the temple), *femoral pulse* (located on either side of the groin), *popliteal pulse* (behind the knee), *posterior pedis pulse* (ankle), and *dorsalis pedis pulse* (in the instep of the foot) (see Figure 3–1 on page 86).

Pulsus paradoxus. The disappearance of a *Korotkoff* sound during blood pressure measurement (see Chapter 3).

Reynaud's phenomenon. Episodes of pallor and numbness of the extremities associated with emotional stress, cold, or smoking.

Rheumatic heart disease. Valvular heart disease or damage to the endocardium after rheumatic fever.

Septum (cardiovascular). The partition between the right and left sides of the heart.

Sinoatrial node (SA node). Site in the right atrium where a heart-beat is initiated; the pacemaker of the heart.

Systole. Contraction phase of the ventricular heart muscle.

Tachycardia. A fast heartbeat.

Tetralogy of Fallot. A syndrome of congenital heart defects which includes a *ventricular septal defect, pulmonary stenosis, transposition of the aorta toward the right, and hypertrophy of the right ventricle.*

Tissue plasminogen activator. A drug, such as streptokinase, used to prevent clotting and improve survival after a myocardial infarction.

Tricuspid valve. Heart valve between the right atrium and ventri-cle which has cusps, or flaps.

Valve. Structures in the heart or veins which close to prevent back-flow of blood. **Valvular abnormalities** or dysfunctions in heart valves can include **atresia** (congenital absence or closure); **pro-lapse** (typically of the mitral valve, where the valve cusp falls back into the atrium during systole); **regurgitation** (an incompetent or *insufficient,* valve allowing backflow); and **stenosis** (stiff and fibrotic valve obstructing passage of blood flow).

Varicose veins. Condition in which valves in the veins fail to pre-vent backflow of blood resulting in abnormally swollen veins, occurring particularly in the legs.

Vasoconstriction. Narrowing of a blood vessel.

Vasodilatation. Widening of a blood vessel.

Vasospasm. Contraction of a blood vessel.

Vegetations. Growths within or on a structure. Damaged heart valves are vulnerable to vegetation growth.

Vein. Blood vessels that carry blood toward the heart.

Venae cavae. The *superior vena cava and inferior vena cava* which carry blood from the upper and lower body, respectively, to the right atrium of the heart.

Ventricles. Larger, lower chambers of the heart.

Ventricular septal defect (VSD). Congenital heart defect in which there is a partial or complete absence of the ventricular septum.

B. Cardiac and Circulatory Abbreviations

AAA. Abdominal aortic aneurysm

ACG. Angiocardiography

AD. Aortic dissection (also see Chapter 10)

AHA. American Heart Association

AI. Aortic insufficiency

AIF. Aorto-ileo-femoral (graft)

AMI. Acute myocardial infarction

AS. Aortic stenosis

ASD. Atrial septal defect

ASH. Asymmetrical septal hypertrophy

ASHD. Atherosclerotic heart disease

AST. Aspartate aminotransferase

AV. Atrioventricular

BBB. Bundle branch block

BP. Blood pressure

BPM. Beats per minute

CABG. Coronary artery bypass graft

CAD. Coronary artery disease

CC. Coronary catheterization

CCA. Circumflex coronary artery

CCU. Coronary care unit

CHF. Congestive heart failure

CK. Creatine kinase

CO. Cardiac output

CPB. Cardiopulmonary bypass

CPR. Cardiopulmonary resuscitation

CVP. Central venous pressure

DVTs. Deep vein thromboses

ECC. Extracorporeal circulation

EKG/ECG. Electrocardiogram

ESR. Erythrocyte sedimentation rate

FHS. Fetal heart sounds

G1, G2, G3, G4, G5, G6. Grade one, grade two, and so on (referring to extra heart sounds)

HDL. High density lipoproteins

IHSS. Idiopathic hypertrophic subaortic stenosis

JVD. Jugular venous distention

KVO. Keep vein open

LA. Left atrium

LADA. Left anterior descending artery

LAP. Left atrial pressure

LBBB. Left bundle branch block

LD. Lactic dehydrogenase

LDL. Low density lipoproteins

LHF. Left heart failure

LMCA. Left main coronary artery

LV. Left ventricle

MI. Myocardial infarction

MS. Mitral stenosis

MVP. Mitral valve prolapse

NSR. Normal sinus rhythm

OHS. Open heart surgery

PAC. Premature atrial contractions

PAT. Paroxysmal atrial tachycardia

PDA. Patent ductus arteriosus

PMI. Point of maximal impulse

PPS. Postperfusion syndrome

PTCA. Percutaneous transluminal coronary angioplasty

PVC. Premature ventricular contraction

RA. Right atrium

RAE. Right atrial enlargement

RCA. Right coronary artery

RHF. Right heart failure

RV. Right ventricle

S1,S2, S3, S4. Sound one, sound two, and so on (basic heart sounds)

SA. Sinoatrial

SBE. Subacute bacterial endocarditis

SCD. Sudden cardiac death

SGOT. Serum glutamic-oxaloacetic transaminase

tPA. Tissue plasminogen activator

TEE. Transesophageal echocardiogram

2-D echo. Two-dimensional echocardiogram

VCG. Vectorcardiogram

VLDL. Very low density lipoproteins

VSD. Ventricular septal defect

C. Fundamental Principles in Cardiology

1. **Circulation.** The heart is a fist-sized organ with four chambers which pumps deoxygenated blood to the lungs and oxygenated blood to the tissues of the body. The two upper chambers of the heart are the **atria**; the two lower chambers are the **ventricles**. Deoxygenated blood enters the right atrium from the *inferior and superior venae cavae*, where it is pumped through the **tricuspid valve** into the right ventricle. From the right ventricle, the blood is pumped into the *pulmonary arteries* to the lungs for oxygenation and removal of carbon dioxide. Blood returning from the lungs enters through the *pulmonary veins* into the left atrium. It then passes through the **mitral** (or bicuspid) **valve** into the left ventricle and is then pumped through the **aortic valve** into the aorta and on to the body. Figure 7–1 illustrates the circulation of the heart.

2. **Conduction.** The excitation of a heartbeat and maintenance of rhythmic *contractions* (**systoles**) and *relaxations* (**diastoles**) are regulated by neuroelectrical nodes within the myocardium. These impulses originate from the parasympathetic and sympathetic nerves of the autonomic nervous system, primarily from the Vagus nerve (CN X).

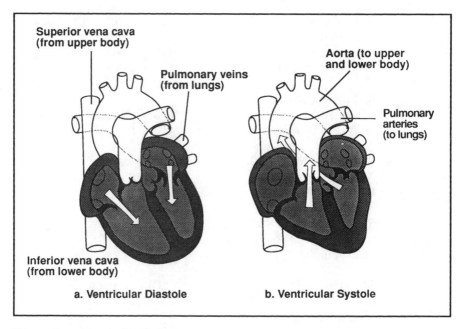

Figure 7–1. Heart circulation

The sinoatrial (SA) node, or pacemaker of the heart, is located in the right atrium near the superior vena cava. The SA node stimulates simultaneous contractions of the atria. Electrical impulses from the SA node are projected to the **atrioventricular (AV) node** located in the interatrial septum. Impulses from the AV node are then directed to a region deep in the ventricular wall, the *Bundle of His*, or **atrioventricular bundle**, which elicits contractions of the ventricles. Ventricular contraction is called the *systole*, and ventricular relaxation is called the *diastole*. Figure 7–2 illustrates the locations of these nodal impulses. Damage to the heart causing an interruption in the conductive impulses arising from the AV node and extending to the right ventricle is called a *right bundle branch block* (RBBB); damage in the conduction of impulses from the AV node extending to the left ventricle is called a *left bundle branch block* (LBBB).

3. **Electrocardiographs.** The electrocardiograph (EKG, ECG) is a recording of the neuroelectrical **conduction** activity across the heart muscle. The EKG has five characteristics in its wave pattern, which are designated by the letters **P, Q, R, S,** and **T,** representing phases in conductive activity. The "P" wave

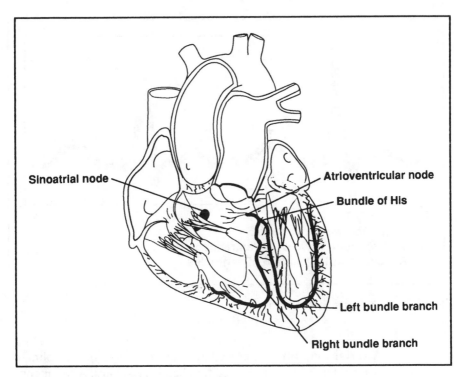

Figure 7–2. Heart conduction

occurs with depolarization of the atria, as the impulse passes from the SA to the AV nodes. The "Q," "R," and "S" waves, or *QRS complex*, represent the spread of excitation elicited by the Bundle of His, causing contraction of the ventricles. The "T" wave represents repolarization, or the relaxation, of the ventricles. Figure 7–3 illustrates a normal EKG tracing.

D. Cardiac Procedures and Studies

(See Chapter 2, Section 111, A, for cardiac enzymes and other laboratory studies.)

Anastomosis. Two vessels attached together, usually referring to a surgical procedure.

Angiogram. Radiographic study using a contrast medium to reveal dimensions of the heart and its vessels.

Angioplasty. Surgical correction of a blood vessel.

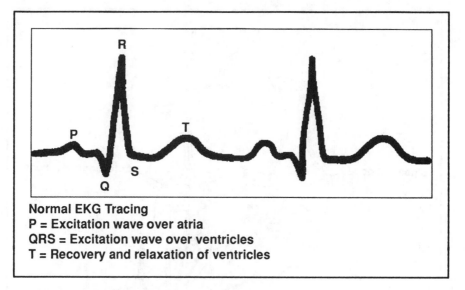

Normal EKG Tracing
P = Excitation wave over atria
QRS = Excitation wave over ventricles
T = Recovery and relaxation of ventricles

Figure 7–3. Normal EKG tracing

Arterial puncture. A procedure used for blood gas sampling or when arterial blood is needed for chemistry studies. Arterial puncture involves using a heparinized needle to aspirate blood from the radial, femoral, or brachial arteries.

Artificial pacemaker. An electronic device implanted to provide rhythmic electrical stimulation of the heart.

Cardiac monitor. An electronic device which monitors and reveals heart functions and permits detection of arrhythmias. **Hardwire monitoring** involves the use of a three- or five-lead EKG cable attached to a bedside, hardwire monitor connected to a computerized central monitor. **Telemetry monitoring** involves continuous monitoring of cardiac rhythm through the use of a portable transmitter in the ambulatory patient, *who stays within the vicinity of the monitor* to document cardiac dysrhythmias. "**Holter monitoring**" refers to the trade name of an ambulatory cardiac monitoring device with which a cardiac rhythm recording is made while the patient is involved in his or her normal activities, usually *away from the hospital*, for an extended period of time. The information recorded in the monitoring device is later transferred to a computer for analysis.

Cardiocentesis. A surgical puncture into the heart.

Cardiopulmonary bypass. A technique for diverting blood temporarily from the heart so the surgeon can operate directly on the heart or its vessels.

Cardiopulmonary resuscitation. Revival of cardiac and respiratory functions through rescue techniques, mechanical means, drugs, or electrical stimulation.

Cardioversion (defibrillation). Application of direct electrical current to the chest to correct abnormal rhythms back to normal sinus rhythms.

Coronary artery bypass grafts (CABG). Surgery to improve the blood supply to the heart by anastomoses (joining together) of other arteries to the coronary arteries. The notations "CABG $\times$ 2," "CABG $\times$ 3," "CABG $\times$ 4," "CABG $\times$ 5," and so on, refer to the number of *bypass grafts* done, not to the number of *vessels* operated on. In other words, a single coronary vessel can have more than one graft.

Doppler echocardiogram. Ultrasound study of cross valvular pressure gradients and blood flow patterns; part of the work-up for valvular disease.

Doppler flow and pressure assessments. An evaluation of peripheral vascular disease and routine blood pressure measurements. This assessment uses a Doppler flow monitor and blood pressure cuff.

Echocardiography, transesophageal echocardiography (TEE), two-dimensional echocardiography (2-D echo). Diagnostic techniques for studies of the heart's structure and activity using ultrasound.

Electrocardiography (ECG, EKG). A measurement of the electrical and conductive activity of the heart muscle (see Section C above).

Endarterectomy. Surgical removal of fatty deposits (atheromas) along the walls of arteries.

Percutaneous transluminal coronary angioplasty. A procedure using a balloon catheter to expand the lumen of a blood vessel to the heart to improve blood flow.

Scalp monitoring (internal). A method for assessing fetal heart rate patterns during labor to determine if there is fetal distress.

Stress test. A study of the heart's activity (along with blood pressure and respiratory rate) during physical exertion, such as jogging on an inclined treadmill.

Valve replacement. Surgical removal of a stenotic or incompetent valve and replacement with either a valve from a normal cadaver or a prosthetic valve.

Venipuncture (phlebotomy). Needle puncture into a vein.

Venoclysis. Intravenous drip; injecting medication or other fluids into a vein.

II. PULMONARY FUNCTIONS AND DISEASES

A. Pulmonary Terminology

Abscess (pulmonary). A localized area of necrosis and suppuration of the lung tissue.

Actinomycosis of the sinus. Fungal infection of the nasal sinus.

Acute respiratory failure (ARF). A sudden, life-threatening condition characterized by difficulty breathing and excessively low levels of oxygen and excessively high levels of carbon dioxide in the blood.

Adult respiratory distress syndrome (ARDS). A form of pulmonary edema resulting from marked, widespread damage to the alveolar-capillary membrane.

Aerophore. A device for inflating the lungs of stillborn infants.

Aerosolization. Suspending droplets of water into a gas.

Airway. The passages through which air passes in and out of the lungs.

Alveoli. Air sacs at the end of bronchioles in the lungs.

Anoxia. Lack of oxygen.

Apex (pulmonary). Top of the lung.

Aplasia (pulmonary). Lack of lung development.

Apnea. Temporary cessation of breathing.

Asphyxia. A depletion of oxygen from the blood.

Aspiration. The movement of material from one cavity to another, or in or out of a cavity, by means of suction. Secretions or other substances in the hypopharynx can be aspirated, or drawn into the lungs. Aspiration can also refer to the removal of substances out of the body by means of a vacuum suction machine.

Asthma. Bronchial airway obstruction.

Atelectasis. Collapsed, airless portion of the lung; lack of pulmonary dilation.

Atomization. Suspending and spraying large droplets into the air.

Bag-mask. Face mask for resuscitation equipment.

Base (pulmonary). Lower portion of the lung.

Bennett respirator. Trade name for a popular model of mechanical ventilation device.

Bird respirator. Trade name for a popular model of mechanical ventilation device.

Bronchi. Branches of the trachea passing into the lungs. The mainstem bronchi are the initial (left and right) branches into the lungs.

Bronchial hyperactivity. Reactive airway disease.

Bronchiectasis. Bronchial dilatation.

Bronchioles. Smallest branches of the bronchi.

Bronchitis. Inflammation of the bronchi.

Bronchogenic carcinoma. Lung cancer originating in the mainstem bronchus.

Bronchopulmonary dysplasia (BPD). A progressive lung disease seen in infants who have received high concentrations of oxygen during mechanical ventilation.

Bronchopulmonary segment. One of the divisions of the lungs. The right lung has ten divisions; the left lung has nine.

Carina. Point at which the trachea branches into the right and left bronchi.

Cheyne-Stokes respiration (CSR). Rhythmic breath cycles followed by periods of apnea lasting from 10 seconds to 1 minute before breathing resumes.

Choana. Opening of the nasal cavity into the pharynx.

Choanal atresia. A rare condition identified in infants in which there is a partial or complete obstruction of the posterior nasal cavity causing respiratory distress.

Cilia. Hairs lining the mucous membranes of the respiratory tract.

Complemental air. The amount of air that can be forcibly inspired beyond normal inspiration; also referred to as *inspiratory reserve.*

Coryza. Common cold.

Cracking. A technique used by respiration therapists and nurses which involves releasing a burst of oxygen into a tank for the purpose of clearing particles from the outlet.

Crepitus. Crackling sounds (in the lungs or joints).

Croup. Acute respiratory obstruction resulting from infection, allergy, or a foreign body in the glottis; characterized by respiratory distress, hoarseness, and a "barking" cough.

Cuff pneumometer. Gauge for measuring the pressure within an inflated tracheostomy cuff (balloon).

Cystic fibrosis. An inherited condition affecting the respiratory system as well as the pancreas and sweat glands.

Dyspnea. Difficulty with breathing.

ECMO. Extracorporeal membrane oxygenation.

Edema. Swelling, fluid retention in the tissues.

Effusion. Dispersement of fluid into a tissue.

Emphysema. A chronic progressive pulmonary disease marked by a loss in elasticity of lung tissues eventually causing the bronchioles to become obstructed with mucus. Emphysema is often related to smoking and exposure to industrial hazards.

Endolaryngeal carcinoma. Malignant epithelial cancer of the laryngeal structures.

Epiglottis. Cartilaginous covering of the trachea located at the base of the tongue, providing aspiration protection during swallowing.

Epistaxis. Nosebleed.

Eupnea. Normal or good respiration.

External respiration. Gas exchanges within the lungs.

Fremitus. A vibration, or "thrill sound"; heard during auscultation of lung sounds or felt with touch (*tactile fremitus*).

Functional residual capacity. The air left in the lung after normal expiration.

Glottis. Opening into the trachea. The *rima glottis* refers to the space between the true vocal folds.

Hemothorax. Blood in the chest cavity.

Histoplasmosis. A fungal disease sometimes associated with the formation of calcifications in the pulmonary tissues.

Humidification. Adding moisture to the air.

Hypercapnia, hypercarbia. An excess of carbon dioxide in the blood. The abnormally high carbon dioxide tension causes overstimulation of the respiratory center in the medulla.

Hyperpnea. Rapid respirations.

Hypoplasia of the epiglottis. Incomplete development of the epiglottis.

Internal respiration. Gas exchanges within the tissue cells.

Kussmaul's breathing. A respiratory pattern associated with metabolic acidosis in which there is a deep gasping breathing pattern, also called "air hunger."

Lobes (pulmonary). Referring to lung divisions. The right lung has three divisions (right upper lobe, right middle lobe, and right lower lobe). The left lung is smaller, to accommodate the heart, and has two divisions (the left upper lobe and the left lower lobe).

Mediastinum. Chest cavity between the lungs.

Mesothelioma. A malignant tumor of the serous membrane of the pleural sac.

Minimal air. Air remaining in the alveoli.

Narcosis. A reversible state of sleepiness or incomplete unconsciousness due to reduced oxygenation or anesthesia.

Nares. Nostrils. One nostril is called a "naris."

Nebulization. Transforming liquid into a fog or mist.

Orthopnea. Inability to breathe comfortably unless sitting up.

Oxyhood. A head box used to deliver oxygen to infants requiring oxygen therapy.

Paranasal sinuses. Cranial sinuses above the nasal cavity; includes the *ethmoidal sinus,* the *frontal sinus,* the *maxillary sinus,* and the *spheroid sinus.*

Parietal pleura. Outermost fold of the pleura lying close to the ribs.

Paroxysmal nocturnal dyspnea (PND). Respiratory difficulties occurring at night usually associated with heart disease.

Perichondritis. Inflammation of the perichondrium, the fibrous connective tissue surrounding the trachea.

Persistent fetal circulation (PFC), persistent pulmonary vascular obstruction of the newborn (PPVON), progressive pulmonary hypertension in the newborn. A group of related cardiopulmonary disorders in newborn infants.

Pertussis. Whooping cough.

Phthisis. (Pronounced /tɪs-ɪs/) wasting of tissue, usually referring to *pulmonary* phthisis related to **tuberculosis**. Phthisis is often preceded by an adjective, such as *renal* phthisis or *diabetic* phthisis. Lung sounds are described as *phthisic* (**tɪz**-ɪk) when there is an asthmatic condition related to lung tissue wasting.

Pleura. Double folded sac surrounding the lungs.

Pleural adhesions. Fibrosities binding the visceral pleura to the parietal pleura.

Pleural effusion. Fluid in the pleural spaces.

Pleural exudate. Serum or pus in the pleural spaces.

Pleurisy. Inflammation of the pleura.

Pleuritic pain. Intercostal pain.

Pneumonia. Inflammation with exudation of the lung tissues. *Nosocomial* (hospital acquired) pneumonias are usually caused by gram negative organisms, discussed in Section VIII, Chapter 6.

Pneumothorax. Air in the chest cavity.

Pollinosis. Hay fever.

Pulmonary edema. Fluid in the lungs.

Pulmonary interstitial emphysema (PIE). A condition that sometimes occurs in infants who have received mechanical ventilation.

Pulmonary parenchyma. Cells of the lungs.

Pyothorax. Infection with pus in the chest cavity.

Rales. Crackling or bubbling sounds heard during auscultation of the lungs.

Respiratory acidosis. A condition in which blood pH is below 7.35 due to a deficiency in respiratory ventilation most often caused by emphysema, obstructions, or pneumonia.

Respiratory alkalosis. A condition in which blood pH is above 7.45 due to an increase in respiratory ventilation most often related to anxiety hyperventilation, elevated temperature, or drug intoxication.

Retinopathy of prematurity (ROP). A complication of long-term oxygen therapy with newborns in which there is obliteration of the retinal vessels after hyperoxia.

Rhinorrhea. Drainage from the nose.

Rhinovirus. One of the viruses causing a common cold.

Septum (nasal). Partition between right and left sides of the nasal cavity.

Siderosis. Inflammation of the lungs due to inhalation of iron oxide causing chronic bronchitis and emphysema.

Silicosis. Industrial disease due to inhalation of silica dust.

Speaking trach valves. Devices which can be attached to tracheostomy tubes to permit phonation by allowing air to be directed through the glottis (see Figure 7–8 on page 255).

Status asthmaticus. Prolonged state of severe asthma.

Stridor. Sound heard when there is obstruction of the upper (laryngeal) airway.

Supplemental air. The amount of air that can be forcibly expired following normal expiration; *expiratory reserve.*

Tachypnea. Rapid breathing.

Total lung capacity (TLC). The maximal volume of air in the lungs after maximal inspiration.

Tracheoesophageal fistula (TEF). An opening between the esophagus and the trachea.

Tracheopleural fistula (TPF). An opening between the trachea and the pleura (sometimes the result of pressure necrosis from an inflated tracheostomy cuff).

Ventilator. Respirator; mechanical device providing assistance with breathing. Ventilator machines used in most hospitals are equipped with *breathing circuitry*, a heated *humidification* and sterile *water distribution system*, *oxygen* and *air sources*, *oxygen analyzer* (*oximeter*), *manual resuscitator, stethoscope, sphygmomanometer,* and *suction machine*. Ventilator controls regulate and measure *tidal volume, respiratory rate,* and the percent of *concentration of oxygen.* Audible and visible alarms are activated when respiratory parameters are outside of the control settings (due to a change in the patient's respiratory status, a problem with the machine, or during any disconnection process).

Ventilator dependent. Requiring mechanical support to breathe.

Visceral pleura. Innermost fold of pleura lying close to lung tissues.

B. Pulmonary Abbreviations

A. Alveolar (gas)

a. Arterial (gas)

ABGs. Arterial blood gases

AFB. Acid fast bacilli

ARD. Acute respiratory disease

ARDS. Adult respiratory distress syndrome

BH. Bronchial hyperactivity

BPD. Broncho-pulmonary dysplasia

BS. Breath sounds

c. Capillary

CDAP. Continuous distending airway pressure

CF. Cystic fibrosis

CNH. Central neurogenic hyperventilation

COAD. Chronic obstructive airway disease

COLD. Chronic obstructive lung disease

COPD. Chronic obstructive pulmonary disease

CPAP. Continuous positive airway pressure

CPTPD. Chest physiotherapy and postural drainage

CXR. Chest X ray

D. Dead (space gas)

E. Expired (gas)

ERV. Expiratory reserve volume

ET. Endotracheal

ETT. Endotracheal tube

F. Fractional (concentration of)

FEF. Forced expiratory flow

HBOT. Hyperbaric oxygen therapy

H & L. Heart and lungs

HMD. Hyaline membrane disease

I. Inspired (gas)

IMV. Intermittent mandatory ventilation

IPPB. Intermittent positive pressure breathing

IRDS. Infant respiratory distress syndrome

IRV. Inspiratory reserve volume

MBC. Maximal breathing capacity

MW. Minimal voluntary ventilation

OTB. Old tuberculosis

P. Pressure (in blood gases)

PAP. Pulmonary artery pressure

PEEP. Positive end expiratory pressure

PFT. Pulmonary function test

PIE. Pulmonary interstitial emphysema

PND. Post nasal drip

PPD. Purified protein derivative

ppd. Packs (of cigarettes) per day

R. Respiration

RD. Respiratory disease

RDS. Respiratory distress syndrome

RLF. Retrolental fibroplasia

SIDS. Sudden infant death syndrome

SIMV. Synchronous intermittent mandatory ventilation

SOB. Short of breath

T. Tidal (gas)

T & A. Tonsillectomy and adenoidectomy

TB. Tuberculosis

TLC. Total lung capacity

URI. Upper respiratory infection

V. Volume (of gas)

VC. Vital capacity

V/Q. Ventilation-perfusion

C. Fundamental Principles in Pulmonology

1. **Respiratory tract.** The respiratory tract begins with the nasal and oral cavities where air passes into the nasopharynx, pharynx, and hypopharynx (see Figure 7–4). The **nares**, or nostrils, of the nose open into two chambers divided by the nasal septum. Within these cavities are three passages, the **superior,**

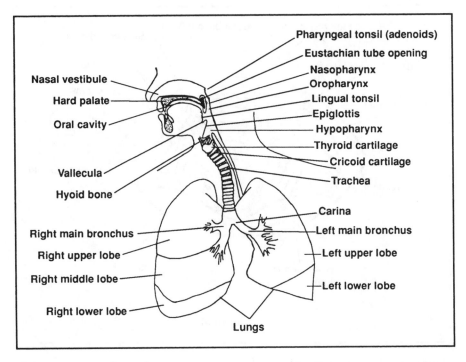

Figure 7-4. Respiratory tract

inferior, and **middle meati** which are connected to the middle ears through the eustachian tube, to the paranasal sinuses, and to the pharynx. The respiratory tract is sometimes called the *aerodigestive tract*, because oral, pharyngeal, and some laryngeal structures are shared by these systems. The **epiglottis** is a laryngeal cartilage located at the base of the tongue. It is part of the protective mechanism for venting food and liquid away from the airway toward the esophagus and preventing aspiration. The recesses on either side of the epiglottis are the **valleculae**; the recesses just lateral to the glottis are the **pyriform sinuses** (see Figure 7-5). Pooling and/or stasis of material in these recesses are recognized as indicators for risk of aspiration.

Entry into the lungs begins at the **larynx**. The elevation and rotation of the larynx and constrictive closure of the endolaryngeal musculature during swallows serve to prevent unwanted material from passing into the airway. Coughing helps to clear material from the larynx, trachea, and endolaryngeal mucosa. The

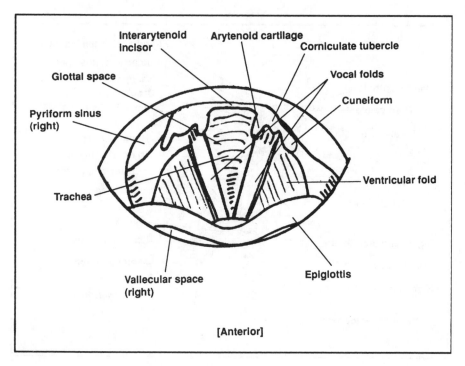

Figure 7–5. Superior view of the glottis

endolarynx has three divisions, *supraglottic* (above the vocal folds), *subglottic* (below the vocal folds), and *glottic* (at the level of the vocal folds). The **rima glottis** refers to the space between the vocal folds.

The **trachea**, attached to the larynx at the cricoid cartilage, is a flexible tube of 18 to 20 C-shaped cartilages. It is about 1 inch in diameter and 4 to 5 inches long. The trachea terminates in a bifurcation, called the **carina**, where it opens into the two **mainstem bronchi** of the lungs. The bronchi branch into progressively smaller **bronchioles** terminating in the **alveolar sacs**. The alveoli are the tiny air sacs that contain pulmonary capillaries which bring air into contact with blood, allowing for the exchange of oxygen and carbon dioxide. This exchange of gases within the lungs is referred to as **external respiration. Internal respiration** refers to the process of oxygen and carbon dioxide exchange from *tissue cells through the capillaries.*

The alveoli are supported by the lung's network of elastic tissues. The lungs are enclosed in the *visceral,* or pulmonary, *pleurae* (each lung having its own pleural sac). The right lung is larger than the left which has a medial indentation to accommodate the heart (the **cardiac depression**).

2. **Respiration.** The air inhaled during respiration contains about 21% oxygen and about one fourth of that is taken up by the lungs. Expired air contains about 16% oxygen as well as a small amount of carbon dioxide (about 5%) and moisture. Because expired air retains a fairly substantial percentage of oxygen, **rescue breathing** (in which a rescuer expires his or her own lung air into a stricken person to inflate the lungs when breathing has stopped) can provide ventilatory support during **cardiopulmonary resuscitation (CPR)**. (See Section IV.)

   Respiration is both a neuromuscular and neurometabolic phenomenon. Respiratory centers in the medulla and pons sense changes in oxygen and carbon dioxide levels in the blood and correct any imbalances by activating respiratory musculature.

3. **Respiratory centers.** Respiration is controlled by centers in the brain stem. The **medullary center** is responsible for initiation and maintenance of spontaneous respiration; the **pneumotaxic center** in the pons coordinates respiration cycles. Chemoreceptors in the brain's respiratory centers work together to monitor and correct metabolic abnormalities. Respiratory failure can be the result of a variety of extrapulmonary causes, including *respiratory muscle weakness, upper airway obstruction, efferent disruption of impulses to respiratory musculature chest wall disorders,* and *dysfunction of the respiratory centers.* Neurogenic causes of efferent disruption of impulses to the *diaphragm* via the *phrenic nerve* include *high spinal cord lesions* (C2, C3), which can diminish or abolish innervation to the diaphragm and intercostal muscles. Other neurogenic causes of disruptions in respiration include *anterior horn cell disease* (such as amyotrophic lateral sclerosis), *peripheral neuropathies* (e.g., Guillian-Barré syndrome), and *neuromuscular junction disease* (e.g., myasthenia gravis). Obstructive causes include *obesity-hypoventilation syndrome* (Pickwickian syndrome, see Chapter 3); *pleural disease: skeletal abnormalities*; and *upper airway obstructions* (paralysis, foreign body obstructions, tracheal stenosis or malacia, and obstructive apnea).

4. **Respiratory patterns.** Examination of respiratory patterns is helpful in determining the extent and location of disorders of the brain stem. Large (usually deep and bilateral) supratentorial lesions or metabolic disturbances give rise to a breathing pattern

termed *Cheyne-Stokes respiration* (CSR), in which there is a pattern of rapid respirations followed by *apnea* (cessation of breathing) lasting 10 seconds or longer. The CSR phenomenon is attributed to disruption of controls from the cerebrum to the brain stem's respiratory centers causing hyperventilation. Hyperventilation causes the carbon dioxide levels in the blood to drop, and this drop is sensed by the respiratory centers which then are stimulated to stop breathing to correct the imbalance. CSR may also be related to the effects of low levels of oxygen in arterial blood in conditions such as congestive heart failure. Lesions in the upper pontine tegmentum and lower midbrain may cause *central neurogenic hyperventilation* (CNH), in which there is an increase in both rate and depth of respiration, potentially leading to respiratory alkalosis. (See discussion of **blood gases** and **I.C.U. monitoring** in Chapter 3.)

Basilar artery occlusion causing low pontine lesions sometimes produces *apneustic breathing*, which may be called *"short cycle"* respirations (SCRs) characterized by short pauses after deep inspirations. In some cases, the patterns include intermittent quick shallow breaths; in other cases, there is an occasional omission of breaths (*respiration alternans*). Lesions in the dorsimedial region of the medulla may cause each breath to vary in rate and depth. This pattern is variously described as *Biot breathing*, "chaotic breathing," and sometimes—inappropriately—"ataxic breathing."

5. **Neurolaryngologic Factors.** The inspiratory contractions of the glottic opening, especially the posterior cricoarytenoid (PCA) muscle activity, are controlled by laryngeal innervation through the branches of the vagus nerve and are also influenced by physiologic pulmonary mechanisms. Damage to the nerves innervating the larynx will affect glottal closure (see Cranial Nerve discussions, Chapter 4). Procedures, such as the presence of a tracheostomy, can also cause glottal dysfunction. Tracheostomy can cause tube-induced abrasions and infections and their presence reduces stimulation of the PCA receptors. Patients with prolonged tracheotomies who have experienced reduced respiratory resistance to the glottis sometimes have an inadequate glottal closure initially following decanulation of the tracheostomy tube (see Kirchner, 1991, for discussion). For that reason, it may be necessary to introduce air resistance through the glottis gradually to re-establish phonation following tracheotomies (Kirchner, 1991).

D. Pulmonary Procedures and Studies (also see Chapter 5, Nutrition, Hydration, and Swallowing)

Ambu bag. One of the self-inflating breathing bags and masks used for emergency artificial ventilation of the lungs.

Antrotomy. Removal of the antral wall of the nasal cavity.

Assisted ventilation. A mechanical ventilation technique in which the initiation of each inspiration comes from the patient's own effort.

Bronchial brushing, brush biopsy. Method for establishing a diagnosis in a lung mass in which a radiopaque catheter is passed under fluoroscopic guidance into the bronchial passage where the mass is located. Minute nylon brushes then take scrapings of cells for analysis.

Bronchogram. Radiologic study of the bronchial branches using a radiopaque contrast material.

Cervicomediastinotomy. An excision in the mediastinum of the neck region to obtain a biopsy of the lymph node.

Continuous positive airway pressure (CPAP). A respiratory therapy maneuver producing positive airway pressure throughout the respiration cycle.

Cordectomy, laryngofissure. Incision made to separate the vocal folds or remove part of the vocal folds.

Decanulation. Removal of the tracheostomy tube.

Downsize. Progressively adjusting tracheostomy tubes to smaller sizes.

Extubation. Removal of an endotracheal or tracheostomy tube apparatus.

Fiberoptic bronchoscopy. An endoscopic examination of the right and left mainstem bronchi and the carina.

Fowler's positioning. Placement of the patient in a *sitting position* to facilitate breathing.

Heimlich maneuver. A technique using a brisk, posterior and upward compression of the abdomen subdiaphragmatically (above the naval) of a choking individual to expel an airway obstruction (see Figures 7–lOA 7–lOB, 7–11, and 7–12 on pages 267, 268, and 269). Techniques to expel foreign body obstructions vary depending on the age and consciousness of the stricken individual.

Hemilaryngectomy. Removal of one half of the laryngeal structures.

Incentive breathing spirometers. Devices used in respiratory therapy to prevent atelectasis and improve lung volumes.

Intermittent mandatory ventilation (IMV). Respiration therapy maneuver in which the patient breathes on his or her own with intermittent intervals of ventilator support as part of the weaning process in respiration therapy.

Intermittent positive-pressure breathing (IPPB). Administration of gases or drugs by mechanical means using pressures above atmospheric pressure to force deeper inspirations. This therapy uses commercially available machines which are portable for home use.

Intubation. Insertion of an endotracheal tube (from the oropharyngeal cavity into the trachea) or tracheostomy tube (directly into the trachea).

Laminography. Tomograms, or planigrams, taken of the lung providing a sectional study of lung tissues and the underlying and surrounding structures.

Laryngectomy. Removal of the larynx.

Lobectomy. Complete removal of a pulmonary lobe.

Lung biopsy. Removal of a small specimen of lung tissue to examine for carcinogenic, bacteriologic, or other pathologic conditions.

Lung resection. Partial removal of a portion of the lung.

Needle biopsy, percutaneous needle biopsy. Insertion of a biopsy needle into a lesion, usually through the skin, to aspirate cells to examine for cytologic, bacteriologic, and other pathologic conditions.

Oxygen delivery. Oxygen may be delivered by a mask, oxygen tent, nasal catheter, nasal cannula, or directly into a tracheostomy tube or intubation apparatus (through a T-piece, see Figure 7–9). Oxygen may be piped from a pressurized tank or directly from a wall vent.

An *oxygen flowmeter* is used to control the amount of oxygen delivered at a liter-per-minute rate. These rates are required (by the Joint Commission on Accreditation of Health Care Organizations [JCAHO]) to be converted into equivalent percentages according to the delivery method. For example, a mask delivering 6 liters of oxygen per minute will have a percent equivalent of 60% oxygen flow, whereas a nasal cannula delivering 6 liters of oxygen per minute will have a percent equivalent of 44% oxygen flow. Some masks, such as a Venturi mask, will deliver precise mixes of oxygen and room air. Since oxygen will dry mucous membranes, delivery devices will direct the oxygen gas through a bottle of sterile water which humidifies the oxygen before delivering it to the patient.

Percussion. A technique for loosening lung secretions by rhythmic gentle blows across the chest with a cupped hand.

Positive end-expiratory pressure (PEEP) therapy. A respiratory therapy maneuver used to increase the functional residual capacity of the lungs.

Postural drainage. Technique using positioning to promote gravitational drainage of secretions from areas of the lungs.

Pulmonary function studies. Laboratory studies of the respiratory functions, including lung volumes, ventilation, and oxygen consumption.

Rescue breathing. Mouth-to-mouth (or mouth-to-tracheostoma) artificial ventilation.

Respirometry. Use of a respirometer to measure exhaled tidal volume. This device may be attached to the endotracheal tube of an unconscious patient.

Rhinoplasty. Plastic surgical reconstruction of the nose.

Silverman-Anderson score. System for scoring the degree of respiratory distress.

Sinus lavage. Method for removing purulent material from the sinuses using flushing and suctioning.

Spirometry. Measurement with graphic recording of lung capacities. *Bronchospirometry* measures the relative differences between the two lungs' capacities.

Stroboscopy, videostroboscopy. Method for endoscopic (and usually videotaped) visualization of laryngeal activity using flashes of light in synchrony with the phases of vibratory cycles of the vocal folds.

Suctioning. Suctioning uses a *vacuum* (wall unit or freestanding device), *suction tip,* and *catheter* to clear secretions, primarily from the airway. Suctioning is done to remove secretions that have accumulated when the patient is unable to clear his or her own air passages. Table 7–1 describes suctioning methods.

Thoracentesis. Surgical procedure which involves introducing a tube into the thoracic cavity to remove fluid.

Thoracostomy. Excision of a rib segment to allow for drainage of an empyema (pus filled space).

Thoracotomy. An incision into the chest.

Tracheostomy. An opening into the trachea.

Tracheostomy care. Techniques for cleaning tracheostomy tubes. Usually this is done every 6 or 8 hours (see Table 7–2).

Tracheostomy tubes. Tracheostomy tubes, or "trachs," vary in dimensions and characteristics and are selected based on the ventilatory needs of the patient. Figure 7–6 illustrates the parts and features of a metal (Jackson type) tracheostomy tube. Figure 7–7 illustrates a type of plastic, cuffed, trach tube. Figure 7–8 illustrates some of the devices that can be used to permit phonation when attached to tracheostomy tubes, so-called "speaking trachs and valves." Table 7–3 provides general guidelines for speech-language pathologists training ventilator-dependent patients to use speaking trachs and valves.

Tracheostomy collar, or T-piece. Flexible tubing for humidification or oxygen delivery that may be attached to the trach tube of a tracheostomized patient; sometimes called a *Brigg's adapter* (see Figure 7–9).

Tracheotomy. An incision into the trachea.

Transantral ligation of the maxillary artery. The application of vascular clips to the maxillary artery to control severe, recurrent nosebleeds (epistaxis).

TABLE 7–1. Tracheostomy and oropharyngeal suctioning methods

Step	Procedure
1.	Determine the need for suctioning.
2.	Explain to the patient why and how suctioning will be done.
3.	Assemble the necessary equipment.
4.	Turn on the suction machine and set the pressure gauges. **Suction vacuum settings** usually are around: **80–120 mmHg** for *adults*, **80–100 mmHg** for *children*, and **60–100 mmHg** for *infants*.
5.	Place the patient in a Fowler's (sitting) or semi-Fowler's position (leaning back between 45–60°), or lying on the side if unconscious.
6.	Remove the sterile catheter without contamination.
7.	Don sterile or clean gloves.
8.	Turn on the suction machine with the nondominant hand.
9.	Test the suction in normal saline solution.
10.	Lubricate the tip with a water soluble lubricant.
11.	Introduce the suction catheter into the tracheostomy or toward the base of the pharynx; patient may want to and should be encouraged to cough.
12.	Occlude the catheter vent or one end of a Y-tubing connector with the gloved thumb to create a vacuum in the catheter lasting about 10–15 seconds.
13.	Rotate and twist the catheter as it is being withdrawn to collect additional secretions.
14.	Remove the thumb from the catheter vent when ready to release the suctioned material into a collection basin.
15.	Continue until the suctioning process is completed; remove the glove while holding the catheter, pulling the glove off inside out, and dispose of the catheter and the glove in the appropriate receptacles.
16.	Reassess status of the patient and record procedure in the medical chart.

Source: Adapted from Lewis, L. W., & Trimby, B. K. (1988). *Fundamental skills and concepts in patient care* (4th ed.). Philadelphia: J. B. Lippincott; and Persons, C. G. (1987). *Critical care procedures and protocols.* Philadelphia: J. B. Lippincott.

TABLE 7–2. Tracheostomy care

Step	Procedure
1.	Assemble equipment, including a basin of hydrogen peroxide, a basin of sterile water, and a receptacle for soiled items.
2.	Wash hands thoroughly and don sterile gloves.
3.	Remove the stoma dressing.
4.	Swab the stoma area with sterile hydrogen peroxide followed by sterile water.
5.	Unlock and remove the inner cannula and clean it thoroughly with a brush and hydrogen peroxide before placing it in sterile water.
6.	Dry the inner cannula with sterile gauze and resecure.
7.	Reapply a sterile dressing and tie the tracheostomy tube in place avoiding knots that might press on the neck.
8.	Dispose of all contaminated items.

Source: Adapted from Lewis, L. W., & Trimby, B. K. (1988). *Fundamental skills and concepts in patient care* (4th ed.). Philadelphia: J. B. Lippincott; and Persons, C. G. (1987). *Critical care procedures and protocols*. Philadelphia: J. B. Lippincott.

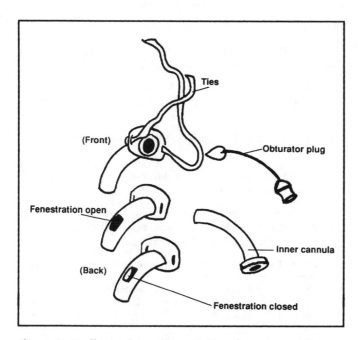

Figure 7–6. Illustration of a metal tracheostomy tube

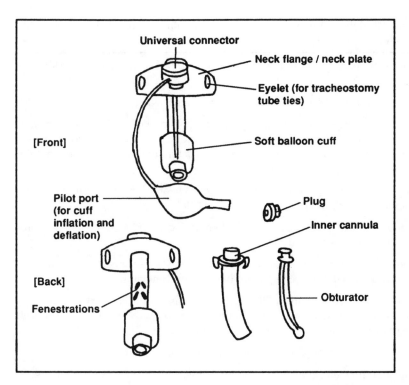

Figure 7-7. Illustration of a fenestrated, cuffed plastic tracheostomy tube

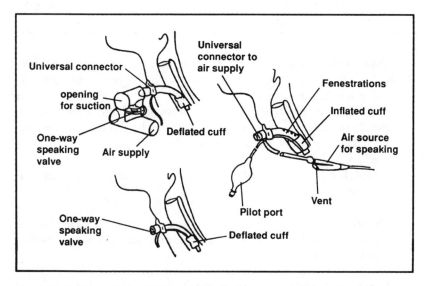

Figure 7-8. Illustration of three methods of speech with tracheostomy tubes

TABLE 7–3. Guidelines for working with the ventilator-dependent patient using speaking valves

☐ Inform the primary nurse and/or respiratory therapist (R.T.) of your session and plans.

☐ Encourage the primary nurse to observe how the speaking valve functions.

☐ Check oximeter level and take precautions to ensure that adequate oxygen saturation in the blood is maintained throughout the session (recommended level is 88% or above). it is prudent to use an oxygen saturation monitor throughout the sessions.

☐ Take a resting heart rate. If pulse increases to 20 beats above the resting rate, the patient may be in distress.

☐ *High pressure alarms* may be triggered when tubing is occluded, coughing is present, or suctioning is needed.

☐ *Low pressure alarms* may be triggered if the tubing is disconnected or if the circuitry is disconnected from the patient or from the ventilator.

☐ If the speaking valve requires deflating the cuff, as with a Passy-Muir valve, the low pressure alarm will be triggered. The respiratory or therapist or nurse will need to assist with any changes in the pressure settings.

☐ Check with the nurse and/or R.T. before deflating the trach cuff.

☐ Cuff inflation pressures are usually recommended to be 24 cm water pressure.

☐ Document your observations and the results of the session in the medical chart. Be sure to note any concerns that may affect prognosis for using the device successfully or adjustments that may improve the patient's potential for using the device without compromising ventilatory status.

Tuberculin (TB) skin tests. Tests of exposure or sensitization to tuberculosis. TB tests include the *Mantoux* (an interdermal tuberculin test using purified protein derivative [PPD]); *Tine test* (interdermal test using a four pronged device, dipped in attenuated TB, for puncturing the skin); *Heaf test* (uses multiple punctures for interdermal TB testing); and *Mono-Vacc* (screening test using multiple punctures).

Ventilatory management. Use of a machine to provide adequate ventilatory support

Vibration. Loosening lung secretions using firm, circular motions applied to the chest with open hands to produce wavelike vibrations within the chest.

Water-seal drainage management. In cases where drainage of accumulated fluids in the lungs is necessary, a water-seal drainage

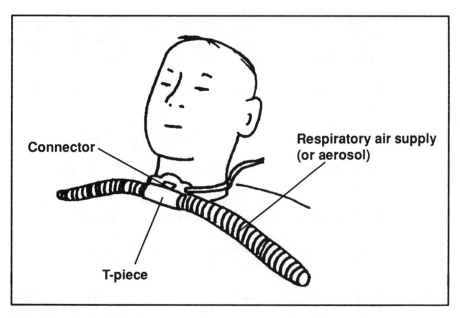

Figure 7–9. Illustration of a T-piece

system is used to ensure air is not permitted to contact the fluids being drained. Hospitals normally use a commercially available system, such as a "Pleur-evac" (Deknatel Corporation).

Weaning. Gradual elimination of mechanical support for respiration.

III. HEMATOLOGIC FUNCTIONS

A. Hematologic Terminology

ABO typing. An international system for typing the main blood groups.

Acquired immune deficiency syndrome (AIDS). A condition in which the patient's immune defenses are compromised allowing opportunistic infections. (See discussion of the Human Immunodeficiency Viruses [HIV] in Chapter 6.)

Albumin. A blood protein. The measurement of albumin levels in the blood, or **serum albumin**, aids in determining nutrition status.

Anemia. Low red blood cells.

Antibodies. Proteins synthesized by lymphoid tissue in the presence of antigens (foreign or invading substances) which destroy or inactivate the antigens that have stimulated its formation.

Anticoagulant. A substance that inhibits the formation of blood clots.

Antigens. Substances causing the formation of antibodies.

Autohemotherapy. The use of a patient's own blood for his or her treatment.

B-cells. Lymphocytes that are capable of forming antibodies.

Bilirubin. Orangish-yellow pigment derived from the hemoglobin in blood; released by the liver after red cell destruction.

Bleeding time. Time taken for a wound to form platelets and clot. Bleeding time is clinically determined by measuring the time required to stop the flow of blood following a puncture (usually done on the earlobe or forearm).

Chyle. Fats in lymph fluids that are absorbed from the small intestine.

Coagulation time. Time taken for the formation of a clot in the bloodstream.

Corpuscle. Blood cell.

Creatinemia. Excessive creatine in the blood.

Disseminated intravascular coagulation (DIC). A group of disorders with accelerated coagulation and activation of the fibrinolytic mechanisms resulting in both hemorrhages and thromboses.

Electrophoresis. Use of an electric force to separate out proteins in plasma.

Embolus. Clot, air bubble, or particle that has migrated within the circulatory system; a potential cause of blockage.

Erythrocyte. Red blood cell.

Erythrocytosis. Condition in which there is an abnormally high number of red blood cells.

Erythropoiesis. Formation of red blood cells.

Exchange transfusion. Removing and replacing blood with fresh, whole blood from a donor.

Extravasation. A condition in which fluids have escaped into surrounding tissues.

Fibrin. Threads of protein causing blood to clot.

Globulin. Plasma proteins which include *alpha, beta*, and *gamma* types.

Hematocrit. A blood test that uses a centrifuge to separate solids from plasma.

Hematoma. A mass of blood.

Heme. Iron-containing portion of the hemoglobulin molecule.

Hemochromatosis. A blood disease in which there is a buildup of iron in the skin tissues and damage to the liver, pancreas, and heart due to a lack of iron metabolism.

Hemoglobin. The iron-containing portion of red blood cells.

Hemolysis. Red blood cell destruction.

Hemophilia. A sex-linked, inherited blood disease in which there is a tendency to bleed due to a prolonged coagulation time. Individuals with **hemophilia A** have a deficiency in blood factor VIII; individuals with **hemophilia B** have a deficiency in factor IX.

Hemorrhage. Gushing, excessive flow of blood.

Hemostasis. Stopping the flow of blood. In surgery, hemostats are instruments used to stop blood flow.

Hypercapnia. Elevated levels in the pressure of arterial carbon dioxide ($PaCO_2$). A respiratory acid-base imbalance can develop, referred to as *acidosis*.

Hyperglycemia. Excessive amounts of glucose in the blood.

Hyperlipidemia. Excessive amounts of lipids (fats) in the blood.

Immunoglobulin (Ig). Blood proteins that act as antibodies (IgA, IgD, IgE, IgG, and IgM). Increases or decreases in Ig indicate disease.

Leukemia. A blood condition which may be malignant, acute, or chronic, characterized by an overproduction of white blood cells (leukocytes).

Leukocytopenia. A lack or diminished number of white blood cells.

Lymph. Clear liquid made up of water, salts, sugar, metabolic waste (such as urea and creatinine), lymphocytes, monocytes, platelets, and erythrocytes, circulating in lymphatic vessels.

Lymph node. Collection of lymph tissue.

Lymphadenopathy. Enlarged or inflamed lymph glands.

Lymphedema. Accumulation of lymph due to poor tissue drainage, most often the result of surgery or radiation.

Mononucleosis. A higher than normal number of mononuclear white blood cells in the blood.

Multiple myeloma. Malignant tumors of the bone marrow.

Neutropenia. A decreased number of neutrophilic white blood cells.

Packed cells. Blood component therapy in which most of the plasma has been removed; used after marked blood loss.

Pernicious anemia. A blood disease characterized by a reduction in red blood cells, reflecting a deficient absorption of vitamin B_{12}.

Phagocytes, histocytes. Cells that engulf and remove bacteria.

Plasma. The fluid part of the blood. **Serum** is the fluid that separates from a blood clot.

Plasmapheresis. A technique performed by circulating the blood extracorporeally through a centrifuge to separate the plasma; used as a therapy for Guillian-Barré syndrome.

Pneumocystis pneumonia, *Pneumocystis carinii* **pneumonia (PCP).** A form of pneumonia prevalent among individuals with severe immunodeficiencies, especially patients with HIV, caused by a protozoan infection.

Polycythemia, polycythemia rubra vera. A condition in which there is a greater than normal number of red blood cells.

Septicemia. Bacteria in the blood.

Seroculture. Bacterial blood culture.

Sickle-cell anemia. An inherited blood disease found predominantly in individuals with African heritage, characterized by hemolysis and sickle-shaped erythrocytes.

Sideropenia. Lack of iron in the blood.

Spleen. Organ involved in blood cell production, storage, and elimination.

Splenomegaly. Enlarged spleen.

T-cells. Lymphocytes produced by the thymus gland; infection-fighting cells important to the body's immune defense system.

Thalassemia. An inherited, anemic condition occurring primarily in individuals with Mediterranean or Southeast Asian heritage.

Thrombocyte. Blood platelet, or clotting cell.

Thrombotic thrombocytopenic purpura (TTP). A group of clinical syndromes characterized by thrombocytopenia, hemolytic anemia, fever, renal dysfunction, and fluctuating neurologic abnormalities.

Thrombus. A blood clot formed around plaque deposits along blood vessel walls; a thrombo-embolic clot refers to a thrombus particle that has dislodged (become an embolus) and moved into the blood stream. (Further discussion can be found in Chapter 9.)

Thymoma. Tumor of the thymus gland.

Thymus. One of a pair of endocrine glands, located just above the kidneys, important to fetal and early childhood growth, and a part of the lymphoid system; manufactures T-cells.

Tonsils. Lymphoid tissues located in the pharynx that aid in the formation of white blood cells. The tonsils include the *palatine* tonsils, *nasopharyngeal* (adenoidal) tonsils, and *lingual* tonsils.

Universal donor. Person with type O negative blood, the blood type having no agglutinogens to other blood types.

Universal recipient. Person with AB positive blood.

B. Hematologic Abbreviations

AABB. American Association of Blood Banks

Ab. Antibody

ACD. Acid-citrate-dextrose

ADO. Blood groups

Ag. Antigen

AHF. Antihemophilic factor VIII

AHG. Antihemophilic globulin (factor) VIII

AIDS. Acquired immune deficiency syndrome

AIHA. Autoimmune hemolytic anemia

ALL. Acute lymphoblastic leukemia

BAC. Blood alcohol concentration

Basos. Basophils

CBC. Complete blood count

CLL. Chronic lymphocytic leukemia

CML. Chronic myelocytic leukemia

diff. Differential (count)

EBV. Epstein-Barr virus

ELISA. Enzyme-Linked Immunosorbent Assay

ESR. Erythrocyte sedimentation rate

FDP. Fibrin-fibrinogen degradation products

FR. Fibrin-fibrinogen related

FSP. Fibrin-fibrinogen split products

HAI. Hemagglutination-inhibition immunoassay

HCT, Hct, crit. Hematocrit

Hgb. Hemoglobin

HIV-1, HIV-2. Human immunodeficiency viruses

Ig. Immunoglobulin

ITP. Idiopathic thrombocytopenia

Lymphs. Lymphocytes

PA. Pernicious anemia

MCH. Mean corpuscular hemoglobin

MCHC. Mean corpuscular hemoglobin count

MCV. Mean corpuscular volume

monos. Monocytes

PCP. *Pneumocystis carnii* pneumonia

Polys, PMN. Polymorphonuclear (leukocytes)

PT. Prothrombin time

PTT. Partial thromboplastin time

RBC. Red blood cell (count)

Rh. Rhesus (factor)

RIA. Radioimmunoassay

SCA. Sickle cell anemia

Segs. Segmented(s) (mature red blood cells)

WBC. White blood cell (count)

C. Fundamental Principles in Hematology

1. **Blood and lymph formation.** Blood and lymph circulation occurs through separate but interconnected vascular systems. The average person's blood volume is approximately 6 liters. Blood is made up of 40% "formed elements" and 60% plasma. The formed elements are the blood's cells, including *erythocytes* (red blood cells formed in the red bone marrow); *thrombocytes* (also called platelets); and *leukocytes*, which include *granulocytes* (neutrophils, basophils, and esophils), *monocytes*, and *lymphocytes*. Lymph contains two types of leukocytes, lymphocytes, and monocytes. Blood cells carry oxygen, hormones, and nutrients to body tissues.

   Lymph transports proteins that have seeped out of the blood circulation (capillaries) back into the veins. Lymph absorbs fat from the small intestine and carries it to the bloodstream. The lymph system also provides the body's immune responses and responses to pathogens. The following section describes some of the studies of immune mechanisms as well as blood counts and blood cell morphology. Such studies are key indicators of infectious processes, cardiopulmonary status, and oncologic and hematologic diseases.

D. Hematologic Procedures and Studies

Also see the list of Commonly Ordered Laboratory Studies, Chapter 3.

1. **Antinuclear antibodies (ANA) test.** Blood test for antibodies present in autoimmune diseases.

2. **Aspirin therapy, ASA therapy.** A prophylactic anticoagulation therapy to diminish risk factors for stroke and heart attack.

3. **Blood gases.** Measurements of blood to examine for indicators of deficiencies in tissue perfusion and lung function. Blood gas

measurements include the **pressure**, or tension, of **carbon dioxide** (*PaCO$_2$ for arterial measurements and PvCO$_2$ for venous measures*), **blood acidity** (pH), and **pressures of oxygen** (PaO$_2$ and PvO$_2$).

4. **Blood typing.** Blood test to determine Rh factor (Rh– or Rh+) and blood type (A, B, AB, and O).

5. **Bone marrow aspiration, bone marrow biopsy.** Removal of cells from the bone marrow to diagnose blood-related diseases or for donor purposes.

6. **Complete blood count (CBC).** A blood analysis that includes a *white blood cell count* (WBC); *red blood cell count* (RBC); *hemoglobin* (Hg, Hbg); *hematocrit* (HCT, Hct, Crit., Hemocrit.); *mean corpuscular hemoglobin* (MCH); *mean corpuscular hemoglobin count* (MCHC); *mean corpuscular volume* (MCV); and the *red cell distribution.*

7. **Coumarin derivative therapy.** The use of an anticoagulant drug to act as an antagonist to the coagulating properties of vitamin K.

8. **(Erythrocyte) sedimentation rate (ESR), "sed rate".** A blood test measuring the depth to which red blood cells settle in a vertical tube following a specified time delay. Increased "sed rates" indicate pathologic conditions, such as infectious processes, inflammation, myocardial infarction, endocarditis, and neoplasm.

9. **Heparin therapy.** The use of an anticoagulant drug to inhibit platelet aggregation as a prophylactic treatment to prevent clotting.

10. **Immunoglobulin (Ig) analysis.** Serologic test to examine for the presence of immunoglobulin.

11. **Partial thromboplastin time (PTT).** A test of the time required for clotting in plasma; helps to determine heparin levels and to diagnose clotting disorders.

12. **Red blood cell (RBC) count and morphology.** Measurement of the number of *erythrocytes* present in the blood and identification of any abnormalities in cell characteristics (shape and maturity); useful in diagnosing liver diseases, anemias, and other hematologic conditions.

13. **White blood cell (WBC) count and morphology.** Measurement of the number of *leukocytes* in the blood and their cell characteristics (shape and maturity); useful in diagnosing blood diseases, such as leukemias and anemias, and other conditions such as infections.

IV CARDIOPULMONARY RESUSCITATION (CPR)

A. Life Support Training

1. **Completion of CPR Training.** *Basic life support* (BLS) training involves learning the techniques of **cardiopulmonary resuscitation (CPR)** for *emergency cardiac care* (ECC). The purpose of this training is to prevent circulatory or respiratory arrest and subsequent damage to the central nervous system. Basic life support training and *Advanced Cardiac Life Support* (ACLS) training are obtained through programs conducted and/or sanctioned by the American Heart Association. These classes involve lectures, readings, and hands-on practice in **foreign body airway management** and **cardiopulmonary resuscitation** of infants, children, and adults. Minimum performance criteria and knowledge are required for "successful completion" of the AHA-approved course by an AHA-affiliate certified instructor. Completing an AHA-approved BLS training program does not indicate that an individual is "licensed" or "certified" in CPR. Furthermore, biannual reviews and updates are required for any person who has completed a CPR course.

2. **Codes.** Most health care facilities have emergency paging procedures, or *codes*, that are known by all staff and will elicit a swift response in an emergency. For example, "code 9" or "code 99" may refer to a cardio-respiratory emergency; "code blue" may refer to a respiratory emergency, "code red" may refer to a fire emergency, and so forth. Patients who have required emergency cardiopulmonary management may be said to have been "coded."

Clinicians should be familiar with how to initiate a "Cardiac Code" or a "Respiratory Code" in the facility(ies) where they work. Any clinician who works with patients with cardiac disease in a location or setting that is remote from staff trained in CPR emergency management should complete basic life support training to be prepared to respond to a cardiopulmonary emergency. In some settings, speech-language pathologists are required by the privileging guidelines or hospital policies to have this training.

3. **Cardiac arrest, respiratory arrest, and airway obstruction.**
   When sudden "cardiac death," or cardiac arrest, has occurred, respiration will cease; and after 4 minutes of **hypoxia** irreversible
   damage to the brain begins. Exceptions to this can be found in
   cases of near-drownings or other conditions in which hypoxia
   occurs in association with extreme cold (when metabolic rate is
   slowed). When the heart has ceased to beat and no ventilation is
   apparent, **clinical death** has occurred. This state is potentially
   reversible. **Biological death**, however, will occur *unless oxygen
   perfusion is initiated immediately.* Consequently, even though the
   probability of needing to use CPR rescue efforts might be small,
   clinicians should be prepared for the possibility. Similarly, familiarity with the *subdiaphragmatic abdominal thrust,* or the so-
   called "Heimlich maneuver," is important for health care personnel and lay persons alike; and it is an especially important safety
   technique when working with patients at risk for foreign body
   aspiration (see Figures 7–10A and 7–10B, 7–11, and 7–12).

4. **ABCs of CPR.** The sequence of emergency measures used during CPR is based on three basic skills: *Airway, Breathing, and
   Circulation*, referred to as the ABCs of CPR. Sometimes CPR is
   described as an ABC and **D** procedure, in which "D" refers to
   Definitive therapy, meaning direct cardiac care management.

   Before initiating CPR, the rescuer **first determines if the strick-
   en individual is *responsive* and *conscious*.** Next he or she *will*
   call for help, if possible, to obtain *Emergency Medical Service.*
   If it has been determined that the person is *not breathing*, the rescuer will **position the head so that the tongue and epiglottis
   are not obstructing the airway**. This may require tilting the
   head and pulling the jaw forward, or pulling the jaw up and forward with a "**jaw thrust**" maneuver. If the individual has not
   resumed breathing after the airway is cleared, the rescuer begins
   rescue breathing (see definition above). Rescue breathing can
   require mouth-to-mouth, mouth-to-nose (with the mouth closed),
   or mouth-to-stoma (with laryngectomees) ventilation. These
   techniques need to be learned from a trained instructor, because
   inadequate or excessive rescue ventilation can be problematic.

   Following airway clearance and initiation of rescue breathing,
   the rescuer **determines the need for assistance with circulation**. Following two rescue ventilations, the resuscitator will feel
   for *pulselessness* by palpating for the carotid pulse. If no pulse is
   palpable, chest compressions will be initiated. Chest compres-

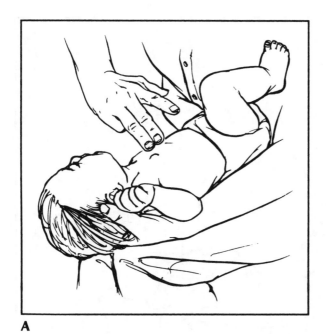

A

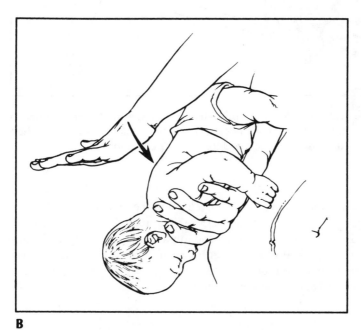

B

Figure 7-10. Illustrations of chest compression and foreign body airway management techniques for infants (From *Healthcare provider's manual for basic life support*, copyright © 1988, American Heart Association, reproduced with permission)

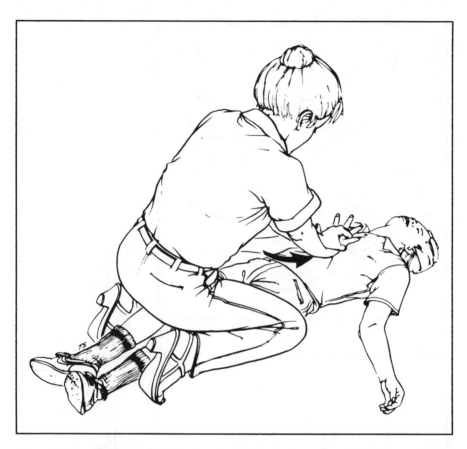

Figure 7–11. Illustration of foreign body airway management with an uncon-scious person (From *Healthcare provider's manual for basic life support*, copyright © 1988, American Heart Association, reproduced with permission)

sion and rescue ventilation cycles will then continue until emergency medical personnel arrive. The techniques used in CPR need to be well-understood and implemented correctly, and without delay. **Training is essential** to a positive outcome because knowledge, confidence, and immediacy in implementing each step can determine survivability.

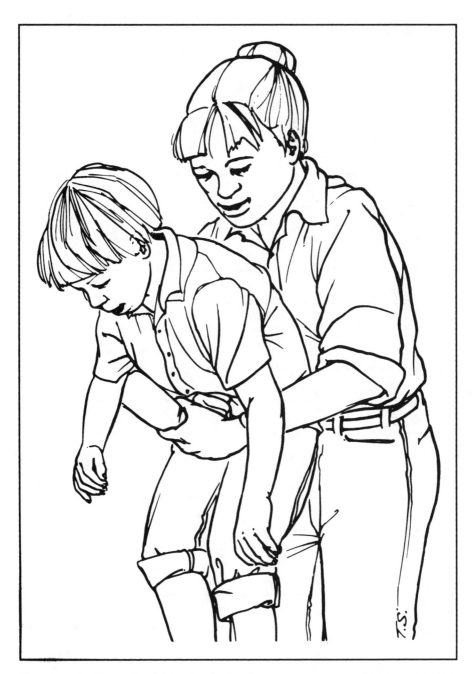

Figure 7–12. Illustration of foreign body airway management with the "Heimlich maneuver" (From *Healthcare provider's manual for basic life support,* copyright © 1988, American Heart Association , reproduced with permission)

V. NOTES

VI. REFERENCES

Albarran-Sotelo, R., Flint, L. S., & Kelly, K. J. (1988). *Healthcare provider's manual for basic life support.* Dallas, TX: American Heart Association.

Ayres, S. M., Schlichtig, R., & Sterling, M. J. (1988). *Care of the critically ill* (3rd ed.). Chicago: Yearbook Medical Publishers.

Bleile, K. M. (1993), *The care of children with long-term tracheostomies.* San Diego: Singular Publishing Group, Inc.

Budassi, S. A., & Barber, J. M. (1981). *Emergency nursing: Principles and practice.* St. Louis: C. V. Mosby.

Fein, I. A., & Strasberg, M. A. (1987). *Managing the critical care unit.* Rockville, MD: Aspen.

Hirano, M., Kirchner, J. A., & Bless, D. M. (Eds). (1987). *Neurology: Recent Advances.* San Diego: Singular Publishing Group, Inc.

Kirchner, J. A. (1987). The larynx-lung relationships. In M. Hirano, J. A. Kirchner, & D. M. Bless (Eds.), *Neurology* (pp. 160–166). San Diego: Singular Publishing Group, Inc.

Lewis, L. W., & Trimby, B. K. (1988). *Fundamental skills and concepts in patient care* (4th ed.). Philadelphia: J. B. Lippincott.

Persons, C. G. (1987). *Critical care procedures and protocols.* Philadelphia: J. B. Lippincott.

Tobin, M. J. (1989). *Essentials of critical care medicine.* New York: Churchill Livingstone.

CHAPTER

8

Imaging Studies and Radiologic Oncology

Speech-language pathologists are often involved in radiologic studies that evaluate oro-pharyngeal, laryngeal, and esophageal structures and their function. They are also interested in the results of neuroradiologic studies. This chapter reviews terminology encountered in radiologic studies and various diagnostic imaging (radiologic) procedures and therapies encountered in medical speech-pathology practice. Conditions frequently diagnosed by radiologic studies are also found in Chapters 5, 9, and 10.

I. TERMINOLOGY

Abdominal decubitus (position). Position in which patients are examined lying flat.

Acute abdominal series (AAS). Includes KUB and X rays for acute (sudden) abdominal disorders.

Adhesions. Abnormal fibrous bands between structures.

Adynamic. Not moving.

Aerated. Filled with air.

Aerophagia. Swallowing excessive amounts of air.

Air-barium double contrast (ABDC), air contrast barium enema (ACBE). Techniques used when examining the gastrointestinal tract which involve giving the patient both barium and effervescent (gas producing) crystals to swallow or by enema allowing for better examination of the mucosa than is possible with barium alone.

Air-space disease. Lung disease involving the alveolar sacs.

Alopecia. Hair loss.

Alpha ray. Least penetrating form of radiation; positively charged particles of helium.

Analog. In PET scanning, a radiopharmaceutical agent that is biochemically equivalent to a natural body compound.

Anechoic. Structures that fail to respond to internal echoes in sonography.

Anger camera. Instrument used for recording the distribution of gamma-emitting radioactivity, named for its inventor, Hal Anger.

Angiocardiogram. An x-ray study using radiopaque contrast medium to examine the heart and its vascularities as well as its great vessels.

Angiogram. An x-ray study using bolus radiopaque contrast medium to examine blood vessels. Various rapid series studies are used for cardiac, pulmonary and cerebral angiography. *Digital subtraction angiography* (DSA) uses a minimal contrast load.

Aortogram. An x-ray study using radiopaque contrast medium to examine the aorta.

Aplasia of the lung. Incomplete development of the lung.

Aplastic anemia. A type of anemia caused by bone marrow destruction resulting from chemotherapy or radiation therapy effects.

Arteriogram. An x-ray study using radiopaque contrast media to study arteries.

Arthrogram. An x-ray study using radiopaque contrast media to study joints.

Artifact. An artificially produced image, as in "movement artifact."

Ascites. An accumulation of fluid into the abdominal (peritoneal) spaces.

Atelectasis. Collapsed, airless portion of the lung.

Barium swallow, esophagram. Fluoroscopic study used to examine the swallowing mechanism, esophagus, and esophageal peristalsis. (Also see Chapter 5, Section II.)

Barrett's esophagus, Barrett's metaplasia. A condition characterized by metaplastic epithelium occurring in the lower esophagus following peptic ulcer disease.

Basilar skull fracture. Fracture at the base of the cranium.

Beta rays. Radiation capable of penetrating body tissues for a few millimeters.

Betatron. A machine used to deliver high energy radiation for *megavoltage* radiation therapy.

Bezoar. Hair mass or a collection of foreign bodies in the gastrointestinal tract.

Blowout fracture. Fracture of the floor of the orbit with possible entrapment of the orbital contents; hemorrhage into the maxillary sinuses is usually present.

Bone Scan. Used for metastatic work-up of bony structures.

Brachytherapy. Radiation therapy where a source of radiation is inserted near the area of the body being treated.

Bronchogram. An x-ray study using radiopaque contrast medium for examination of the bronchi.

Bucky grid. A grid placed between the x-ray machine and the patient to absorb ambient radiation and to reduce blurs on the film.

C-spine. X-ray study of all seven cervical vertebrae for trauma, neck pain, and neurologic disorders involving the upper spine.

Calcification. Deposits of calcium salts in tissues.

Calculus. Abnormal accumulation of mineral salts usually forming a stone-like body.

Carrier. Nonradioactive element or compound with the same chemical properties as a radioactive molecule.

Cassette. The covering of x-ray film providing protection from light exposure and containing a grid to enable the use of a lesser amount of radiation to obtain a desired result.

Cavitary lesions. Lung cavities seen with abscesses, cancer, and tuberculosis.

Cesium-137. Radionuclide used to study vaginal cancer.

Cholangiogram. An x-ray study using contrast medium to examine the bile ducts.

Cholecystogram. An x-ray study using contrast medium to examine the gall bladder and its contents (i.e., gall stones).

Cineradiography. Radiologic studies using motion picture film for recording; this term may be applied to videotape recording.

Cisternogram. An x-ray study of the base of the brain.

CM line, OM line. Canthomeatal, or orbitomeatal, line defined by an imaginary line from the lateral canthus of the eye to the meatus of the ear.

Cobalt-60. Radionuclide used in radiation therapy.

Coin lesion. Circular-shaped pulmonary lesions seen with granulomas and some carcinomas.

Collimator. The device in an x-ray machine that restricts diffusion of x-ray beams and focuses the beam at a desired area on a crystal detector.

Communicating hydrocephalus. A condition where there is increased cerebrospinal fluid in the brain despite the existence of a normal egress between the CSF and ventricles; communicating hydrocephalus is due to a problem with the resorption of CSF. (See Chapter 9 for additional discussion of hydrocephalus.)

Consolidation (pulmonary). Solidification of the lung, as found with pneumonia.

Contra coup. Referring to an injury to the brain occurring on the side opposite to the traumatic blow.

Contrast medium. Compounds, usually having iodinated organic molecules, that are injected or imbibed for the purpose of obtaining better delineation of structures during x-ray.

Curie. A unit of radioactivity.

Cyclotron. A machine capable of producing megavoltage external radiation by creating accelerated, charged particles electromagnetically.

Decubitus. Lying down.

Degenerative joint disease (DJD). Osteoarthritis.

Density. Compactness.

Depressed skull fracture. Fracture of the cranial bones with depressed fragments of bone.

Diaphanogram. Infrared photographic examination.

Diffuse esophageal spasm. An esophageal contraction that occurs in response to thermal stimulants (hot or cold) and/or gastroesophageal reflux.

Digital subtraction. The use of a computer to subtract x-ray images instantaneously from low doses of contrast medium within a vessel.

Discrete. Well-defined.

Disseminated idiopathic skeletal hyperostosis (DISH). Extensive anterior hypertrophic spurs of the cervicothoracic spine.

Dosimetrist. Technical specialist in calculating radiation dosage.

Dry CT. A computed tomogram taken without contrast medium.

Dysmotility. An impairment in the normal peristaltic activity of the esophagus or intestines.

Echoencephalogram. An ultrasound study of the brain used to examine for tumors and other masses.

Electrokymogram. An x-ray study of the dynamic movements of the heart or other organs.

Enhanced CT. A computed tomogram taken after introduction of a contrast agent.

Epiphysis. The articulated end of bone where growth has occurred.

Extrinsic masses. Growths that are outside of the bowel but exert pressure on the gastrointestinal tract.

Fibrosis. Where normal tissue has been replaced with fibrous tissue.

Film. A light-sensitive, thin cellulose sheet used for recording x-ray images.

Film badge. A badge containing a strip of material sensitive to ionizing radiation used to detect exposure to beta and gamma radiation.

Fluoroscopy. An x-ray study using a fluorescent surface to view the shadows of structures of the body after they are exposed to an x-ray beam.

Fractionation. Administration of radiation therapy in measured doses over a period of time to diminish radiation effects on normal tissues.

Gamma rays. Electromagnetic waves emitted from the atoms of radioactive elements. Gamma rays may be used in diagnostic scanning or radioactive implant therapies.

Gastraview, Gastragrafin study. Referring to the trade names for contrast agents used most often in radiologic studies prior to abdominal surgery when barium residues are not desired.

Gray units. Preferred units for quantifying radiation dosage. One unit of gray (Gy) equals 100 rads, thus 1 cGy = 1 rad.

Half-life. The time required for half of the radioactivity in a radioactive substance to disintegrate.

Hiatus hernia; hiatal hernia. Protrusion of the wall of the stomach through the hiatus (esophageal opening) of the diaphragm.

Hilum. The triangular depression on the medial surface of the lung which contains the hilar lymph nodes and through which blood and lymph vessels, nerves, and bronchi pass (left should be 2–3 cms higher than right).

Infiltrates. Radiodensities in the lungs indicating permeation of substances into the lung spaces.

Inflammatory joint disease (IJD). Referring to rheumatoid arthritis, gout, and pseudo-gout.

Interstitial pulmonary disease. Pulmonary disease of the tissues between the air (alveolar) spaces.

Intrathecal, thecal space. Within a sheath; usually pertaining to the space within the covering of the brain or spinal cord.

Intravenous pyelogram. An x-ray study using an injected contrast agent excreted from the bladder for examination of the urinary tract.

Intrinsic mucosal mass. Benign or malignant growths within the mucosa.

Intrinsic nonmucosal mass. Mural, or wall, tumors; benign or malignant growths covered by normal mucosa.

Ionization. Separating stable molecules into their charged particles, called ions.

Ionmeter. A device used to measure radiaton.

Iridium-192. A radionuclide used in internal radiation therapy.

Irradiation treatment. Therapeutic use of radiation beams and radionuclides.

Kilovolt. One thousand volts.

Kilowatt. One thousand watts.

Kyphosis, cervicothoracic kyphoscoliosis. Humpback; an abnormal anterior convexity of the cervicothoracic spine.

Linear accelerator. A device capable of generating megavoltage radiation dosage.

Linear skull fracture. Fracture line across the skull.

Luxury perfusion. Increased blood flow around the margins of a brain lesion.

Lymphangiogram. An x-ray study using a contrast medium to examine the lymph glands and lymphatic ducts.

Magnetic resonance imaging (MRI). An imaging technique that uses magnetic movements of atomic nuclei to delineate tissues. Radiowaves are directed toward a body area contained in an external magnetic field. When the radiowaves are turned off, the hydrogen nuclei emit microwaves and weak radiowaves which are detected and interpreted by a computer to construct transsectional images (tomograms) (See Chapter 4 and Section III, G of this chapter for further discussion of MRIs.)

Mammogram. An x-ray or xeroradiographic study of the breast tissue for early detection of tumors.

Megavolt. One million volts.

Myelitis. Inflammation of the bone marrow.

Noncontrast computed tomogram (nc CT). Computed tomogram taken without a contrast agent; dry CT.

Oblique. Positioning at approximately a 45° lateral angle from the x-ray beam.

Obstruction hydrocephalus. A condition where there is an excessive accumulation of cerebrospinal fluid (CSF) in the brain due to a blockage of the egress of CSF from the ventricular system, usually due to stenosis or obstruction of the Sylvian aqueduct.

Orthovoltage. Low to medium voltage energy used in radiation therapy (140–450 kV) as palliative treatment for cancer.

Osteoma. Tumor arising from bone tissue.

Osteomalacia. Softening of bone tissue due to calcium depletion associated with pain, tenderness, and muscle weakness; usually the result of a vitamin D deficiency.

Osteopenia. Lack of bone tissue.

Osteoporosis. Abnormal demineralization of bone tissue.

Panorex. Trademarked name for a radiologic procedure using two axis of rotation to obtain a panoramic radiograph of the dentition and dental arches.

Portable chest film. Use of a portable x-ray machine to examine a patient unable to be transported to the radiology suite.

Positron emission tomography (PET) and single proton emission computed tomography (SPECT). Two types of emission computed tomography that permit imaging of metabolic activity from measurements of radioactivity within body sections.

Radiodermatitis. Skin inflammation due to radiation exposure.

Radiolucent. Structures or substances that permit the passage of radiation beams (appearing dark on an x-ray film).

Radionecrosis. Tissue death caused by radiation exposure.

Radiopaque. Structures or substances that restrict the passage of radiation beams (appearing light on an x-ray film).

Rarefaction. Decreased density.

Reticular infiltrates. Interstitial lung infiltrate pattern.

Roentgen. The international term for a unit of exposure to x-ray doses. This eponym refers to Wilhelm Roentgen, the German physicist who discovered X rays.

Scan. General term for methods of visualizing organs, structures, and transverse body sections obtained through computed tomography, ultrasonography, scintigraphy, and other forms of diagnostic imaging.

Scintilligraphy. Studies that involve producing two-dimensional images from the scintillations emitted by radionuclide material administered internally.

Scintiscan. Radionuclide study used to detect scintillations produced when a radioactive substance is introduced into the body. In dysphagia evaluation, scintiscans are used to examine gastric reflux, esophageal motility, and aspiration.

Scoliosis. Curvature of the spine.

Sella, sella turcica. A shallow depression in the sphenoid bone at the base of the brain.

Shield. In radiology, a protective structure or garment containing lead used to prevent the passage of radiation.

Sialogram. An x-ray study of the salivary ducts and the secreting portion of the gland feeding the duct.

Spondylitis. An inflammation of the vertebrae.

Sternal wires. Surgical staples closing a suture in the sternum which are left in place following chest surgeries.

Tertiary waves, tertiary peristalsis. A condition usually found in the elderly in which there are multiple regions of dilation and narrowing of the esophagus during swallow; also called *corkscrew esophagus* and *presbyesophagus.*

Thermography. Recording of heat patterns within body structures; used to detect breast cancer and other inflammatory conditions.

Thyroid scan. Technetium 99 scan to evaluate thyroid function.

"Tics." In radiology, referring to diver*ti*cula.

Tomography. Diagnostic radiographic studies in which images of single planes across tissues are produced in a series at different depths of an organ or area of the body.

Ultrasonography. Diagnostic studies using high-frequency sound waves that are projected and detected as they strike tissues of varying densities. These data are analyzed by a computer to create a series of images of the structure.

Valsalva maneuver. Procedure for increasing oral, pharyngeal, and nasal cavity pressures by holding the nose and mouth closed during forced exhalation against a closed glottis.

Venogram. An x-ray study of the veins, using a radionuclide contrast agent.

Wedge angle. In Doppler flow ultrasonography, the scanner is usually held at a "wedge" angle, rather than perpendicular, to the vessel being studied.

Xenon-127. Radioactive gas inhaled in ventilation x-ray studies of the lungs.

Xeroradiography. Dry radiologic techniques in which the x-ray image is made on a powdered surface and transferred photographically to specially treated paper.

II. ABBREVIATIONS USED IN RADIOLOGIC STUDIES AND THERAPIES

AAS. Acute abdominal series

Abd. CT. Abdominal computed tomogram

AM. Auditory meatus

AP. Anteroposterior

AU-198. Radioactive gold

AXR. Abdominal x-ray

Ba. Barium

B/K. Bladder/kidney (scan)

CAT, CT. Computed or computerized axial tomogram/tomography, computed or computerized tomogram/tomography

C CT. Contrast computed tomography

cGy. Centi-grays

Ci. Curie; mCi millicurie; μCi, microcurie; nCi, nanocurie; pCi, picacurie

CM. Costal margin, canthomeatal (line)

CPB. Competitive protein binding

C-spine. Cervical spine (study)

CT. Computed tomogram

CXR. Chest x-ray

EMI. Electronic Musical Instruments (British company which built the first computed tomographic scanner, then called an "EMI scanner")

ERCP. Endoscopic retrograde cholangiopancreatogram

ERT. External radiation therapy

ESR. Electron spin resonance.

G. Glabella.

GA-167. Gallium-167; radioactive gallium (used in whole body scanning studies

I-131. Iodine-131; radioactive iodine (used in liver, kidney, and thyroid studies)

IC. Iliac crest

IRT. Internal radiation therapy

IVC. Intravenous cholangiogram

IVP. Intravenous pyelogram

KUB. Kidney, urethra, bladder (study)

kV. Kilovolt

kW. Kilowatt

LCBF. Local cerebral blood flow

LL. Left lateral

MAMA. Trademark name of a videofluoroscopic positioning chair used with children under 60 pounds

MFG. Manofluorogram

MRI. Magnetic resonance imaging

MUGA. Multigated acquisition (heart scan)

nc CT. Noncontrast computed tomogram

NMR. Nuclear magnetic resonance

OCG. Oral cholecystogram

OM. Orbitomeatal (line)

P-32. Phosphorus-32; radioactive phosphorus (used for palliative treatment of hematologic disorders)

PA. Posterior-anterior

PET. Positron emission tomogram

PTHC. Percutaneous trans-hepatic cholangiogram

Ra. Radium

Rads. Radiation absorbed doses

rCBF. Regional cerebral blood flow

RISA. Radioiodinated human serum albumin

RL. Right lateral

ROI. Region of interest

RPG. Retrograde pyelogram

SBFT. Small bowel follow through

SN. Sternal notch

SP. Symphysis pubis

SPECT. Single photon emission computed tomogram

TBI. Thyroxine binding index

TC. Thyroid cartilage

Tc-99m. Technetium-99m; radioactive technetium (used in tracer studies of the brain, skull, lungs, spleen, liver, thyroid, and bony structures)

TEE. Transesophageal echocardiogram

TRF. Thyrotropin releasing factor

TRH. Thyrotropin releasing hormone

TSH. Thyroid stimulating hormone

2-D echo. Two-dimensional echocardiogram

U. Umbilicus

UGI. Upper GI

VCUG. Voiding cystourethrogram

V/Q. Ventilation-perfusion (lung) scan

XP. Xiphoid process

III. FUNDAMENTAL CONCEPTS

A. Contrast Agents and Barium Sulfate

It is sometimes desirable to change the radiodensity of the tissues being examined by injecting drugs containing iodine, called **contrast media**, or *contrast agents*. *Barium sulfate* is also introduced to delineate hollow structures better. Other non-barium contrast agents, such as "Gastraview" or "Gastragrafin" may be used to examine for fistulae prior to abdominal surgery. The latter agents are used when barium residues are not wanted.

During special studies, such as **cerebral angiography**, a water-soluble radioactive contrast agent is introduced percutaneously through catheterization of the femoral artery up to the major brachiocephalic arteries of the brain to enhance blood vessels prior to radiography. Sometimes the contrast agent is injected directly into the internal carotid arteries.

Some patients have an adverse response to contrast media. These allergic reactions include feeling hot, having a metallic taste in the mouth, developing hives, angina, bronchospasm, and nausea and vomiting. In severe cases, irreversible shock results in death.

B. Plain (Still) Film Studies (Radiographs)

Plain film studies are used for a variety of purposes, including examination of nasogastric feeding tube placement; for screening purposes in chest, cardiac, abdominal, gastrointestinal, renal, and skeletal examination; and in lymphangiography, cisternography, venography, sialography, and vascular studies, including cerebral angiography. Radiography uses x-ray produced images recorded on film. X-ray photons directed toward body structures will be either absorbed or deflected as they pass through the electrons of the structures in their path. A radiographic image is a reflection of the electron density differences within the tissues the X ray has encountered in its path. The factors that affect electron density are the thickness of the structure and its physical state (gas, liquid, or solid).

C. Fluoroscopic Studies

Fluoroscopy permits immediate and continuous viewing of the x-ray image by using a phosphor screen. The resulting image is then magnified and transferred to a monitor for viewing and, in some cases, video-recorded for review. Rapid series radiographs are sometimes taken during fluoroscopy to provide a permanent record, or "still film." *Videofluoroscopy* refers to recording the fluoroscopic study on videotape. Videofluoroscopy of barium swallows (e.g., *modified barium swallow*) and air contrast studies (described earlier) are used to evaluate swallowing ability and esophageal and LGI motility. Cinefluoroscopy (motion picture filmed recordings) can be used in a manner similar to videotaping and has some advantages because it provides a frame-by-frame analysis with images superior to videotape.

Manofluoroscopy is a technique that combines computerized manometry (see description of manometry in Chapter 5) and fluoroscopy to measure intrapharyngeal and esophageal pressure differences as they relate to bolus flow. Fluoroscopy studies are often used to evaluate cardiac motion, structural and dynamic features of the gastrointestinal tract and pulmonary abnormalities, and to identify optimal positioning for radiography (still films).

D. Angiography

To obtain an x-ray image of blood vessels, a drug containing iodine is injected into the vessel either directly by needle or by a catheter passed percutaneously through the femoral or axillary arteries. Angiography is used for arterial, venous, and lymphatic circulation studies.

E. Pneumoencephalography

The pneumoencephalograph (PEG) is occasionally used to delineate the cisterns and the ventricular system. The PEG is especially useful for the evaluation of the posterior fossa, suprasellar, and third ventricular tumors.

F. Tomography

Tomography is a technique that permits imaging of a section or layer of the body. A **computed** (or computerized) **tomogram** (CT) is an image produced by a computer after processing x-ray data fed from detectors. To perform the scan, an x-ray tube is rotated in a complete circle allowing X rays to pass through the patient at overlapping, multiple intervals. The x-ray detectors provide data on these multiple measurements of a body section to the computer which then calculates the radiodensities of the structures and creates a corresponding image.

The radiodensities ascribed to a *volume* of tissue in the body are called **voxels**, for *volume el*ements. A voxel is the smallest unit of tissue volume that can be imaged by a CT scan. A **pixel**, for *pic*ture *el*ement is the smallest unit of surface the computer can display. Since the thickness of the voxel is usually larger than the size of the pixel, the CT's reconstructed image will lack the precise detail found in MRIs.

CT images are made in transverse (axial) sections of about 1 to 10 mm (see Figure 8–1 for an illustration of brain CT scans). After the CT image data are stored in the computer, radiodensities can be selectively adjusted, or exaggerated, to provide a larger "viewing window." Adjusting the "viewing lever" and "viewing width" controls allows the desired tissues to be visualized better. The introduction of rapid intravenous infusion of iodinated contrast media also assists in examination of intracranial structures. CTs are taken **without contrast** ("dry") followed by **with contrast** ("enhanced") scans. Due to the disruption of the blood-brain barrier, a mechanism that normally prevents certain substances from passing from the

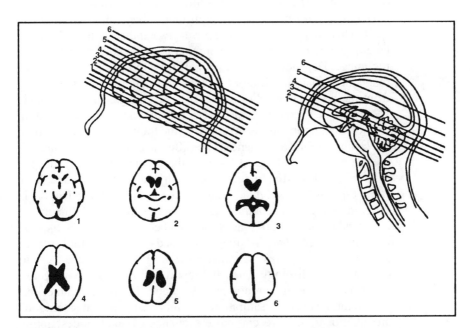

Figure 8–1. Illustration of brain CT scan sections (Adapted from Naeser, M. A., & Hayward, A. 1978. Lesion localization in aphasia with cranial computed tomography and the Boston Diagnostic Aphasia Exam. *Neurology, 28,* 545–551.)

blood into brain tissue, the contrast medium will be "taken up" in areas where pathologic processes exist. These areas will be shown to be "enhanced" (appear lighter) on the CT scan. "Enhancing" lesions are usually vascular and "nonenhancing" lesions are avascular.

G. Magnetic Resonance Imaging

The *magnetic resonance image* (MRI), or *functional magnetic resonance imaging* (fMRI) (see Chapter 4, page 157–158) provides detailed images of the brain and spinal cord and is particularly useful in the evaluation of posterior fossa abnormalities and demyelinating diseases. MRI does not use X rays and can provide higher resolution images than CT scans; however, CT scans are considerably less expensive studies than MRIs and are usually sufficient for diagnostic purposes.

The MRI is based on principles of *magnetism* and *electromagnetic radiation*. To produce a magnetic resonance image, hydrogen atoms in the water substrate of the body are exposed to a strong magnetic field which aligns the atoms. Radio frequency electromagnetic waves are then introduced. These sound waves disrupt the alignment of the atoms. After the waves are turned off, the atoms release electromagnetic energy as they realign themselves with the magnetic field. This energy, termed *"magnetic resonance"* is then detected, localized, and measured by a computer to reconstruct a corresponding image. Depending on the methods used to sequence the electromagnetic radiation, different images and patterns will be elicited from the body's magnetic resonance. The changes in the magnetic vectors of the nuclei are measured as **T-1** (the longitudinal relaxation time of changes in the z axis) and **T-2** (the transverse relaxation time for changes in the x, y plane). The differences between T-1 and T-2 measurements are the data used by the computer to construct the MRI image. The MRI image photograph and report will state the T weightings as "T-1 weighted images" (the image is dependent on T1 differences for visual contrast) or "T-2 weighted images" (the image is dependent on T-2 differences for visual contrast). In *T1 images the ventricles appear dark*. T-1 images are used to delineate **anatomy**. In *T-2 images the ventricles appear white*. T-2 images are used to demonstrate **pathology**. The MRI report will also specify the *pulse sequence*. The most common pulse sequence is termed "spin echo." "Inversion recovery," "saturation recovery," and "partial saturation" are additional, more recent, pulse sequences. Usually a description of the computation values will be designated on the MRI "hard copy" (photographic image) or in the radiologist's report (e.g., "T-1-weighted, repetition time 500–600 ms; echo time 20–30 ms").

The usual positions for MRI scans are *transverse, saggital, oblique*, and *coronal*. The saggital plane is frequently used to examine for posterior fossa and spinal cord abnormalities (refer to Figure 4–8, page 158). Although dental fillings and prostheses are not considered a problem during MRI, vascular clips, pacemakers, and cochlear implants are contraindicated, as the magnetism will cause them to displace. Biochemical *spectral analysis* is also possible from MRI data.

H. Sonography

The sonogram uses high-frequency sound waves promulgated through a body structure and reflected back to a crystal transducer. Sound waves will be stopped by either air or bone (anechoic); thus, sonography is best suited for soft tissue studies. Systems for ultrasonography include *real time scanners, phased-arrayed systems,* or *linear array systems*. Different methods for recording images include **A mode** (creates a linear graph), **B mode** (creates a two-dimensional image), and **M mode** (demonstrates the motion of a structure of the body, such as the motion of a heart valve). In *echocardiography*, the image is usually recorded in the **M** mode. Two-dimensional echocardiography (**2-D echo**) is a study in the motion mode in which a wedge or sector of cardiac activity can be viewed.

I. Tracer and Emission Imaging

Diagnostic imaging uses *radiotracers* (Technetium-99m, Iodine-131, Xenon-133, Thallium-201, and Gallium-167) to image or treat diseases. These radioactive drugs can be used to mimic nonradioactive drug activity or to examine metabolic activity (as in thyroid studies). For example, Xenon-133 gas distributes in the lungs in a manner similar to nitrogen and, thus, permits imaging of respiratory functions in pulmonary ventilation and perfusion scans. Tracer imaging provides metabolic, physiologic, and anatomic information.

Most of the radionuclides used in tracer imaging are gamma ray emitters. Images are detected by a *rectilinear scanner* or a *gamma camera*, also called an Anger camera after Hal Anger, the inventor. Positron emitters are also used for imaging, as with **positron emission tomography (PET)** and **single proton emission computed tomography (SPECT)**. After positrons interact with the electrons in their path, measurements can be made of the radioactive decomposition. These data are analyzed by a computer which then generates an image. When images are formed by external detection of radiation emitted from an internally administered radioactive compound, the study will be called an **emission scan. Emission computer**

tomography (ECT) is the study of a *slice* across a variety of planes (transaxial, coronal, or saggital).

The radionuclides used in tracer scans and tomograms mimic metabolic activity. Thus, tracer scanning and emission tomography can allow the neuroradiologist to look directly at cerebral glucose metabolism (how rapidly glucose is used by neural cells). This is the principle underlying PET scanning. This technique uses radioactive *Fluorine*, F-18, attached to an altered glucose molecule (*deoxyglucose*) which is injected into a vein. The radioactive *fluorine* emits a positive electron, or positron, which combines with a negative electron to produce gamma rays. These rays are then read by radiation detectors to construct dynamic (changeable) tomograms of the brain. Similarly, **regional cerebral blood flow (rCBF)** and **local cerebral blood flow** (LCBF) studies use the radioactive gas Xenon-133 injected into the carotid artery allowing for gamma radiation detection from the brain's surface. PET, SPECT, and rCBF studies are particularly useful in research examining neuronal metabolic activity under various stimulus conditions and in the clinical evaluation of cerebral dysfunction. Abnormalities in blood flow and brain metabolism can be revealed in brains appearing structurally intact by CT scanning. (See Chapter 4, Section V. C for additional discussion and a review of functional MRIs.

IV. RADIATION ONCOLOGY

A. Methods

Radiologic Oncology refers to the treatment of cancerous or other undesirable tissues with alpha, beta, gamma, or X rays while attempting to preserve *healthy tissues.* **Internal radiation** methods can include either sealed (implantation of sealed containers near the tumor) or *unsealed* (intravenous administration of radionuclides) techniques. Sealed-type radiotherapy, termed *brachytherapy*, uses radioactive rods, pellets, or beads or interstitial needles, sutures, or wires. Unsealed types of *infusion therapies* use intravenous or intracavitary infusion of radioactive Phosphorous-32. Intravenous injections are absorbed by bone marrow and are effective agents in the treatment of leukemia and polycythemia. Intracavitary methods are not absorbed by bone marrow. Oral ingestion of Iodine-131 is used to treat hyperthyroidism.

External radiation, or *teletherapy*, administers doses calculated by the size, site, and depth of the lesion for maximal destruction of malignant cells. To accomplish external radiotherapy a Cobalt 60 teletherapy unit, 2 MeV Van de Graaf generator, or a *low megavolt-age linear accelerator* will be used.

The radiotherapy treatment regimen for cancer will vary by site and tissue type. Radiotherapy for glottic carcinoma, for example, generally ranges from 6000 to 7000 rads with dosage calculated in *fractions* over 6½ weeks. Preferred dosages are determined depending on the size, location, and type (histopathology) of the tumor. The field of radiation can be altered with techniques such as **wedge filters** and **rotations**. The site of maximal radiation is precisely determined, and *isodose curves* are computed based on the dosage, size of the *portal* (width of the beam), and treatment technique used. For example, wedges are used to enhance radiation to a particular area and to eliminate "cold spots," areas receiving insufficient doses of radiation.

Radiation therapy is often an **adjuvant therapy** used prior to or after surgery and/or chemotherapy (refer to Chapter 11).

B. Problems and Side Effects

To achieve a therapeutic, cumulative dose of radiation, unwanted side effects sometimes result. These can include **induration** (hardening) of the radiated soft tissues, **anorexia** (loss of appetite), **alopecia** (loss of hair), **necrosis** (death) of the bone, **diarrhea, vomiting, erythema** (reddening), **stomatitis** (irritation of the mouth), **xerostomia** (dry mouth), **mucositis** (irritation of the mucous membranes), and **malaise** (generally feeling weak and ill).

Radiation to the laryngeal area can, although rarely, cause *radiochondronecrosis* when the dosage has exceeded 7000 rads. Transient edema of the arytenoids occasionally occurs following laryngeal radiation, and subcutaneous fibrosis with telangiectasis (dilatation of a group of capillaries) may occur.

Radiation treatment for brain tumors will be affected by the "radio resistance" of neoplastic (tumor) cells. *In vitro* studies of hypoxic cells have shown them to be less sensitive to radiation than normally oxygenated cells. To overcome the hypoxic condition, biologically enhanced doses of radiation have been applied to treat brain tumors, such as malignant astrocytomas. Enhancement methods have included the use of **hyperbaric oxygen chambers, whole body hyperthermia**, and **bromodeoxyuridine**.

V. NOTES

VI. REFERENCES

Freeman, M. (Ed). (1988). *An introduction to clinical imaging*. New York: Churchill Livingston.

Jones, B., & Downs, M. W. (1991). *Normal and abnormal swallowing: Imaging in diagnosis and therapy*. New York: Springer-Verlag.

Juhl, J. H., & Crummy, A. B. (1987). *Paul and Juhl's essentials of radiologic imaging* (5th ed.). Philadelphia: J. B. Lippincott.

Kirkwood, J. R. (1995). *Essentials of neuroimaging* (2nd ed.). New York: Churchill-Livingston.

Naeser, M. A, & Hayward, R. W. (1978). Lesion localization in aphasia with cranial computed tomography and the Boston Diagnostic Aphasia Exam. *Neurology, 28,* 545–551.

Plausic, B. M., Robinson, A. E., & Jeffrey, R. B., Jr. (1992). *Gastrointestinal radiology: A concise text*. New York: McGraw Hill.

Rice, D. H., & Spiro, R. H. (1989). *Current concepts in head and neck cancer.* New York: The American Cancer Society.

Shapshay, S. M., & Ossoff, R. H. (Eds.). (1985). Squamous cell cancer of the head and neck. *The Otolaryngologic Clinics of North America* (Vol. 18). Philadelphia: W. B. Saunders.

Squire, L. F., & Novelline, R. A. (1988). *The fundamentals of radiology* (4th ed.). Cambridge, MA: Harvard University Press.

CHAPTER

9

Neurologic and Psychiatric Disorders

Speech-language pathologists who work in medical settings need to consider how a patient's *physical* state (disease, surgery, medication, neurologic status, etc.) and *emotional* state might affect communication and swallowing. In this chapter, specific attention is given to neurologic and psychiatric conditions. Neurologic conditions can have a direct impact on processes of primary concern to speech-language pathologists. Psychiatric conditions may be revealed, in part, by the patient's verbal statements, and psychiatric status can cloud diagnostic workup or complicate communication therapies.

This chapter provides a brief descriptive outline of various neurologic and psychiatric disorders and diseases. As in previous chapters, the goal of this review is to provide basic descriptions and explanations; thus, it includes both diseases (e.g., cerebrovascular diseases) and conditions associated with those diseases (e.g., hemiparesis). It is beyond the scope or intent of this chapter to describe the etiology, pathology, clinical features, or treatment of each of the disorders listed. Related terminology, abbreviations, descriptions of procedures, and the features of the mental status and neurologic examinations are found in Chapter 4. Infectious diseases that cause neurologic damage are discussed in Chapter 6, and some of the conditions likely to require intensive care are described in Chapter 10.

I. NEUROLOGIC DISORDERS

A. Mobility Disorders

In this section, disorders affecting mobility are listed under the broad headings *paralysis* and *paresis* and *extrapyramidal disorders*. Disorders causing paralysis and paresis include lesions in the motor cortex, pyramidal tract (cortico-spinal tract), cortico-bulbar tract, and bulbar and spinal motor nuclei. **Paralysis** refers to an absence of voluntary motor functions, and **paresis** refers to the partial existence of voluntary motor functions.

Extrapyramidal disorders primarily include lesions and disorders involving the *subcortical gray structures*, or *basal ganglia*, and the *cerebellum*. Cerebellar disorders include lesions within the cerebellum itself and lesions involving cerebellar relay nuclei in the brain stem (midbrain, pons, and medulla). The cerebellum coordinates skilled movements and controls muscle tone, posture, and gait. Mobility disturbances associated with peripheral neuropathies, including neuromuscular diseases, are discussed later in this chapter.

1. Paralysis and paresis

Flaccidity. Lower motor neuron paralysis results from destruction of the anterior horn cells and their axons, causing flaccidity. When muscle tone during passive movement and in response to *myotactic*, or stretch, reflexes is lacking, muscles are said to be flaccid, or *hypotonic*.

Hemiplegia. Paralysis of one side of the body. The location of a lesion producing hemiplegia may be anywhere along the cortico-spinal tract, and the level of lesion is determined by the neurologic examination (see Chapter 4).

Monoparesis or monoplegia. Weakness or paralysis, respectively, of one limb.

Paraparesis or paraplegia. Weakness or paralysis, respectively, of both legs, usually following spinal cord injuries or diseases.

Quadriparesis or tetraparesis, quadriplegia or tetraplegia. Weakness or paralysis, respectively, of all four extremities.

Spasticity. Spasticity is associated with upper motor neuron lesions and is characterized by a state of heightened stretch reflexes and muscular tone. Spasticity is more discrete following spinal cord lesions than lesions higher up the cortico-spinal tract. Following an **acute lesion** there is usually an initial flaccidity and areflexia (*spinal shock*) which evolves to hypertonicity and exaggerated reflexes for muscles innervated below the level of injury. Flaccidity followed by hypertonicity and exaggerated reflexes may also be seen *acutely* after cortical strokes.

Spasticity results from the interruption of descending inhibitory innervation and the reticulo-spinal and vestibulo-spinal influences. The *"clasp knife"* phenomenon illustrates the effects of these combined influences. A clasp knife reaction is seen when a hemiplegic limb is passively extended in a brisk manner eliciting an abrupt catch followed by a degree of release allowing further extension.

It is important to consider that upper motor neuron paralysis is *not absolute paralysis*, as is the case with LMN destruction, and that upper motor paralysis *involves muscle groups* rather than individual muscles. Occasionally, hemiplegia with UMN lesions will be described as *flaccid* with no discernible EMG activity, except in response to reflex testing. After UMN lesions there may be occasional involuntary activation of the "paralyzed" muscle, called *synkinesis*, occurring when the patient coughs, yawns, or moves the contralateral limb.

2. Extrapyramidal disorders

Akathisia. Referring to the *motor unrest*, such as that observed in patients receiving neuroleptic drugs, in which there is restlessness and a compulsion to move about.

Asterixis. A disorder observed with hepatic encephalopathy and other metabolic and toxic conditions in which rhythmic, flexion movements of the hands are seen when the arms and hands are extended and dorsiflexed; "liver flap."

Ataxias. Cerebellar ataxia is characterized by a wide-based gait with irregular steps, swaying of the trunk, and unsteadiness. **Sensory ataxia** indicates a disturbance in joint position sense. This disturbance can result from *bilateral, parietal lobe* *lesions; posterior column damage* in the spinal cord, or *damage to the afferent fibers or posterior roots* of peripheral nerves. During the neurologic examination, a "positive Rhomberg" sign may be reported (swaying and falling with the eyes closed but not with the eyes open). **Friedreich's ataxia** is an autosomal recessive trait associated with spinocerebellar degeneration. **Olivopontine cerebellar degeneration** (OPCD) is characterized by ataxia and dysmetria due to degeneration of the pontine cerebellar relay nuclei and inferior olives.

Ballism, ballismus. Ballism refers to a condition associated with an abrupt onset of flinging motions of the extremities. *Hemiballism* involves only *one side of the body; monoballism* involves only *one limb*. This condition seems to result from a lesion in the subthalamic nucleus and/or its connections.

Blepharospasm. A persistent tonic spasm occurring around the eyes during which the patient maybe unable to keep his or her eyes open. The spasm may be limited to the muscles of the eyelids or may involve other facial musculature. Treatment can involve nerve sectioning or injection of a neurotoxin, such as botulinum toxin.

Cerebellar incoordination, intention tremor, and hypotonia. A complex of movement disorders associated with lesions to the cerebellar hemispheres or the middle and inferior cerebellar peduncles and brachium conjunctivum. Cerebellar signs are ipsilateral to the lesion, except for very rare lesions of the contralateral red nucleus (decussation of the superior cerebellar peduncle).

Choreas. Choreiform movements are abrupt, irregular, writhing movements of short duration. Various forms of chorea have been identified in association with basal ganglia lesions and degeneration. **Huntington's disease** (*Huntington's chorea*) is a hereditary, autosomal dominant disease characterized by a progressive onset of restlessness, choreiform movements, and dementia. Neurochemical deficiencies in Huntington's disease lead to atrophy of the caudate nucleus. **Rheumatic**, or *Sydenham's* **chorea** has been associated with group A streptococcal infections. With this type of chorea, dysarthria has an explosive quality, due to the sudden contractions of respiratory muscles.

Senile chorea is one of the movement disorders described with basal ganglia degeneration in the elderly and in patients with known Alzheimer's disease. Patients with *hemichorea* exhibit unilateral choreiform movements. This condition has been seen following a unilateral, small vascular lesion (stroke) to the posterior ventrolateral nucleus of the thalamus.

Choreoathetosis, *or paroxysmal, kinesiogenic choreoathetosis,* is a condition that begins in childhood and is characterized by sudden attacks of choreoathetoid movements, occurring frequently and without warning. These bizarre contortions may be a variant of a seizure disorder, since they are diminished with anticonvulsant therapies.

Dyskinesias. Dyskinesias include a group of movement disorders of varying etiologies. **Involuntary dyskinesia** is associated with phenothiazine (tranquilizer) therapy. Patients who have long-term neuroleptic therapies may develop *dystonias of the face and mouth, parkinsonian rigidity and tremors, tardive dyskinesia and dystonia,* and *akathisia.* **Tardive dyskinesia** is a syndrome characterized by involuntary movements of the mouth, lips, and tongue and, in most cases, dystonic postures of the neck, trunk, and upper extremities. The repetitive movements of the mouth usually include lipsmacking or sucking motions. A condition termed *rabbit syndrome* has been associated with long-term neuroleptic use. This condition is diagnosed by eliciting fine, rhythmic contractions of the upper lip when the examiner taps his or her finger just above the patient's upper lip. Another complication of neuroleptic therapy is **malignant neuroleptic syndrome**, in which severe *rigidity*, high fever, and autonomic dysfunction result from high doses of neuroleptics.

Dystonia musculorum deformans, or torsion spasm. A dystonia involving limb and axial musculature on one or both sides of the body. This condition can be progressive, but in some cases, spontaneous remission occurs. Juvenile onset of this disorder has been described, and there may be hereditary factors in some cases. Lesions of the caudate nucleus, putamen, and globus pallidus have been associated with torsion spasms.

Gilles de la Tourette syndrome. A syndrome associated with multiple tics, compulsive snorting, barking, sniffing, and involuntary repetitive movements and verbal behavior, sometimes including **palilalia** (compulsive repetitions of the same words or phrases) and **coprolalia** (compulsive expressions of obscenities and scatologies). Haloperidol can be an effective therapy.

Hepatolenticular degeneration, Wilson's disease. Wilson's disease is an autosomal recessive condition associated with accumulations of copper in tissues and present in the urine, often occurring with an associated liver failure. Copper deposits in the basal ganglia damage the globus pallidus, thalamus, subthalamic nucleus, red nucleus, and claustrum. This disease presents with either choreiform or dystonic movements and behavioral disturbances. These patients are dysarthric and dysphasic and may become aphonic.

Meige syndrome, Breughel's syndrome, focal cranial dystonia, oro-lingual-facial-mandibular dystonia. These terms refer to dystonia syndromes involving the lingual and oromandibular musculature. These **action dystonias** (dystonia elicited by the initiation of movement and not present at rest) may occur in one or more muscle groups and there may be an associated *blepharospasm* (involuntary eye blinks) and *writer's cramp*.

Nothnagel syndrome. A brainstem syndrome associated with a tumor in the tectum, affecting the superior cerebellar peduncles, and associated with a gaze paralysis and cerebellar ataxia.

Palatal and facial myoclonus. A type of rhythmic myoclonus seen with lesions of the contralateral dentate nucleus or superior cerebellar peduncle, or the ipsilateral inferior olivary nucleus, and central segmental tract.

Parkinson's disease and parkinsonism. *Parkinson's disease* is a syndrome characterized by resting tremors, bradykinesia, and rigidity occurring in association with impaired or reduced activity of the neurotransmitter dopamine. Neuropathologic studies at autopsy of patients with Parkinson's disease have found multiple areas of neuronal loss in the cortex, basal ganglia, and thalamus, and a notable focal neuronal loss in the substantia nigra. *Parkinsonian signs* may be found in association with infarctions in the basal ganglia, **arteriosclerotic parkinsonism**. Other types of parkinsonism include **drug-induced parkinsonism** (resulting from the use of phenothiazine or butyrophenone); **toxic parkinsonism** (resulting from environmental toxins and gases); **post encephalitic parkinsonism** or **encephalitis lethargica** (possibly the result of a "slow virus" following viral encephalitis); **parkinsonism secondary to infectious disease** (symptoms co-occurring with conditions such as viral encephalitis and treated tuberculosis); and **parkinsonism in association with other degenerative neurologic diseases** (such as olivopontinecerebellar degeneration, Alzheimer's disease, Creutzfeldt-Jakob disease, Wilson's disease, and Huntington's disease).

Spasmodic laryngeal dystonia, spasmodic dysphonia. A dystonia limited to the laryngeal muscles, causing adductor or abductor spasms, and treated by sectioning or disrupting the recurrent laryngeal nerve, injection of a neurotoxin, such as botulinum toxin, and/or voice therapy.

Spasmodic torticollis. A dystonia limited to the shoulder and neck muscles treated by sectioning the spinal accessory nerve or by a neurotoxin (e.g., botulinum) injection.

Tremors. In general, tremors are regular, rhythmic movements of a body part. **Parkinsonian tremors**, or resting tremors, are localized tremors of one or both hands and, infrequently, involve the jaw, lips, or tongue. Parkinsonian hand tremors are rhythmic flexion-extension motions with "pill rolling" adduction-abduction motions of the thumb. During voluntary movements, such as reaching for a cup, the tremor is absent or diminished. Conversely, **intention tremors**, **ataxic tremors**, or **rubral tremors** are not obvious at rest but occur during performance of fine, skilled actions. **Action tremors** resemble the tremors characteristic of intense fear or anxiety. Such tremors are seen with hyperthyroidism, alcohol or drug abuse withdrawal, and toxic conditions. Most action tremors are rapid and rhythmic; however, **kinetic tremors** are a coarser type of action tremor usually involving the hands, voice, or head. This coarser type of action tremor is sometimes described in association with *demyelinative polyneuropathy.*

Other action tremors include **essential tremors**, or benign *familial tremors*, which appear in adulthood and usually are limited to the upper extremities or head. Head tremors are characterized by nodding or side-to-side movements. **Orthostatic tremor** refers to an essential tremor limited to the legs.

Writer's cramp. A type of focal dystonia occurring during fine motor activity, particularly writing, characterized by a cramping dystonia of the hand.

B. Seizure Disorders

Individuals who have more than a single seizure during their lifetime will usually be diagnosed to have *epilepsy*, or a **seizure disorder.** When a seizure, or convulsion, occurs, it is proper to state the patient is "seizing," not "seizuring." Seizures are abnormal, electrical discharges emanating from *living cells* in an area of the cortex. Diagnosis of the type of seizure disorder is made based on the time of onset, extent of loss of consciousness, and the characteristic motor pattern during the seizure. Seizures may occur with rare types of *hereditary diseases* and *inborn errors* of metabolism, such as Sturge-Weber syndrome, trisomy D, tuberous sclerosis, leukodystrophies, lipidoses, aminoacidurias, phenylketonuria, maple syrup urine disease, and glucagon storage diseases.

Prenatal and neonatal seizure disorders may be found in association with *teratogenic agents* (environmental agents damaging the developing fetus). Infections such as cytomegalovirus, rubella, toxoplasmosis, and syphilis and exposure to substances such as alcohol or trimethadione are teratogens associated with neonatal seizures.

Atonic seizures. A form of generalized seizure characterized by a sudden onset of akinesis, "rag doll" muscle tone, with no loss of consciousness and rapid recovery.

Complex partial (partial complex) seizures. See Partial Seizures, Chapter 4, page 127.

Febrile convulsion. A grand mal, *tonic-clonic* type seizure occurring in association with a fever, usually related to a viral illness.

Grand mal seizure. A generalized tonic-clonic seizure characterized by an initial loss of consciousness followed by rigidity (tonic phase), rhythmic jerking (clonic phase), sweating, and incontinence. Grand mal seizures usually are not life-threatening unless they are prolonged. Grand mal seizures lasting 20 to 30 minutes require emergency medical assistance, as they are potentially life-threatening (see *status epilepticus*, Chapter 10, page 350).

Infantile spasm. A type of seizure disorder most often associated with the early stages of inherited diseases affecting the nervous system. The spasm involves a series of sudden, "jack-knifing" contractions. This type of seizure disorder usually progresses to a grand mal type in association with progressive mental retardation when widespread nervous system damage has occurred.

Landau-Kleffner syndrome. A syndrome characterized by an acquired aphasia and bilateral temporal lobe epilepsy in childhood.

Lennox-Gastaut seizures. A form of *absence* seizures associated with motoric characteristics which may be varied (tonic-clonic, tonic-only, or myoclonic).). This type of seizure is seen in young children and is often associated with mental retardation syndromes and cerebral palsy.

Petit mal, or absence [æb-sɑns] **seizures.** Condition in which the affected individual momentarily loses consciousness and appears to be staring into space, often without the loss of muscle tone or any tonic-clonic jerks.

C. Dysthymic Disorders

In psychiatry, the term *dysthymic disorder* generally refers to **depression**; in metabolism, a disorder in thymus secretion. Specific depression syndromes are discussed later in this chapter.

D. Syncope and Sleep Disorders

This section reviews several disorders related to alertness, disorders associated with sleep, and disorders occurring when the patient is reclining or attempting to sleep. Disorders affecting mental status are discussed in Section L of this chapter and in Chapter 4.

Acroparesthesia. An unpleasant prickling or burning sensation present upon awakening or after lying or sitting in one position for a prolonged period.

Bruxism. Referring to teeth grinding, especially during sleep.

Cardiac syncope. Referring to syncope of cardiac origin, including *Stokes-Adam type* cardiac syncope, dysfunction of the sinus node (*"sick sinus syndrome"*), syncope related to dysrythmias and myocardial infarction, and the cardioinhibitory syncope due to irritation of the vagus nerve (termed "**vagovagal" faints**).

Cataplexy. A sudden loss of muscle tone with temporary paralysis, often found in association with *narcolepsy*.

Insomnia. A chronic inability to sleep. The term *primary insomnia* is used to describe conditions where sleep is chronically disturbed despite a lack of medical or psychiatric problems. An inability to sleep due to conditions such as pain, anxiety, depression, or pharmacologic agents is called *secondary insomnia.*

Micturation syncope. Lightheadedness or loss of consciousness following urination, seen mainly in the elderly.

Narcolepsy. A condition characterized by sudden attacks of irresistible sleepiness. Patients with narcolepsy may also have episodes of depressed consciousness while awake, during which they engage in automatic behaviors, and will have no memory of the episodes.

Pickwickian syndrome. A condition characterized by obesity, somnolence, hypoventilation, tachycardia, and erythrocytosis; the syndrome name comes from the fat boy in Dickens' *Pickwick Papers.*

Primary autonomic insufficiency. Syncope related to degenerative diseases involving the brain stem autonomic structures or the peripheral autonomic nervous system.

Sleep apnea. A prolonged cessation of breathing during sleep which may be due to a disturbance of the respiratory centers (*central apnea*) or the result of airway obstruction (*obstructive apnea*).

Syncope. A temporary loss of consciousness (fainting) due to diminished blood flow to the brain. The primary causes for syncope are circulatory and cardiac dysfunction, anemia, hypoxia, or emotional disturbances (hysterical fainting).

Syncope related to orthostatic (postural) hypotension. A type of syncope that occurs on standing up or when standing for long periods. This type of syncope is found in patients with chronic orthostatic hypotension, varicose veins of the legs, peripheral neuropathies, hypovolemia, primary autonomic insufficiency, and patients taking drugs such as sedatives, L-Dopa, or antihypertensive agents.

Vagoglossopharyngeal syncope. A reflexive type of syncope elicited by chewing or swallowing in a manner that causes pressure on the afferent pathways of the Glossopharyngeal (CN IX) nerve, which then stimulates the vasomotor centers of the Vagus (CN X) nerve.

Vasodepressor (vasovagal) syncope. Fainting in response to a painful or strong emotion; simple faint.

E. Disturbances in Cerebrospinal Fluid Circulation

Colpencephaly. Ventricular enlargement in underdeveloped brains.

Congenital hydrocephalus. Hydrocephalus occurring during fetal development as a feature of inherited conditions (such as Dandy-Walker syndrome or Arnold-Chiari malformation), defective nervous system development, or the result of fetal or neonatal infections or hemorrhages.

Hydrocephalus. Increased cerebrospinal fluid in the ventricles of the brain. (See **communicating** and **obstructive hydrocephalus**, Chapter 8, pages 276 and 280.)

Hydrocephalus ex vacuo. Ventricular enlargement subsequent to brain atrophy.

Normal pressure hydrocephalus. A condition of chronic hydrocephalus in adults associated with delayed absorption of cerebrospinal fluid and characterized by progressive neurologic deficits (gait disturbances, incontinence, and cognitive deficits). This condition, like other forms of hydrocephalus, may be treated with a **ventriculo-atrial** (V-A) **shunt**, draining from the ventricles into the right atrium of the heart, or a **ventriculo-peritoneal** (V-P) **shunt**, draining from the ventricle into the peritoneal cavity, usually near the liver.

Tension hydrocephalus. A condition in which there is increased pressure in cerebrospinal fluid (CSF) due to a disruption or obstruction of flow between the CSF production sites in the lateral ventricles and the subarachnoid space where it is absorbed. The forms of tension hydrocephalus include **meningeal-obstructive, third ventricle-obstructive**, and **aqueductal-obstructive hydrocephalus**.

F. Toxic, Nutritional, and Metabolic Disorders

This section reviews some of the conditions associated with toxic nutritional, and metabolic disorders. The effects of hazardous chemicals or agents or neurologic complications associated with nonprescription drugs, "recreational" drugs, and prescribed drugs are not discussed. Discussions of the functions of various vitamins and minerals and effects of fluid and electrolyte imbalances are found in Chapter 5, Nutrition, Hydration, and Swallowing.

Alcoholic seizure disorder. Seizure disorders are frequent among alcoholics, possibly related to repeated head injuries or a lowered threshold for seizures caused by the toxic effects of alcohol itself. Seizures may also be a prodromal symptom of alcohol withdrawal.

Diabetic neuropathy. A syndrome of polyneuropathies, focal asymmetric mono- or polymononeuropathies, and/or autonomic neuropathies.

Dialysis dementia. Progressive encephalopathy seen in patients who have undergone long-term hemodialysis for end-stage renal disease.

Disequilibrium syndrome. A syndrome characterized by nausea, vomiting, headache, and disorientation.

Marchiafava-Bignami disease. A nervous system disease sometimes found in chronic alcoholics characterized by degeneration of the corpus callosum.

Nonmetastatic effects of carcinoma. Central nervous system dysfunction can result from carcinoma remote from the brain without frank metastases. The causes of nonmetastatic effects of carcinoma, characterized by gliosis and/or demyelination in the CNS, are not known, although possible factors include an autoimmune dysfunction elicited by tumor antigen, viral infection, and metabolic or endocrinologic problems.

Protein-calorie malnutrition (PCM) syndrome. Two overlapping syndromes of malnourishment in children (diagnoses are sometimes used with adults) are included as forms of PCM, **kwashiorkor syndrome** and **marasmus**. *Kwashiorkor syndrome* refers to the severe protein deficiency with edema and ascites and stunted growth found in poorly nourished children; *marasmus* refers to the severe *cachexia* with growth deficiencies in children with inadequate diets (and a history of early weaning or lack of breast feeding). Children with PCM are frequently found to have mental retardation, possibly as a result of decreased myelination. Chapter 5 contains related discussions.

Pseudotumor cerebri, benign intracranial hypertension. Referring to a syndrome of presumed toxic or metabolic etiology causing increased intracranial pressure with papilledema and headache.

Thyroid-related dysfunction. Referring to the range of neurological complications associated with hypo- and hyperthyroidism and hypo- and hyperparathyroidism, including weakness, seizures, mental status changes, paresthesia, and other neurologic problems.

Uremic encephalopathy. Encephalopathy associated with renal failure is characterized by asterixis, seizures, decreased alertness, and apathy and, in the later stages, hallucinations, and agitation.

Uremic neuropathy. The peripheral sensorineural deficits seen in association with renal disease include autonomic disturbances and motor disturbances (e.g., "restless leg syndrome").

Vitamin B$_{12}$ deficiency. Patients with pernicious anemia as a result of vitamin B$_{12}$ deficiency have a number of neurologic manifestations, including irritability, apathy, somnolence, progressive weakness, parasthesias, "pins and needles" tingling, and sensory losses, including visual deficits.

Wernicke's encephalopathy. Wernicke's encephalopathy is thought to be due to a *thiamine deficiency* causing pathologic changes in the periaqueductal gray matter, including petechial hemorrhages, demyelination, degeneration of neurons, and astrocyte formation. The classic syndrome includes ophthalmoplegia, ataxia, and dementia. If there is recent memory loss, poor retention of new information, and confabulation (Korsakoff amnestic syndrome, or psychosis), the patient will be diagnosed to have *Wernicke-Korsakoff syndrome*. (See **Alcoholic dementia**, Chapter 4, page 154.)

Whipple's disease. A disease thought to be the result of a bacterial infection involving the CNS causing inflammation of the hypothalamus, thalamus, and mammillary bodies. Whipple's disease may be found in patients with HIV.

G. Cerebrovascular Disease and Cerebral and Brain Stem Syndromes

Other brain stem syndromes are discussed later in this chapter (see Section J).

Aneurysms. Aneurysms of blood vessels usually occur at the bifurcations, presumably due to developmental defects. "Berry," or saccular, aneurysms are small blisters protruding from the artery walls. *Giant aneurysms* are defects large enough to cause pressure on surrounding structures.

Arteriovenous malformations (AVMs). Arteriovenous malformations refer to abnormal blood vessel tangles in the cerebral arterial and venous system.

Arvellis syndrome. A brain stem syndrome associated with malacia, hemorrhage, or tumor in the tegmentum of the medulla where the spinothalamic tract and pupillary fibers descend, resulting in an ipsilateral paralysis of the soft palate and larynx and contralateral hemianesthesia.

Atherosclerotic thrombotic strokes. Atherosclerosis is a vascular disorder caused by diseases affecting circulation, as well as genetic factors, and life-style factors. Risk factors include hypertension, diabetes, high (LDL) blood cholesterol levels, smoking, and the extent of routine physical activity. *Atheromas,* small lipid deposits, form plaques along vessel linings that become fibrotic and calcified. These plaques can become ulcerated leading to the formation of *mural thromboses.* Thromboses are blood clots made up of agglutinated platelets, white cells, and fibrin. Atheroscleroic thrombotic strokes are characterized by an abrupt onset of neurologic signs sometimes occurring in a saltatory (stepwise) manner over a period of several minutes, hours, or days.

Benedikt syndrome/paramedial midbrain syndrome. A brain stem syndrome associated with malacia, hemorrhage, or tumor in the area of the tegmentum, resulting in oculomotor palsy, cerebellar ataxia, contralateral intention tremor, and corticospinal tract signs.

Binswanger's disease, subcortical arteriosclerotic encephalopathy. Binswanger's disease, frequently listed as a cause for dementia, is associated with arteriosclerotic disease of the penetrating vessels of the cerebral hemispheres, causing multiple subcortical microinfarctions, particularly in the white matter.

Claude syndrome. A brain stem syndrome associated with vascular disease or tumors in the area of the brachium conjunctivum and red nucleus, resulting in oculomotor palsy, contralateral cerebral ataxia, and tremor.

Cranial arteritis. *Temporal arteritis* and *giant cell arteritis* are conditions characterized by severe focal headache and, if untreated, blindness and multiple areas of focal neurologic damage can result. Giant cell arteritis refers to granulomatous microneuropathologic changes in artery walls. Arteritis is treated with corticosteroids.

Déjerine's syndrome, medial medullary syndrome. This syndrome, also called *anterior spinal artery syndrome*, is characterized by ipsilateral flaccid tongue weakness from XIIth nerve involvement, contralateral hemiplegia from damage to the pyramidal tract, and contralateral loss of position and vibration resulting from damage to the medial lemniscus.

Embolic strokes. An embolic stroke occurs when a particle (air, fat, or thrombus) passes into a brain artery and occludes blood flow. Cerebrovascular diseases associated with embolic states are characterized by abrupt deficits that are at their peak at onset.

Foville's syndrome, inferior lateral pontine syndrome. A brain stem syndrome associated with malacia, hemorrhage, or tumor in the region of the anterior inferior cerebellar artery causing an ipsilateral lower motor weakness (both upper and lower face are weak), loss of taste from the anterior two-thirds of the tongue, ipsilateral loss of pain and temperature sense over the face, ipsilateral loss of conjugate gaze, and an ipsilateral Homer's syndrome.

Hematologic disorders. A number of hematologic disorders are associated with cerebrovascular disease, including polycythemia, sickle-cell disease, thrombotic thrombocytopenic purpura, thrombocytosis, and others.

Hemorrhages. There are several forms of intracranial hemorrhages, including hemorrhages occurring outside of the brain's covering, *extradural hemorrhage*; along the surface of the brain, *subdural hemorrhage*; and within the substance of the brain, *intracerebral hemorrhage*. **Hematomas** are "blood tumors," or hemorrhagic masses.

Hypertensive encephalopathy. Prolonged essential hypertension and hypertension secondary to other diseases can lead to multiple small hemorrhages (petechiae) and microinfarcts throughout the brain. Focal neurologic signs may be lacking unless a large vessel hemorrhage has occurred.

Jackson syndrome. A brain stem syndrome associated with malacia, hemorrhage, or tumor in the tegmentum of the medulla where the cortico-spinal tracts, spinothalamic tracts, and pupillary fibers descend, resulting in ipsilateral paralysis of the tongue, soft palate and larynx, and contralateral hemianesthesia.

Lacunar syndrome. Lacunar syndrome refers to small cavities within the brain resulting when the small, penetrating branches of arteries are occluded. These lacunae usually are associated with focal neurologic damage. If a lacuna occurs in the internal capsule, then a *pure motor hemiplegia* or *pure hemisensory* loss may result. Lacunae in the pons may cause ataxic hemiparesis, characterized by the *"dysarthria-clumsy hand syndrome."*

Millard-Gubler syndrome, medial pontine syndrome. A brain stem syndrome associated with malacia, hemorrhage, or tumor located where the cortico-spinal tract passes through the base of the pons, resulting in facial and abducens palsies, a gaze palsy to the side of the lesion, a contralateral hemiparesis, and an ipsilateral loss of conjugate gaze.

Reduced cerebral perfusion. Reduced cerebral perfusion refers to a general diminution in blood supply to the brain, usually the result of impairments in cardiac output or diseases involving the large vessels supplying the brain.

Reversible ischemic neurologic deficit (RIND). RINDs are ischemic events in which the neurologic deficits gradually resolve within a time frame of more than 24 hours up to three weeks post ictus. Persistent neurologic deficits indicate a **completed stroke**.

Steal syndrome. Steal syndromes refer to disturbances in blood circulation that result in diversion of circulation away from one vessel into another.

Superior lateral pontine syndrome. Referring to a brain stem syndrome involving the superior cerebellar artery, producing ipsilateral intention tremor of the arm and leg due to infarction of the superior cerebellar peduncle, an ipsilateral Homer's syndrome caused by the loss of the descending sympathetic tract, and a contralateral loss of pain and temperature sense of the face and body due to destruction of the lateral spinothalamic end ventral ascending tract of the Vth cranial nerve.

Systemic lupus erythematosus (SLE). SLE is an autoimmune disease in which neuropathologic changes are associated with multiple strokes, resulting in multifocal neurologic signs and progressive dementia.

Transient ischemic attacks (TIAs). Episodes of temporary focal ischemia with neurologic deficits lasting no longer than 24 hours. TIAs are considered to be "warning signs" of an impending stroke.

Vertebral basilar artery insufficiency. Reduced blood flow in the vertebral basilar artery circulation will result in deficits in the posterior areas of the brain, including visual deficits and neurologic signs indicative of brain stem and cerebellar ischemia.

Wallenberg syndrome, lateral medullary syndrome. A brain stem syndrome associated with vascular (usually occlusive) disease of the posterior inferior cerebellar artery (PICA) in the lateral tegmentum of the medulla, resulting in an ipsilateral Facial (CN VII), Glossopharyngeal (CN IX), Vagus (CN X), Hypoglossal (CN XII), and Spinal Accessory (CN XI) involvement; Horner syndrome; cerebellar ataxia; and a contralateral sensory loss for pain and temperature. Patients with a lateral medullary syndrome have ipsilateral laryngeal and pharyngeal paralysis (due to damage of the nucleus ambiguous) and a decreased gag response (due to infarction of the nucleus solitarius of the rootlets of CN IX).

Weber syndrome, medial midbrain syndrome. A brain stem syndrome associated with vascular causes or tumors at the base of the midbrain, resulting in an ipsilateral, complete oculomotor (CN III) palsy and contralateral hemiplegia with face and tongue involvement.

H. Degenerative Diseases

Many degenerative diseases are conditions that occur insidiously after a period of normal neurologic status. Some degenerative conditions are apparent during infancy or childhood and are considered hereditary. This section lists some of the more commonly encountered degenerative neurologic diseases, including selected hereditary diseases. Additional congenital diseases are listed later in this chapter. Additional degenerative diseases are found under **Extrapyramidal Disorders** in Section A-2, and elsewhere.

Amyotrophic lateral sclerosis (ALS), motor neuron disease. The cause of ALS is not known although a number of associated disorders and deficiences have been reported (heavy metal intoxication, thyroid disorders, enzyme deficiencies, and metabolic disorders). ALS is associated with progressive degeneration of the motor neurons. Four general forms of ALS are diagnosed depending on the primary area of motor destruction: *bulbar type, primary lateral sclerosis, progressive muscular atrophy*, and a *combined form*. Other forms of motor neuron disease include progressive muscular atrophies and progressive bulbar palsy (PBP).

Ataxia telangiectasia, Louis-Barr syndrome. See congenital disorders in the next section.

Friedreich's ataxia. An autosomal recessive trait associated with progressive damage to the posterior columns, spinocerebellar tract, and corticospinal tract characterized by dysmetria, intention tremor, dysdiadochokinesia, and nystagmus. This condition typically emerges in adolescence or young adulthood. (Also see discussion of ataxias on page 297.)

Creutzfeldt-Jakob disease (CJD). A dementing disease presumably associated with a "slow virus," causing rapid progression of neuronal degeneration and astrocyte proliferation, termed *spongiform encephalopathy*, and characterized by a rapid onset of profound dementia.

Olivopontinecerebellar degeneration (OPCD). A condition thought to be an autosomal dominant trait causing a metabolic dysfunction associated with progressive atrophic changes to the cerebellum characterized by ataxia, nystagmus, intention tremor, titubation of the head, and dysarthria.

Primary progressive dementias (PPD). The primary progressive dementias generally refer to Alzheimer's disease (AD), also called *dementia of the Alzheimer's type* (DAT) and *senile dementia Alzheimer's type* (SDAT), *Pick's disease,* and *Creutzfeldt-Jakob disease* (CJD), just discussed. The etiology of Alzheimer's disease is not known, although there is speculation about abnormalities in the biosynthesis of neurotransmitters, as well as viral, environmental, and genetic factors. The appearance of senile plaques and neurofibrillary tangles (neuronal filament degeneration) and increased aluminum are reported in Alzheimer's disease. In addition, aggregates of amyloid protein are found adjacent to and within cerebral blood vessels. CT scans of patient's with Alzheimer's disease reveal ventricular enlargement with diffuse atrophy, depending on the advancement of the disease. CT scans of patient's with Pick's disease reveal maximal atrophy in the frontal and temporal lobes.

Progressive supranuclear palsy (PSP), Steele-Richardson-Olszewski syndrome. A progressive disease associated with neuronal changes in the basal ganglia, cerebellum, locus ceruleus, substantia nigra, and brain stem and characterized by an initial loss in vertical and then horizontal gaze movements followed by the onset of a parkinsonian-like syndrome with dysarthria, dysphagia, and, occasionally, dystonias.

Shy-Drager syndrome. A syndrome of progressive autonomic neuronal degeneration associated with dry mouth, constipation, impotence, lightheadedness, and ataxia related to hypotension occurring with changes in posture.

I. Hereditary, Teratogenic, and Other Congenital Disorders

Also see Degenerative Diseases.

This section lists syndromes and congenital conditions which have associated neurologic damage. Included in this list are conditions having speech, language, hearing, and cognitive dysfunctions (mental retardation and developmental delays) as notable features of the syndrome complex. Teratogenic causes for fetal dysmorphology cannot be listed entirely here, but it is recognized that exposure to drugs, alcohol, radiation, and infectious conditions (such as rubella and cytomegalovirus) will affect fetal development, depending on the timing and extent of the exposure. It is also beyond the scope of this section to list all of the hereditary conditions associated with profound mental retardation. These conditions are predominantly the autosomal recessive disorders which are characterized by inherited metabolic errors and enzyme deficiencies. Some of the more common of these rare conditions are described here.

Alport syndrome. An hereditary condition (autosomal dominant or sex-linked) associated with nephritis and sensorneural hearing loss.

Anencephaly. An absence of the development of the forebrain and cranium.

Apert syndrome, acrocephalosyndactyly Type I. A congenital disorder though to be the result of an autosomal dominant mutation and characterized by craniosynostosis, synostosis or syndactyly of the feet and hands, strabismus, midline hypoplasia, frontal bossing, speech impairment, and hearing loss.

Arnold-Chiari malformation. A condition often associated with hydrocephalus in which there is an abnormal development of the cerebellum, skull and upper cervical vertebra. In **Chiari Type I malformation**, there is a herniation of the cerebellum below the foramen magnum.

Ataxia-telangiectasia. An autosomal recessive condition occurring relatively frequently in which there is a decrease in immunoglobulin (IgA); a progressive ataxia (dysarthria, grimacing, and choreoathetosis); and characteristic telangiectasias (dilatation of small capillaries forming a variety of angioma) on the ears, neck, nose, cheeks, and wrists.

Ataxic static encephalopathy (ataxic cerebral palsy). A condition associated with congenital damage to the cerebellar motor system as a result of a vascular lesion or in association with cerebellar agenesis syndromes.

Athetotic, or extrapyramidal, static encephalopathy (athetotic cerebral palsy). A form of cerebral palsy characterized by choreoathetoid movements resulting from damage to the basal ganglia. Athetosis is a potentially unfortunate outcome from kernicterus deposits in the basal ganglia caused by high bilirubin levels post delivery in Rh incompatbility.

Attention deficit disorder (ADD). A symptom complex characterized by inattentiveness and specific learning disabilities. When ADD is present along with excessive activity, the term **attention deficit disorder with hyperactivity** (ADD-H) will be applied. This symptom complex has been recognized by educators for many years; however, neuropathologic findings are notably inconsistent. Neurochemical disturbances, particularly for activities involving the *reticular activating system's locus ceruleus*, have been proposed. "Soft" neurologic signs are sometimes, but not invariably, present; a minority of ADD/ADD-H children will have abnormal EEGs.

Autism. A rare condition characterized by delayed and deviant language behavior (usually marked by high pitched, sterotypic, and echolalic utterances) and, in most cases, mental retardation. Autistic children often exhibit ritualistic hand movements and self-injurious behaviors and actively avoid contact with others. If a child is diagnosed prior to 30 months of age, the term *infantile autism* will be applied.

Cerebellar agenesis or dysgenesis. A lack of development of the cerebellum resulting in cerebellar ataxic movement disorders.

Complex plegia, mixed cerebral palsy. A form of static encephalopathy (cerebral palsy) in which more than one motor system is involved (extrapyramidal, pyramidal, or cerebellar).

Congenital nystagmus. An inherited autosomal dominant or sex-linked condition in which nystagmus is present at birth.

Congenital seizure disorders. Referring to seizure disorders that are associated with certain chromosomal abnormalities, such as trisomy D, or disorders that accompany inherited metabolic disturbances, including hereditary hypoglycemias and inherited degenerative disorders such as Sturge-Weber disease, tuberous sclerosis, aminoacidurias, and leukodystrophies.

Craniocleidodysostosis. A rare condition in which there is a failure in the development of the membranous bones of the face and, usually, an associated mental retardation and a seizure disorder.

Dandy-Walker syndrome. A condition in which there is a malformation of the roof of the fourth ventricle, potentially causing hydrocephalus, and a lack of development of the cerebellum.

Diastematolomyelia. A rare condition in which there is a duplication of the spinal cord.

Down syndrome, Trisomy 21. A chromosomal abnormality characterized by developmental delays and mental retardation, hypotonicity, epicanthal folds, Brushfield spots of the iris, upslanted palpebral fissures, flat facial profile, brachycephaly, hyperextended joints, protruded tongue, small auricles, cardiac malformations and duodenal atresia. The degree of mental retardation and dysmorphology may be less in cases of Down syndrome **mosaics**, or incomplete expressions of the chromosomal abnormality.

Duane's syndrome. A congenital oculomotor disorder in which abductor movements are limited or lacking.

Duchenne muscular dystrophy. An inherited, sex-linked, recessive disorder almost exclusively found in young males, due to an inborn error of metabolism resulting in failure of dystrophic synthesis and causing an excessive collagen formation. Duchenne muscular dystrophy eventually leads to contractures, muscle wasting, and deformities.

Fetal alcohol syndrome (FAS). A condition found in the offspring of alcoholic mothers where the teratogen *alcohol* causes characteristic dysmorphology of the eyes, head, and face and alters the child's cognitive development.

Fetal cytomegalovirus (CMV) syndrome. A condition associated with fetal exposure to CMV, a form of the herpes virus, resulting in congenital neurologic damage, microencephaly, obstructive hydrocephalus, chorioretinitis, and profound bilateral sensorineural hearing impairment. As with other teratogenic agents, the range and degree of fetal damage varies, depending on the time of exposure during development.

Fragile X syndrome. A sex-linked hereditary condition characterized by mental retardation, large ears, macroorchidism, prominent jaw, delayed speech and motor development, and, in some cases, autism.

Hypertelorism. A condition characterized by a greater than normal distance between the orbits resulting from a disproportionately larger growth of the lesser wings of the splenoid compared to the greater wings of the splenoid. This condition is frequently, but not invariably, associated with mental retardation.

Klippel-Fiel syndrome. A condition in which there are cervical vertebral fusion(s) in association with other congenital abnormalities.

Laurence-Moon-Biedl syndrome. An autosomal recessive condition characterized by polydactyly, hypogonadism, obesity, retinitis pigmentosa, and mental retardation.

Lysosomal storage diseases. Referring to a group of genetic diseases in which storage of certain metabolites occurs within lysosomes due to a specific enzyme deficiency. Lysosomal storage diseases include *Niemann-Pick* disease, *Krabbe's* disease, *Fabry's* disease, *Gaucher's* disease (adult and child form), *Hurler-Scheie* disease, *Wolman's* disease, *mucopolysaccharidoses*, *Sanfilippo's* syndrome, *Marateaux-Lamy* syndrome, and other disorders.

Macroencephaly. An enlarged cranium usually associated with hydrocephalus or bony growth abnormalities, such as *osteogenesis imperfecta.*

Maple syrup urine disease and its variants. These conditions are associated with autosomal recessive traits which have resulted in *inborn metabolic errors* in amino acid catabolism often leading to seizures. With some of these conditions, restrictive diets allow normal neurologic development.

Microencephaly, microcephaly. Abnormally small cranium. A number of genetically linked conditions are associated with microencephaly, or microcephaly, as are intrauterine infections (including rubella, cytomegalovirus [CMV], encephalitis and meningitis, and trauma).

Moebius syndrome. A congenital condition of heterogeneous etiology, characterized by weakness of the facial muscles (facial diplegia) and bilateral inability to abduct the eyes.

Neural tube defects. Neural tube defects result from incomplete closure of the neural tube during embryonic development. Such disorders include *anencephaly, spina bifida,* and certain forms of *hydrocephalus.* In spine bifida, there is a failure of closure of the vertebral laminae which could result in a *spinal meningocele (myelomeningocele).* A fissure of the spinal column is sometimes referred to as a *rachischisis.*

Neurofibromatosis. An autosomal dominant disorder characterized by abnormal pigmentation (café au fait spots), freckling in the axilla, neurofibromas (dysplastic tumors), and, in some cases, *acoustic neuromas.*

Pendred syndrome. A congenital condition characterized by sensorineural hearing loss and goiter.

Peroneal muscular atrophy, Charcot-Marie-Tooth syndrome. An inherited condition in which there are chronic, symmetrical neuropathies with demyelination and neuronal loss of the anterior horn cells.

Phenylkentonurias (PKUs). Variants of an autosomal recessive disorder in which there is a fundamental biochemical deficiency of the hepatic enzyme phenylalanine hydroxylase. Early institution of low phenylalanine diets will, in the majority of cases, avert neurologic damage.

Pigmentary degeneration of the retina. Degeneration of the retina may occur as a feature of Lawrence-Moon-Biedl syndrome, Refsum's disease, and Kearn-Sayre syndrome (sometimes called *homocarcinosis*).

Prader-Willi syndrome. An inherited condition characterized by hypotonicity, obesity, small hands and feet, almond-shaped palpebral fissures, hypogonadism, delayed speech development, and mental retardation.

Refsum syndrome, phytanic acid storage disease. An autosomal recessive condition characterized by polyneuropathies, cerebellar ataxia, sensorineural hearing loss, retinitis pigmentosa, and chronic polyneuritis.

Rubella syndrome, congenital rubella, Gregg syndrome. A condition characterized by congenital heart defects, patent ductus arteriosus (see Chapter 7), hearing impairment, microcephaly, and central nervous system damage.

Sacrococcygeal dystrophy. A condition in which there is a defect in the development of the sacrum and coccyx along with other spinal abnormalities.

Spasmus nutans. This relatively rare condition is characterized by a nystagmus, often accompanied by head bobbing or head tilting. Spontaneous resolution within a year of onset is common.

Spastic (pyramidal) diplegia, or quadriplegia, spastic cerebral palsy. A form of static encephalopathy (cerebral palsy) associated with bilateral damage to the corticobulbar or corticospinal tracts.

Spastic (pyramidal) hemiplegia. A form of static encephalopathy (cerebral palsy) resulting from unilateral damage to the motor cortex.

Tay-Sachs disease. An autosomal recessive disease mainly found in the offspring of Jewish parents of eastern European descent, associated with a basic enzymatic deficiency for hexosaminidase A. This metabolic deficiency leads to an accumulation of gangliosides causing pervasive nervous system damage.

J. Cranial Nerve, Lower Motor Neuron Disorders, Neuromuscular Disorders, and Peripheral Neuropathies

Carpal tunnel syndrome. Pain, numbness and paresthesia of the hand due to pressure on the median nerve in the wrist.

Cerebellopontine angle (CPA) tumors. Acoustic neuromas or meningiomas affecting the Vestibulo-Cochlear (CN VIII), Facial (CN VII), and Trigeminal (CN V) nerves, or tracts located at the cerebellopontine juncture.

Cranial nerve neuropathies. Cranial nerves may be damaged focally as a result of ischemic lesions, hemorrhage, neuromas, trauma, focal infections, and some viral inflammations that are prone to involve bulbar nerves. *Bulbar palsy syndromes* and *multiple cranial nerve palsies* refer to conditions where multiple nerves are affected. A number of specific brain stem syndromes and cranial nerve syndromes (several are listed separately in this section) result from medullary and pontine tumors, ischemia, or hemorrhages (also see Section G). Some viruses have a proclivity for damage to particular cranial nerves.

Neuropathies of cranial nerves III, IV, and VI cause oculomotor palsies, such at that found in Moebius syndrome (see above). *Trigeminal neuralgia,* or *tic douloureux*, is characterized by severe lancinating (stabbing) pain in the distribution of the Trigeminal (CN V) nerve. Carbamazepine treatment has been used with some success. **Bell's palsy**, or VIIth (Facial) nerve palsy, is characterized by unilateral facial paralysis resulting from a viral infection involving the geniculate ganglion. *Ageusia*, a loss of taste, is sometimes found in association with Bell's palsy. *Geniculate neuralgia* is associated with severe, spasmodic pain in the region of the external auditory canal and ear. *Facial myokymia* is a condition seen in some cases of multiple sclerosis, brain stem gliomas, and Guillain-Barré syndrome, in which fine, irregular contractions are observed on one or both sides of the face.

Neuropathies of the vestibulocochlear (CN VIII) nerve can result from the toxic effects of drugs, especially the "-mycin" varieties. Streptomycin and gentamicin can affect the vestibular branch of the VIIIth nerve, and drugs such as vancomycin, neomycin, and streptomycin are known to have toxic effects on the auditory branch. Balance testing, MRI, and BAER (see Chapter 4) are used to diagnose the site of lesion with VIIIth nerve dysfunction. Acoustic neuromas are tumors of the auditory branch of the VIIIth nerve. A tumor or aneurysm in this area may be referred to as a "*space occupying lesion*" at the cerebellopontine angle area.

Glossopharyngeal nerve (CN IX) *neuralgia* is rarely described, except in association with Vagus (CN X) and Accessory (CN XI) nerve involvement, resulting from ischemia or tumors located at the posterior fossa. Tumors and aneurysms in the posterior fossa may be referred to as *Vernet syndrome.*

Laryngeal neuralgia, associated with inflammation of the superior branch of the Vagus (CN X) nerve, is characterized by lancinating pain over the side of the neck. Tumors, hematomas, or ischemic damage near the jugular foremen can cause ipsilateral damage to the areas innervated by the Vagus (CN X), Spinal Accessory (CN XI) and Hypoglossal (CN XII) nerves. *Retroparotid space* tumors may be referred to as *Villaret syndrome, MacKenzie syndrome*, or *Tapia syndrome.* Tumors of the p*osterior lateralcondylar spaces* are usually referred to as *Collet-Sicard syndrome.*

Diphtheria. Neuropathy of the palatal musculature, dyspnea, aphonia, and dysphagia may be associated with diphtheria, an infectious disease and inflammatory toxicosis occurring in the presence of *Corynebacterium diphtheriae.*

Foix syndrome. Cranial nerve syndrome associated with sphenoid bone tumors, affecting the Abducens (CN VI), Trigeminal (CN V), Trochlear (CN IV), and Oculomotor (CN III) nerves.

Gradenigo syndrome. Cranial nerve syndrome associated with tumors of the petrous bone, affecting the Trigeminal (CN V) and Abducens (CN VI) nerves.

Guillain-Barré syndrome, postinfectious polyneuritis. Guillain-Barré syndrome is an ascending polyneuritis (with weakness progressing from the legs up to the bulbar muscles), occurring shortly (1–8 weeks) following a viral infection. It is thought to be due to lymphocytic sensitivity to peripheral nerve antigens that cause inflammation and demyelination of the peripheral nerves. (See Chapter 10 for additional discussion.)

Herpes zoster (shingles). Herpes zoster is a systemic illness involving the varicella virus. The viral activity is located predominantly in the sensory ganglia of the cranial nerves and spinal cord.

Jacod syndrome. Cranial nerve syndrome associated with tumors of the middle cranial fossa, affecting the Optic (CN II), Oculomotor (CN III), Trochlear (CN IV), Trigeminal (CN V), and Abducens (CN VI) nerves.

Mononeuropathy. Dysfunction of one peripheral nerve, a condition that can occur following trauma, infarction of peripheral nerves, or in association with diabetes mellitus.

Myasthenia gravis. A mostly bulbar neuromuscular junction dysfunction characterized by a progressive weakening with exertion (also see Chapter 10).

Nutritional neuropathies. Peripheral neuropathies are found with a number of nutritional deficiencies, including *thiamin neuropathy* (Beriberi), caused by a chronic lack of vitamin B_1, and sometimes seen in vegetarians and alcoholics. (See Chapter 4 and Toxic, Nutritional and Metabolic Disorders in this chapter.)

Oculopharyngeal dystrophy. An inherited autosomal dominant trait that presents late in life (between age 40 and 50 and is characterized by a slow, progressive ptosis, dysphagia, and hoarse, weak phonation).

Parinaud syndrome. A brain stem syndrome associated with hydrocephalus, pinealoma, or other lesions of the dorsal midbrain in the area of the periaqueductal gray matter, resulting in an upward gaze paralysis and fixed pupils.

Plexitis. Inflammation of a nerve plexus.

Poliomyelitis. An acute, viral infection characterized by headache, stiff neck, vomiting, and sore throat which, in the major form, may result in central nervous system damage with atrophy of a muscle group (bulbar and/or spinal neurons may be affected).

Polyradiculitis. Inflammation of several nerve roots.

Restless legs syndrome. A condition with symptoms including leg discomfort and prickling or burning dysesthesias. The cause is unknown in many cases, but in some patients it may be related with peripheral neuropathies.

Stiff-man syndrome. A syndrome of motor neuron dysfunction characterized by persistent muscle cramping, stiffness, and spasm that are relieved during sleep.

Viral or bacterial myositis. Inflammatory, neuromuscular disorder caused by infectious agents and resulting in weakness and tenderness.

K. Demyelinating Diseases

Acute disseminated encephalomyelitis. Referring to a group of allied demyelinating disorders, including *postinfectious, postexantrem,* and *postvaccinal encephalomyelitis* and *acute perivascular myelinoclasis.*

Acute necrotizing hemorrhagic encephalomyelitis. A condition almost invariably associated with a respiratory infection and characterized by abrupt onset of a fulminant variant of demyelinative disease.

Central demyelination of the corpus callosum, Marchiafava-Bignami disease. A condition almost exclusively found in chronic alcoholics and associated with central demyelination (revealed by MRI).

Multiple sclerosis (MS). A disease of unknown cause associated with a periodic autoimmune response directed at the ogliodendrocytes and creating irregular patches of demyelination. MS is characterized by "waxing and waning" neurologic deficits. Restoration of myelin can occur, with a corresponding functional improvement, or the formation of gliosis can occur leaving scars and destruction of white matter (axons).

Progressive multifocal leukoencephalopathy (PML), Schilder's disease. Relatively rare demyelinating disease in which dementia is a prominent feature. PML is usually associated with an underlying malignancy, most often lymphoma.

L. Disorders Related to Mental Status

For a discussion of the mental status examination and disorders, see Chapter 4.

Acute confusional states. Referring to an inability to think with the usually expected degree of clarity, coherence, and speed. Confusional states usually reflect diffuse cortical dysfunction and can occur as a stage in the evolution of central nervous system diseases leading to somnolence, stupor, and, eventually, coma.

Amnestic states and syndromes. Impairments in memory may be present as a feature of *delirium* (as a result of faulty perceptions of the environment); *dementia* (related to damaged cognitive processes for interpreting, retrieving, or encoding information); or as a feature of specific *amnestic states* and the *amnestic syndrome* (*Korsakoff amnestic syndrome*). Korsakoff amnestic syndrome is diagnosed in the patient who is alert and responding appropriately to others but has a notable anterograde amnesia (impairment in learning new information) despite relatively intact immediate and remote, or retrograde, memory. Some patients with Korsakoff psychosis are found to confabulate, perhaps, in part, to compensate for faulty recollection of recent events.

Another amnestic disorder, *transient global amnesia*, is characterized by a period of confusion and bewilderment lasting for a few hours during which the patient is alert and shows no notable impairment in consciousness or lack of awareness of the environment.

Amnestic states are also found in association with bilateral hippocampal infarctions, infarctions of the basal forebrain, trauma, hypoxic states, herpes simplex encephalitis, spontaneous subarachnoid hemorrhage, and tumors involving the base and walls of the third ventricle and limbic system.

Coma. See Chapter 4, Section V.

Delirium. Delirium is sometimes referred to as a "clouded sensorium," in which patients may misinterpret their environment, experience hallucinations, and verbalize in an incoherent, nonsensical manner.

Dementia. Dementia is a behavioral diagnosis indicative of a generalized intellectual deficit. Dementia is not a disease per se, rather it is a sign of pathology. Dementia may be irreversible or reversible, thus, the underlying cause needs to be diagnosed. Dementia can result from structural lesions, diffuse inflammatory processes, metabolic disturbances, progressive central nervous system diseases, chronic intoxications from drugs and/or alcohol, and as a related feature of psychiatric disorders (hysteria, hypomania, schizophrenia, and depression).

Persistent vegetative state. A stabilized condition of incomplete recovery from coma in which responsiveness is limited to postural and reflexive movements of the extremities and eyes.

Pseudocoma. Referring to a neurologic state caused by lesions in the basis pontis, sparing somatosensory pathways and ascending neuronal pathways for arousal and wakefulness, while interfering with cortiobulbar and corticospinal pathways. Thus, the patient is motionless but fully aware. This syndrome has been referred to as *"locked in"* syndrome, *coma vigil,* or a *de-efferented state.*

M. Neurologic Tumors

Arachnoid cysts. Encapsulated cysts containing cerebrospinal fluid in the arachnoid space.

Astrocytoma, Grade 1, 2. The most common form of brain neoplasms in children, these grades of astrocytomas are slow growing tumors arising from the astrocytes. Cerebellar and pontine astrocytomes are the most common posterior fossa tumors. Astrocytomas are usually diagnosed in the third and fourth decades of life and are found more frequently in the frontal lobes than elsewhere. Treatment involves excision or radiation, including brachytherapy (the temporary implantation of high energy radiation) and combined radiation-chemotherapy (see Chapter 8).

Cerebellar astrocytoma. Histologically and biologically benign cystic infratentorial tumors arising from astrocytes.

Chordoma. A congenital neoplasm arising from notochordal tissue in embryologic development.

Choroid plexus papilloma. A low grade neoplasm arising from the choroid plexus and causing overproduction of cerebrospinal fluid. Complete excision and reversal of the hydrocephalus is usually possible.

Craniopharyngioma. A benign tumor of congenital origin occurring in the suprasellar region potentially with extension into the hypothalamus, third ventricle, optic chasm, and circle of Willis making total surgical removal of the mass difficult to achieve.

Ependymoma. Neoplasms arising from the ependymal lining of the ventricles, posterior fossa, or spinal cord; treated by surgical resection and radiation therapy.

Glioblastoma multiforme; astrocytoma Grade 3, 4; spongioblastoma multiforme. A malignant, invasive and rapidly progressing neoplasm occurring most often in the fifth decade of life. Treatment may include surgical decompression, Decadron to reduce cerebral edema, and chemotherapy.

Medulloblastoma. Highly malignant tumors more commonly found in children and usually developing in the cerebellar vermis. These tumors tend to "seed," leading to recurrence.

Meningioma. Benign, slow-growing tumors arising from the meninges; treated by surgical excision followed by radiation if complete excision is not possible.

Metastatic neoplasms. Tumors arising from distant extracranial neoplasms, usually through the arterial or lymphatic system.

Neurilemomas. Slow-growing, benign tumors originating in the Schwann cells. These tumors are most commonly found on the vestibular portion of the VIIIth cranial nerve, referred to as an *acoustic neuroma*.

Neuroblastomas. Tumors usually arising in the cerebral hemispheres and most often in the medial temporal lobes of children.

Neurofibromatosis, von Recklinghausens's disease. Condition characterized by multiple neurofibromas and cutaneous dark spots (café au lait spots).

Ogliodendrogliomas. A slow-growing form of glioma arising from ogliodendrocytes; treated by surgical excision and radiation therapy.

Pineal region tumors. Neuroectodermal germ cell. Tumors in the pineal region are more frequent in children (10–20 years of age).

N. Head Trauma

Axonal injury. An axonal shear, or diffuse axonal injury, occurs when rotational forces are associated with brain impact, causing stretching and tearing of the gray and white matter interfaces.

Basal fractures and CSF fistulae. Basal skull fractures refer to injuries to one or more of the five bones that make up the base of the skull, including: the orbital portion of the frontal bone, sphenoid bone, petrous squamous portion of the temporal bone; cribiform plate; and ethmoid bone. A severe fracture could cause a CSF fistula into the sinuses.

Cerebral contusion. Contusions range from small, largely reversible injuries, sometimes called a "cortical bruise," to a major brain lesion involving multiple cortical and subcortical areas. Contusions are the common post-traumatic brain lesion consisting of varying amounts of necrosis, edema, and hemorrhage. Contusions are typically present at the site of primary injury and distant in the classic *contre coup* location. Most contusions are found in the frontal and temporal lobes.

Epidural, extradural hemorrhage. A collection of blood between the bony skull and the dura is relatively rare and may resorb; consequently, epidural hemorrhages are not treated surgically unless they enlarge rapidly and compress the brain.

Extracerebral subdural hematoma (SDH). A collection of blood within layers of the dura. *Acute subdural hematomas* may occur from a spontaneous rupture with an arteriovenous malformation (AVM). Patients with an acute SDH usually have an underlying brain contusion. A *subacute SDH* is an injury becoming evident or occurring several days (3 to 20) following a head injury. A *chronic SDH* is one that is present after more than 20 days. Chronic SDHs are occasionally found in the elderly during CT scanning when a SDH has gone clinically unrecognized at the time the injury occurred.

Herniation. Herniations are displacements of brain tissue through the brain covering's openings. *Uncal herniations* are the result of lesions of temporal lobe in which the medial portion of the temporal lobe is forced medially and downward into the ipsilateral tentorial hiatus and the brain stem is then displaced contralaterally (resulting in an ipsilateral compression of cranial nerve III). Also see Chapter 4, page 123.

Infarction from artery injuries. Injuries that cause compression on the major vessels of the brain can cause cerebral infarction. The regions affected depend on the vessels affected, but usually include the "watershed" areas of the parietal lobes; pericallosal regions; MCA regions; and occipital lobes. Injuries following trauma to the blood vessels can also produce "pseudoaneurysms" requiring surgical correction.

Intracerebral hematoma. Well-defined hemorrhages within the brain parenchyma, usually located in white matter and typically the result of a rupture of a major perforating artery following a rapid acceleration and deceleration of the head.

Intracranial pressure and brain swelling. Intracranial pressure is normally below a mean of 15 mmHg. The balance of flow of CSF is intricately managed by fluid dynamic mechanisms within the cisterns, ventricles, and vascular system of the brain. Following brain trauma, these systems can be overwhelmed and disturbed causing fluid accumulations and swelling within the substances of the brain itself. Increases in intracranial pressure can interfere with the mechanisms that allow intracranial blood flow; ultimately, brain death will occur. Swelling of the brain can occur with any type of head injury and can be difficult to control. On CT scans, the cisterns, ventricles, and cortical sulci will be diminished and correction is initiated to avoid brain herniation and death.

Subarachnoid hemorrhage (SAH). Small perforating vessel ruptures can cause hemorrhages to collect under the arachnoid covering of the brain and result in increased intracranial pressure.

Subdural hydroma. Collection of CSF in the subdural space can occur after trauma or rapid decompression of a ventricular system following shunting.

O. Brain Infections

Brain abscess. An encapsulated collection of pus in the brain.

Cerebritis. A regional infection and inflammation of brain tissue without necrosis (tissue death).

Encephalitis. Inflammation of the brain tissues.

Meningitis. An inflammation of the meninges (arachnoid and pia) or cerebrospinal fluid.

Metastatic brain abscess. Chronic infections of the lungs or pleura, or dental infections can enter the blood stream and be transferred to the brain.

Pyogenic infections. Pus-forming bacterial infections of the cerebrospinal fluid.

Septic embolism. Sepsis refers to an infection within the blood; A thromboembolism can be transferred into the brain in conditions such as *subacute bacterial endocarditis* (SBE) and an infection or abscess in the brain may occur.

HIV infections. Neurologic complications with HIV are often associated with various viral and bacterial infections. HIV is associated with *subacute encephalitis, cytomegalovirus, herpes simplex encephalitis, progressive multifocal leukoencephalopathy,* and *varicella-zoster encephalitis.*

II. PSYCHIATRIC DISORDERS

A. Psychiatric Diagnoses

DSM-IV categories. Psychiatric diagnoses are based in large part on observations and reports of the patient's behavior. Thus, to achieve consistency in classification, the *Diagnostic and Statistical Manual of Mental Disorders* was published by the American Psychiatric Association in 1980 (refer to Table 4–6 in Chapter 4). This work was predicated on the DSM-I manual published in 1954 with revisions in 1968 and 1974. Its third edition was referred to as the *DSM-III-R* (revised). The current version is DSM-IV. The DSM-IV codes guide the categorization of psychiatric disorders in a manner compatible with the *International Classification of Disease* ICD-9) codes. The DSM-IV diagnostic categories should be applied only by professionals with extensive clinical experience and knowledge about psychiatric conditions and the DSM-IV categories and "decision trees" (e.g., psychiatrists, psychiatric social workers, psychiatric nurse practitioners), refer to Table 4–6, page 162.

Psychiatric diagnoses. Descriptions of psychiatric disorders and conditions which may be encountered in a patient's medical history, psychiatric consultation summaries, or elsewhere. Most, but not all, of these diagnoses are classified by DSM-IV.

It is not unusual to find inaccurate and indiscriminate use of psychiatric labels in medical records. In general, speech-language pathologists should avoid making psychiatric diagnoses themselves, and if a psychiatric diagnosis is included in the speech-language pathology report, the date and source of that diagnosis should be stated (e.g., "Patient was diagnosed to have a post traumatic stress syndrome by his attending psychiatrist during a Psychiatric admission at this Medical Center in August of this year").

Descriptions of psychiatric disorders sometimes refer to *"organic"* psychiatric conditions, *"personality disorders,"* *"neurotic disorders,"* and *"psychotic disorders."* These terms do not refer to exclusive categories of psychiatric problems. Depression, for example, may be discussed as a result of or a response to organic cerebral disease or as a preexisting disorder. Further, some individuals might be described as having a "depressive personality type," while others might be said to have a "neurotic depression." The psychiatrist applies the DSM-IV codes using **multiple axes** to describe the emotional disorder, any related disorders, the etiology(ies) (including codes to indicate if the cause cannot be specified), related life stressors, and the level of functioning (see Table 4–6).

In psychiatry, it is generally felt that certain personality types are predictive of, or associated with, particular **neurotic disorders** and particular **psychotic disorders**. For example, an individual with an obsessive-compulsive pesonality type might have a related major depressive episode.

Neurotic disorders are usually discussed as either *anxiety disorders* (including phobias, panic states, etc.) or *somatiform disorders* (including hypochondriasis, hysterias, etc.). *Psychoses* can include conditions such as schizophrenias, paranoia, affective disorders with psychotic features (manic-depressive, or bipolar, states and major depressive states). Psychiatrists may refer to *confusional-delirious states* and certain behaviors *associated with focal and multifocal cerebral lesions* (i.e., organically caused delusions, hallucinations, or major mood disorders) as types of **psychoses**. Several of the psychiatric labels and therapies encountered in medical reports are listed in the next section.

B. Personality Disorders

Antisocial behavior. Referring to behaviors characterized by poor interpersonal relationships, frequent conflicts with others, impulsiveness, selfishness, low frustration tolerance, and tendencies to blame others.

Asthenic disorder. Referring to behaviors that indicate easy fatigability, and chronic weakness.

Cyclothymic personality. Referring to personality characteristics that include periods of high energy, ambition, and optimism followed by periods of hopelessness, pessimism, and despair. When mood swings are extreme, ranging from *severe depression* to *mania*, a **bipolar disorder** may be diagnosed.

Dependent personality. Referring to personality characteristics that suggest excessive dependence on others, a lack self-confidence, and a tendency to seek approval from others.

Explosive personality. Referring to individuals who display sudden outbursts of aggressive behavior usually followed by regret.

Histrionic personality. Referring to individuals with tendencies to be overly dramatic and displaying immaturity, sexualized relationships, and dependency.

Immature personality. Referring to individuals with poor adaptation to social, psychological, and physical stressors.

Inadequate personality. Referring to individuals with a tendency toward dependency (on others or institutions) and with an inability to address the demands of everyday living.

Obsessive-compulsive personality. Referring to individuals who are overly meticulous, perfectionistic, and concerned about standards (as applied to themselves and others).

Paranoid personality. Referring to individuals with tendencies to be suspicious and wary of others who display hypersensitivity and envy and have a heightened sense of self-importance.

Passive-aggressive personality. Referring to individuals who display obstructive and stubborn behaviors, particularly in response to authority.

Schizoid personality. Referring to individuals who are reclusive, secretive, and detached from others, and who may demonstrate an inability to express feelings and ideas.

C. Neurotic Disorders

Anxiety disorders. The term anxiety usually refers to a feeling of fearfulness and distress in response to stress. Anxiety disorders include panic attacks and may be a related feature of phobias. Anxiety, or panic, states generally begin with a feeling of foreboding or a sense of unreality followed by autonomic disturbances (palpitation, difficulty breathing, and diaphoresis).

Hypochondriasis. Hypochondriasis refers to an excessive preoccupation with health and an exaggerated concern for imagined illness(es). Hypochondriasis can be found in association with other psychiatric conditions, thus, psychiatrists might examine for conditions such as depression when treating hypochondriasis.

Hysterias. Hysterias include **conversion reactions** (in which there may be nonphysical symptoms of blindness, mutism, amnesia, weakness, etc.), and **hysterical neuroses.** *Briquet's disease* often refers to female hysteria. Male hysteria is sometimes termed "compensation neurosis." Hysteria is typically polysymptomatic and can include hysterical pain, vomiting, seizures, paralysis, tremors, and amnesia. A condition termed *globus hystericus* refers to nonorganic inability to swallow. A condition called *Ganser's syndrome* refers to patients who pretend to be insane. When individuals are consciously and deliberately feigning illness or disability to attain a desired goal, they are said be **malingering**. Malingering is frequently seen in association with hysteria and sociopathic personality disorders. A form of sociopathic malingering increasingly recognized by the medical profession is called *Munchausen's syndrome,* a factitious disorder with physical symptoms. Such patients feign or embellish medical conditions for no obvious motive other than to obtain medical and surgical treatment, and ultimately have innumerable hospitalizations, diagnostic procedures, and surgeries. *Munchausen's-by-proxy* refers to parentally induced illness in children designed to elicit medical attention and sympathy for the parent.

Neurotic depression. There is less than universal agreement about the use of this term; however, in general, neurotic depression refers to a depression occurring in patients who previously had symptoms of anxiety or other neuroses.

Obsessive-compulsive disorders. *Obsessions* refer to thoughts (not delusions) or impulses that intrude upon consciousness. *Compulsions* refer to acts that result from obsessions. These can be single acts or ritualized behaviors. A condition termed "obsessional slowness" refers to patients who exhibit extremely slow execution of everyday living tasks due to time-consuming rituals, compulsions, and checking behaviors.

Phobias. Phobic neuroses are considered to be anxiety disorders that are characterized by obsessive fears. Phobias include *panic states* (see anxiety neuroses, page 330) and specific fears such as *agoraphobia* (fear of open spaces), *acrophobia* (fear of heights), *claustrophobia* (fear of enclosed places), *social phobia* (fear of eating in public, speaking in public, using public restrooms), and so forth. Phobic patients usually recognize that their fears are irrational but feel they are powerless to overcome them.

D. Psychoses

Delusional or paranoid state. Paranoia refers to a psychosis characterized by persecutory delusions without hallucinations, dementia, or mood disorders. Delusional states are divided into *erotomanic type, grandiose type, jealous type, persecutory type, somatic type,* and *unspecified type.*

Depression (major). A *major depressive episode* refers to a prolonged state (at least 2 weeks duration) of a depressed mood and apathy, without delusions or hallucinations. A major depressive episode in the elderly is a frequent response to illness or bereavement and also maybe a prodromal sign of dementia. Usually, major depressive episodes are characterized by weight changes, insomnia or hypersomnia, feelings of worthlessness, inability to concentrate, and recurrent thoughts of suicide.

Depression generally is described as having two forms, an *endogenous type* (having no apparent external cause) and an *exogenous type* (occurring as a reaction to loss or other forms of life stressors). **Psychotic depression** is characterized by faulty reality testing and impaired functioning. Psychomotor retardation and agitation may be present and the patient may express delusional themes related to guilt, doom, or shame.

Neurotic depression, depressive neurosis, and **dysthymic disorder** are terms sometimes used to refer to milder depressive states.

Reactive psychoses. A stress-induced condition characterized by a brief duration (a few hours to 1 month) of loose associations, incoherence, hallucinations, delusions, catatonia, or disorganized behavior.

Schizophrenia. Schizophrenia is categorized into subtypes, including *simple, undifferentiated schizophrenia* (the individual who exhibits a blunt affect, social withdrawal, and a thought disorder); *acute schizophrenia* (characterized by a rapid onset of schizophrenic psychosis, possibly related to toxic, metabolic, or endocrine causes); *hebephrenic schizophrenia* or *disorganized schizophrenia* (in which the individual has delusions, hallucinations, marked emotional swings, and, at times, stereotypic mannerisms); *catatonic schizophrenia* (a condition in which there is no response to the environment, some psychiatrists feel catatonia maybe a feature of manic-depressive disease rather than a form of schizophrenia); *paranoid schizophrenia* (a condition in which the delusions, hallucinations, and thought disorder have persecutory features), and *childhood schizophrenia* (psychosis in childhood characterized by hallucinations and thought disturbances).

E. Other Psychiatric Disorders and Conditions

Anxiety disorders of childhood. Include separation anxiety and avoidant personality type in childhood.

Disruptive behavior. Includes behavioral conduct disorders, such as oppositional, defiant behavior; aggressive behavior; and hyperactivity attention-deficit disorders (in children).

Eating disorders. Include *anorexia nervosa, bulimina nervosa, pica, and rumination disorder of infancy.* The latter refers to the tendency to regurgitate a portion of food immediately after swallowing.

Endocrine psychoses. Include psychotic behaviors associated with hyper- and hypothyroidism, Cushing syndrome, adrenal insufficiency, or psychosis in response to ACTH and cortisone therapy.

Gender identity disorders. Include transsexualism, and gender identity disorders of childhood, adolescence, and adulthood.

Impulse control disorders. Include explosive disorder, pathologic gambling, kleptomania, pyromania, and trichotillomania (impulse to pull out one's own hair).

Organic mental disorders. Include primary degenerative dementia (P.D.D.), or primary progressive dementia (P.P.D.) of the Alzheimer type; multi-infarct dementia; and the dementias and other psychiatric impairments that are the result of brain dysfunction or damage.

Postpartum (puerperal) psychoses. Referring to the postpartum depression, delirium, or schizofreniform-behavior observed in mothers from within hours to months following childbirth.

Sexual dysfunction. Includes hypo- and hyperarousal disorders and paraphilias (exhibitionism, pedophilia, masochism, sexual sadism, and fetishism).

Sleep disorders. Include parasomnias (e.g., sleepwalking), insomnia, and hypersomnia. (See Syncope and Sleep Disorders in this chapter.)

Substance-induced organic mental disorders. Include intoxication withdrawal delirium, alcohol-related amnestic disorder, alcohol-related dementia, and intoxication from other drugs (amphetamine, cannabis, cocaine, opiates, hallucinogens, sedatives, hypnotics, etc.).

F. Psychiatric Therapies

Abreaction. A type of psychotherapy which involves re-experiencing a painful or repressed situation in a therapeutic setting with the goal of gaining insight and a release of painful emotions.

Activity therapy. Treatment utilizing activities that are directed toward a therapeutic goal, such as music therapy, recreational therapy, occupational therapy, bibliotherapy (providing written materials with a psychological benefit), and educational therapy.

Behavioral therapy. A therapeutic approach based on operant learning (conditioning) principles.

Biofeedback. A therapeutic approach in which the patient observes special monitors of his or her own biophysiologic functions (e.g., brainwave activity, blood pressure, nerve conduction activity in muscles) with the goal of learning to exert a conscious control over an autonomic or involuntary function.

Child Life Therapy. Referring to play therapy activities to help ill children cope with their illness and the medical setting.

Cognitive therapy. An approach to psychotherapy which attempts to "break down" existing negative thoughts (cognitions) and replace them with positive and more functionally adaptable thoughts.

Electroconvulsive therapy (ECT). ECT is considered an effective treatment for some patients with major depression. During ECT electrodes are placed over each temple and an alternating current is passed between them for 0.1 to 0.5 seconds. Usually, the patient receives a total course of 6 to 14 treatments administered every other day.

Insight-directed therapy. An approach to psychotherapy which involves directing the patient toward an examination of his or her unrecognized motives and feelings.

Interpersonal therapy. An approach to psychotherapy which attempts to improve the quality of the patient's social and interpersonal functioning by enhancing the ability to cope with internal and external stressors.

Milieu therapy. The use of external, or environmental, adjustments and environmental controls to treat mental illness.

Pastoral or spiritual counseling. Referring to counseling provided by a member of the clergy.

Pharmacologic therapy, biochemical therapy. The use of medications to treat psychiatric disorders or their symptoms. Lithium carbonate is used to treat bipolar conditions. Neuroleptic drugs, such as haloperidol, followed by a tricyclic and monoamine oxidase inhibitors (MAOIs) may be therapeutic for depression. Thyroid hormones may be used as an adjunct to tricyclic therapies to treat nonpsychotic depression.

Psychoanalytic therapy. Referring to a form of psychotherapy in which the fundamental concepts are based on the work of Sigmund Freud. Psychoanalysis seeks to bring unconscious emotional conflicts into the patient's awareness so that he or she can gain insight.

Psychotherapy. Referring generally to treatment that uses explanation, encouragement, reassurance, education, support, and advice to allow the patient and significant others to understand and cope with stress, emotional states, and/or psychiatric disorders better.

Rational-emotive therapy. A cognitive and empirical type of psychotherapy directed toward improving controls on emotions by examining the relationship between beliefs about oneself and their influence on emotions and behaviors.

III. NOTES

_____

_____

_____

_____

NOTES *(continued)*

IV. REFERENCES

American Psychiatric Association. (1987). *Diagnostic and statistical manual of mental disorders* (3rd ed., rev.). Washington, DC: American Psychiatric Association.

American Psychiatric Association. (1994). *Quick reference to the Diagnostic Criteria from DSM-IV*™. Washington, DC: American Psychiatric Association.

Andreoli, T. A., Carpenter, C. J., Plum, F., & Smith, L. H. (1990). *Cecil essentials of medicine* (2nd ed.). Philadelphia: W. B. Saunders.

Berkow, R. (Ed.). (1990). *The Merck manual* (15th ed.). Trenton, NJ: Merck, Sharp, and Dohme.

Bonner, J. S., & Bonner, J. J. (Eds.). (1991). *The little black book of neurology* (2nd ed.). St. Louis: Mosby Year Book.

Chenitz, W. C., Stone, J. T., & Salisbury, S. A. (1991). *Clinical gerontological nursing.* Philadelphia: W. B. Saunders.

Jacobs, J. W., Bernard, M. R., & Delgado, A. (1977). Screening for organic mental syndromes in the medically ill. *Annals of Internal Medicine, 86,* 40–46.

Jung, J. H. (1989). *Genetic syndromes in communication disorders.* Boston: College-Hill Press.

CHAPTER

10

Acute and Critical Illnesses

This chapter reviews several of the illnesses frequently found in acute care settings and, in particular, **intensive care units**. The purpose of this review is to provide a brief, descriptive reference for conditions potentially encountered by clinicians working in such settings and for conditions that may be part of the medical histories of patients in extended care or rehabilitation programs.

I. CARDIAC AND PULMONARY DISORDERS

Acute myocardial infarction (MI). A myocardial infarction is a condition in which there has been *death of heart tissue* usually caused by atherosclerotic coronary artery disease (CAD). Typically, patients will have experienced acute, severe substernal chest pain radiating to the jaw, shoulders, and arms associated with shortness of breath, diaphoresis, nausea, vomiting, and syncope when an MI occurs. The diagnosis is made by physical examination, EKG findings, and laboratory analysis for the enzymes that are elevated in association with myocardial infarction (additional discussion of myocardial infarction is found in Chapter 3 and Chapter 7).

Acute pericarditis. Acute pericarditis is a sudden *inflammation of the lubricated sac encasing the heart.* Pericarditis can be idiopathic (of unknown cause) or result from conditions such as infection, connective tissue disease (including scleroderma), uremia, myxedema, neoplasm, drugs, or a post-heart surgery, or post-MI condition.

Adult respiratory distress syndrome (ARDS). Adult respiratory distress syndrome is a clinical condition, not a specific disease, in which there is *acute dyspnea, severe hypoxemia, decreased lung compliance,* and *diffuse infiltrates* on chest X ray. Conditions associated with ARDS include aspiration, sepsis, trauma, multiple blood transfusions, drug overdoses, near-drowning, head trauma, and lung contusions.

Aortic dissection (AD). An aortic dissection is a condition caused by an *intimal* (within layers) *tear in the aorta*, allowing a channel of blood (hematoma) to accumulate within the linings of the vessel. Hypertension and degenerative diseases may be predisposing factors. This condition is usually treated aggressively with antihypertensive and beta-blocking agents and, in some cases, surgery to avoid an *aortic rupture*. Arterial dissections can occur elsewhere, including the carotid arteries.

Arrhythmias. The basic principles of cardiac *impulse initiation and conduction* are described in Chapter 7. Cardiac arrhythmias, such as *tachydysrhythmias* (tachycardia) and *bradydysrhythmias* (atrial and ventricular bradycardias), may require conversion (with shock or drugs) in an acute setting.

Aspiration. When a foreign body or substance enters the airway, respiratory status will be disrupted to varying degrees. If a foreign body occludes the airway, as might happen when choking on food ("café coronary"), sudden and extreme distress can occur, potentially leading to asphyxiation. Aspiration pneumonia can occur as a result of *neurologic disorders* (decreased level of consciousness, oropharyngeal weakness, or decreased sensation of the oropharynx), *gastrointestinal disorders* (esophageal disease, gastric disease, bowel obstruction), or *pulmonary disorders* (e.g., impaired mucociliary clearance and cellular defenses). (Also see Chapter 6 for additional discussion of pneumonia.)

Asthma. A sudden onset of coughing and wheezing can occur in response to a variety of conditions and cause *bronchial resistance.*

Asthma is sometimes referred to as "reversible obstructive pulmonary disease." *Acute severe asthma* may require treatment with drugs (such as epinephrine, aminophylline, and sympathomimetic or parasympatholytic agents); oxygen support; and mechanical ventilation.

Bronchopleural fistula (BPF). A bronchopleural fistula is a condition usually associated with mechanical ventilation coupled with chest tube suction. These conditions contribute to a risk for air leaking into the pleura. When the patient is asked to bear down or to exhale forcibly with the mouth and glottis closed and nose occluded (Valsalva maneuver), a "leak squeak" will be heard as air passes into the pleural space. Spontaneous BPF can occur in association with lung malignancies, suppurative pneumonia, and following pneumonectomy (resection of the lung).

Cardiac contusion. *Nonpenetrating trauma* to the heart can result in petechiae and ecchymoses of the heart muscle (myocardium). More extensive bleeding would be called a "localized cardiac hematoma." Dysrhythmias are common with myocardial contusions.

Chronic obstructive pulmonary disease (COPD). COPD is a condition associated with a *chronic dyspnea* (shortness of breath) and *productive cough*. Related conditions include emphysema, chronic bronchitis, and reversible obstructive pulmonary disease. Extreme conditions may require endotracheal intubation, oxygen support, and/or mechanical ventilation.

Congestive heart failure (CHF). Congestive heart failure refers to a condition in which the heart is unable to pump blood sufficiently for the body's needs. CHF often follows diseases to the *myocardium* (such as myocardial infarction and cardiomyopathy). Patients with CHF will be short of breath and unable to tolerate lying down in a flat, supine position. Patients with severe CHF will have pulmonary edema. Along with drugs acting on the heart itself, CHF is typically treated with diuretic therapies. Diuretic therapies can result in complications, including azotemia, orthostatic hypotension, hyponatremia, hypokalemia, hypomagesia, contraction metabolic acidosis, and related mental status declines.

Endocarditis. Endocarditis refers to an inflammation due to infection of the linings in the *chambers of the heart*. Abnormal heart valves, with defects as a consequence of congenital heart disease or valvular damage, are prone to infection. Vegetations form on the damaged valve and become surrounded by platelets and fibrin, making the normal immune responses ineffective. *Infectious endocarditis* is treated with the antibiotics appropriate to the culture findings.

Hemoptysis. Numerous disorders of the cardiorespiratory system can cause patients to *cough up blood*. The physician needs to determine if the patient has bleeding from the respiratory system **hemoptysis** or has **hematemesis** (blood coming from the esophagus or stomach). Hemoptysis can occur in association with conditions such as tuberculosis, lung cancer, chronic obstructive pulmonary disease, vascular disorders, pneumonia, bronchitis, bronchiectasis, infections, and trauma.

Hypertensive crisis. A hypertensive crisis is a condition in which blood pressure reaches a level high enough to cause damage to vital organs, most notably, intracranial hemorrhages, myocardial infarction, pulmonary edema, aortic dissection, and renal failure. The blood pressure level at which a hypertensive crisis might occur is not fixed; however, so-called *"malignant hypertension"* is usually defined clinically as a sustained diastolic pressure greater than 130 mm Hg.

Pericardial effusion. Fluid accumulating in the pericardial space is referred to as pericardial effusion. **Cardiac tamponade** refers to an accumulation of fluid in the pericardium that is sufficient to cause acute cardiac compression and diminish cardiac output.

Pneumothorax. A pneumothorax refers to air leaking into the pleural space. The cause can be *spontaneous* or the result of *iatrogenic* errors (e.g., an accidental lung puncture during a medical procedure). A pneumothorax also can occur with patients receiving mechanical ventilation, especially when they have aspiration or necrotizing pneumonia, ARDS, or obstructive lung disease (see Chapter 7).

Pulmonary embolism (PE). Pulmonary emboli are most often found in patients who have a history of **deep vein thromboses** (DVTs). When clots from the peripheral venous circulation are dislodged, they may be passed into the right side of the heart and occlude the pulmonary artery (which carries blood from the heart to the lungs to be oxygenated) and lead to tachycardia, pulmonary infarction, pleuritic pain, and lung changes (including atelectasis, pleural effusion, and localized infiltrates).

Unstable angina. Cardiac angina is a condition in which there is pain related to a lack of oxygen perfusion to the heart muscle. *Effort angina* is a condition that occurs during effort, or exercise, when there is an increased demand for oxygen. *Unstable angina* can occur at rest, when there may be no extra demand on the heart, and is brought on by a vasospasm, hemorrhage, or thrombus of the heart vessel causing an intermittent or transient loss of blood supply to the heart muscle.

Upper airway obstruction (UAO). Upper airway obstructions are life-threatening events. An upper respiratory obstruction produces extreme distress, stridor, cyanosis, and loss of consciousness. *Intrathoracic* causes of upper airway obstruction include tracheal stenosis, tracheomalacia, submucosal hemorrhage of the glottis or subglottis (following intubation, biopsy studies, trauma), and compression on the upper airway (related to lymph node enlargement or tumors). *Extrathoracic* causes of airway obstruction include aspiration of a foreign body, hypopharyngeal edema, hypopharyngeal hemorrhage, epiglottitis, acute angioedema, adenoidal hypertrophy, cricoarytenoid arthritis, hypertrophic thyroid disease, and bilateral (abductor type) vocal fold paralysis.

II. HEMATOLOGIC DISORDERS

Anticoagulation disorders. Complications of anticoagulation therapies, chiefly *heparin* and *coumarin derivatives*, are often treated in the intensive care unit. Bleeding is a major risk with heparin and coumarin derivative therapy because these drugs are intended to prevent the formation of thromboses. Anticoagulant therapies are routinely used with patients who have chronic thrombotic disease. Corrective management of anticoagulant complications involves administration of drugs that have a neutralizing effect with careful monitoring of coagulation parameters. Heparin therapy can cause thrombocytopenia, a condition in which there is a reduction in the number of blood platelets. *Thrombocytopenia* is a commonly acquired problem in the critically ill.

Antiplatelet therapy. Unlike anticoagulate therapy, antiplatelet therapy has an effect on the prostaglandins in platelets and inhibits their aggregation. Aspirin is an antiplatelet drug often prescribed as a prophylactic measure, especially following a transient ischemic attack (ITA) or thrombotic or thromboembolic stroke. Aspirin intake is usually discontinued before and immediately following a major surgery.

Disseminated intravascular coagulation (DIC). Disseminated intravascular coagulation is a hemorrhagic condition in which there is gross *intravascular clotting* in association with profuse bleeding.

Hemostatic failure. Hemostatic failure refers to a disruption in the normal processes for blood clotting. Hemostatic failure occurs in association with drugs used for or known to affect bleeding, including coagulation therapies and drugs causing platelet dysfunction (such as aspirin), and with hematologic diseases associated with blood clotting.

Tumor lysis syndrome. Tumor lysis syndrome occurs in response to large masses of tumor cells, in association with conditions such as small cell lung cancer, widespread metastases, lymphocytic cancer, and myeloma. Widespread cell destruction causes the release of metabolites and intracellular ions which overwhelms the kidney, requiring hemodialysis.

III. GASTROINTESTINAL DISORDERS

Acute hepatic failure. Hepatitis can occur when there is a deterioration of a pre-existing liver disease or following sudden damage to liver cells. **Jaundice** (yellowed skin coloring) is associated with liver disease. *Hepatic encephalopathy* may result from hepatitis, in which an initial mental confusion can progress to stupor and coma. Other problems associated with acute hepatic failure include respiratory alkalosis, hypoglycemia; renal failure; and hemorrhagic manifestations, including bleeding *diathesis* (loss of vitamin K stores).

Acute intestinal ischemia. Infarction of the bowel can result from occlusive vascular disease or hypoperfusion of the intestinal tissues.

Lower gastrointestinal (LGI) hemorrhaging. Lower GI bleeding occurs with inflammatory bowel disease, hemorrhoids, carcinoma, hemorrhagic diatheses, radiation colitis, angiodysplasia, and diverticulosis (weakenings of the intestinal wall). LGI bleeding from the rectum is usually described to be bright red blood, called **hematochezia**. Conversely, "black tarry stools" are usually found in association with upper GI (UGI) bleeding.

Peritonitis. Peritonitis is a condition in which bacteria have entered the peritoneal cavity. Peritonitis can occur in association with acute appendicitis, peptic ulcer perforation, or post-surgical complications.

Upper gastrointestinal (UGI) hemorrhaging. Bleeding in the upper GI tract can result from a variety of conditions, including esophageal varices, Mallory-Weiss syndrome (damage to the esophageal mucosa at the gastroesophageal juncture, most often found in alcoholics), peptic ulcers, stress ulcers, an aortoenteric fistula, and an upper GI malignancy. The diagnosis of UGI bleeding includes a *hemoccult test* (stool study examining for a *guaiac reaction*, a test for the presence of blood). Patients usually present with **hematemesis**, vomiting red blood or "coffee ground" appearing blood, and **melena**, black tarry blood, in the stool (feces).

IV. FLUID, ELECTROLYTE, AND KIDNEY DISORDERS

A. Acid-Base Disturbances

Acid-base disturbances refer to imbalances in the intracellular or extracellular fluids that are either excessively *alkaline* or excessively *acidic*. These balances are quantified by the concentration of hydrogen ions, H+, or **pH** (the negative logarithm of hydrogen ion concentration). A normal body pH value is about 7.40 (7.35–7.45). The normal body pH level is maintained principally by the body's carbonic acid buffering system. The ratio between *bicarbonate* HCO_3 and *partial pressures of carbon dioxide in the arterial blood*, $PaCO_2$, determines the H+ concentration. Regulation of these processes occurs with the interaction of alveolar ventilation, affecting $PaCO_2$, and kidney functions, affecting HCO_3. The major forms of acid-base disturbances are **respiratory acidosis** (in which there will be an increase in $PaCO_2$ in blood gases), **metabolic acidosis** (in which there will be an increased HCO_3), **respiratory alkalosis** (decreased $PaCO_2$), and metabolic **alkalosis** (decreased HCO_3). The term *ketoacidosis* refers to metabolic acidosis associated with diabetes mellitus, starvation, and alcoholism.

B. Acute Renal Failure (ARF)

Acute renal failure refers to a syndrome associated with a dramatic decrease in renal function, causing a reduction in the clearance of solutes (wastes) from the blood which leads to an increase in the concentration of **creatinine** and **blood urea nitrogen** (BUN) levels. Retention of water and solutes can cause uremia and fluid, electrolyte, and metabolite imbalances producing neurologic changes (nausea, vomiting, and encephalopathy) and **metabolic acidosis**. ARF can result from diseases of *other organs* (e.g., congestive heart failure, liver disease); *drugs*; damage to the *kidney* itself; and obstructions to, from, or within the kidney.

C. Fluid, Electrolyte, and Metabolites Disturbance

The proper function of the body's cells depends on maintaining a balance between the volume of fluid in the cells and the salts and other *metabolites* in body fluids. The body is about 60% water. About two-thirds of that fluid is within cells; the rest is *extracellular*.

Water balances in the body, referred to as the balance between *fluid depletion* and *fluid expansion*, are monitored and controlled by renal and extrarenal receptors and functions. Conditions associated with *fluid expansion* (**hypervolemia**) include renal disorders, endocrine abnormalities, and conditions causing edema (such as congestive heart disease). Patients who are *hypervolemic* will sometimes be described as "wet," whereas patients who are *hypovolemic* will be described as "dry." Conditions associated with *fluid depletion* (**hypovolemia**) include vomiting, diarrhea, burns, sweating, hemorrhage, diabetes insipidus, chronic renal failure and other renal diseases, and, commonly, the use of diuretics. (See Chapter 5, Nutrition and Hydration, for further discussion of electrolyte and fluid imbalances.)

V. METABOLIC AND ENDOCRINE DISORDERS

A. Adrenal Insufficiency

Acute adrenal insufficiency, or *Addisonian crisis*, usually occurs in patients who have some pre-existing partial insufficiency. Total failure of the adrenal glands is usually fatal. There are numerous causes of damage to the adrenal glands, including hemorrhagic destruction following anticoagulant use, tumors and metastases, tuberculosis, and diseases associated with a polyglandular autoimmune syndrome.

B. Diabetic Coma and Ketoacidosis

Diabetic coma may be referred to as *hyperosmolic nonketotic diabetic coma* (HNDC) in which acidosis is absent or, if present, is due to a coincidental lactate accumulation from poor circulation.

Diabetic ketoacidosis (DKA) refers to a marked insulin deficiency in which there is hyperglycemia, dehydration, and acidosis. Patients with DKA have severe abdominal pain, hyperventilation, and tachycardia, and their breath smells like acetone. HNDC is clinically less specific; and because a stuporous or obtunded mental state is part of the syndrome, it is sometimes initially confused with other conditions in elderly patients (stroke, polypharmacy, and excessive medication) until a blood glucose tolerance test is obtained.

C. Thyroid Dysfunction

Acute hyperthyroidism can cause a thyrotoxic crisis or so-called "thyroid storm." Hyperthyroidism occasionally follows infection, trauma, surgery, and radioiodine therapy. Serious disease can be associated with hyper- or hypothyroidism. Late stage chronic hypothyroidism in the elderly is usually referred to as a *myxedema crisis*, or *myxedema coma*. The state can follow infection, trauma, exposure to cold, and excessive medication.

VI. OTHER DISORDERS

A. Burns

Burns are classified as *moderate* or *major* according to the amount of the body affected, or the **Total Body Surface Area (TBSA)**, and the depth of the burn. The TBSA is measured by an approximation based on the "*rule of nines*," in which the entire head makes up 9%, each arm makes up 9%, each leg makes up 18%, and the front and back of the body each make up 18%.

The **depth of burns** is classified by degrees. *A first degree burn* is the sort associated with sunburn and is superficial, characterized by erythema and dry or blistered, painful skin. A *second degree burn*, or partial thickness burn, is the sort associated with severe sunburn, scaldings, or flash burns (quick duration exposure to extreme heat) and involves the epidermis and extends into the dermis. Second degree burns are painful and are characterized by blistering and weeping bullae. *Third degree burns*, full thickness burns, result from prolonged contact with extreme heat and involve the epidermis and dermis. The skin is white, translucent or charred, and touch sensation is lacking.

Gastrointestinal dysfunctions and *hemolytic anemia* are often associated with severe burns. Treatment of burn patients requires *fluid resuscitation*, physiologic monitoring, topical antibiotics, analgesia and sedation, plastic surgeries, wound management, infection control, and physical therapy. Speech-language pathologists sometimes assist with oral-facial musculature exercises to improve functional recovery after facial burns. Infection prevention is extremely important when working with patients who have severe burns, because sepsis can lead to *multiple organ systems failure* (MOSF).

B. Coma

Coma refers to an extremely reduced state of consciousness associated with damage to or disruption of the cerebral hemispheres and/or the reticular activating system. Coma can result from structural or metabolic causes. Patients who are described to be in a "persistent vegetative state" may or may not be persistently comatose. Coma is discussed in Chapter 4, Section V.

C. Eaton-Lambert Syndrome

Eaton-Lambert Syndrome has been associated with small cell carcinoma. This disorder causes thigh, shoulder, and pelvic weakness, sparing bulbar and ocular muscles. Unlike myasthenia gravis, anticholinergic drugs are not beneficial, but drugs that cause the release of acetylcholine are sometimes helpful.

D. Guillian-Barré Syndrome

Guillian-Barré syndrome is characterized by an acute polyradiculoneuropathy occurring in association with immunologic stresses or challenges, such as a *viral infection, immunization,* or *mycoplasma* (bacterial) *infections.* Clinical features include progressive weakness of the extremities with more proximal than distal involvement, paresthesias, areflexia, cranial nerve involvement, cramping limb pain, and autonomic disturbances. *Plasmapheresis* has been demonstrated to benefit patients with Guillian-Barré syndrome by reducing the number of days of intubation that is required. (Also refer to Chapters 4 and 9.)

E. Head injury

The effects of a trauma to the head are usually discussed with reference to the **primary effects**, or concussive effect of the trauma itself and the **secondary effects**, or resulting edema, hemorrhage, hematoma, infection, hypoxia, hypercapnia, ischemia, and metabolic disturbances. Focal damage can result from the concussive effects of the blow to the brain. A **shearing effect** is often found along the rough surfaces of the frontal and temporal cranium and dural protrusions. **Increased intracranial pressure (ICP)** can cause additional damage; thus, this condition is carefully monitored in the ICU. The extent of secondary metabolic and vascular damage associated with traumatic brain injury plays a major role in the gradient and degree of recovery. Hemorrhaging around or within the brain is among the main concerns for intensive care management. When soft tissues are violently displaced within the cranium, blood vessel tears with hemorrhaging are likely. The types of pooling hemorrhages, or *hematomas*, associated with head injury include **epidural** hematomas (usually due to tears in the middle meningeal artery or vein), **subdural hematomas** (usually related to vessel tears as they pass the superior sagittal sinus), **subarachnoid hematomas** (bleeding between the layers covering the brain), and **intracerebral hematomas** (bleeding into the parenchyma of the brain). (Also see Section N, Chapter 9).

F. ICU Syndrome

The ICU syndrome refers to states of agitation and delirium reported in patients who remain in ICUs for extended periods. This syndrome is considered to reflect both physiologic factors and psychologic factors.

G. Infectious Diseases

Infectious processes can involve vital organs, causing life-threatening acute and critical illnesses. Examples include infections of the heart valves, (*endocarditis*), the lungs (*pneumonia*), and the brain (*encephalitis or meningitis*). (See Chapter 6 for discussion of infectious diseases and their prevention and treatment.)

H. Myasthenia Gravis

Myasthenia gravis is an autoimmune, neuromuscular junction disease in which antibodies are formed to the receptor neurotransmitter acetylcholine. Patients with myasthenia gravis have increased muscle weakness potentially requiring intensive care. An increase in muscle function follows administration of Tensilon, an acetylcholinesterase inhibitor endorphonium chloride. Plasmapheresis has also been found to be therapeutic. (Additional discussion of myasthenia gravis is found in Chapters 4 and 9)

I. Shock

Shock is a state in which there is an acute circulatory failure leading to hypoperfusion of body tissues and damage to organs. The major forms of shock include *cardiogenic* causes (when there is an acute, severe diastolic function loss in the heart); *hypovolemic* causes (fluid loss due to hemorrhage, vomiting, diarrhea, burns, etc.); *distributive causes* (related to sepsis, anaphylaxis, spinal cord injury, adrenal insufficiency, etc.); and *extracardiac* causes (pericardial tamponade, constrictive pericarditis, pulmonary embolisms, or ventilator-related causes). Shock resulting from sepsis (disseminated infection in the blood or tissues) is called **septic shock**.

J. Status Epilepticus

This condition is defined as a seizure lasting approximately 20 to 30 minutes, or a series of seizures lasting at least 30 minutes without a return to consciousness. Prolonged seizure activity can cause damage to neurologic substrate due to cerebral hypermetabolism. (Also see further discussion and description of related seizure disorders in Chapter 9.)

VII. NOTES

NOTES *(continued)*

_____

_____

_____

_____

_____

_____

_____

_____

_____

VIII. REFERENCES

Ayres, S. M., Schlichtig, R., & Sterling, M. J. (1988). *Care of the critically ill* (3rd ed.). Chicago: Yearbook Medical Publishers.

Boggs, R. L., & Wooldridge-King, M. (1993). *AACN procedure manual for critical care (3rd ed.).* Philadelphia: W. B. Saunders.

Fein, I. A., & Strasberg, M. A. (1987). *Managing the critical care unit.* Rockville, MD: Aspen.

Kenner, C. A. (1992). *Nurse's clinical guide: Neonatal care.* Springhouse, PA: Springhouse Corporation.

Persons, C. G. (1987). *Critical care procedures and protocols.* Philadelphia: J. B. Lippincott.

Tobin, M. J. (1989). *Essentials of critical care medicine.* New York: Churchill Livingstone.

Willett, M. J., Patterson, M., & Steinbock B. (1986). *Manual of neonatal care nursing.* Boston: Little, Brown.

Zschoche, D. A. (Ed.). (1980). *Mosby's comprehensive review of critical care* (2nd ed.). St. Louis: C. V. Mosby.

CHAPTER

11

Oncology and Chemotherapy

This chapter defines terminology related to oncology and the treatment of malignancies. Cancer categories and staging of selected tumor sites are outlined. Emphasis is placed on cancers of the nervous system, the head and neck, and the aerodigestive tract. Malignancies and other neoplasms in these areas are of particular concern to the speech-language pathologist. A brief review of antineoplastic therapies, including chemotherapy, is provided. Cancer treatment with radiation oncology is discussed in Chapter 8.

I. TERMINOLOGY

Acoustic neuroma, acoustic schwannoma. Referring to a neurilemoma (tumor) of the eighth cranial nerve; a **facial schwannoma** involves the seventh cranial nerve. Schwannomas are neoplasms of the nerve sheath.

353

Adenocarcinoma. Malignant tumor of glandular epithelium, particularly the breast, bronchi, digestive tract, and endocrine glands; characterized by anaplasia and metastases.

Adenoma. Benign neoplasm arising from glandular tissue.

Adequate margins. Surgical excision of tumors with edges that are histologically free of tumor cells.

Alopecia. Hair loss.

Alpha-fetoprotein (AFP). An antigen tumor marker associated with testicular tumors, liver cancer, and stomach malignancies.

Anaplasia. Undifferentiated cells, often an indication of malignant growth.

Anemia. A condition characterized by a reduced number of erythrocytes and/or reduced hemoglobin in the circulating erythrocytes resulting in a reduction in tissue oxygenation.

Angioma, hemangioma. Benign tumor of the blood vessels.

Angiosarcoma, hemangiosarcoma. Malignant tumor of the blood vessels.

Anorexia. Loss of appetite or desire for food.

Antineoplastic. Anti-cancer.

Astrocytoma. Tumor arising from the star-shaped neuroglia cells, or astrocytes. The "benign" form of astrocytoma (Grade 1, 2) is slow growing but can invade large areas. The malignant type of astrocytoma is called **glioblastoma multiforme**.

Basal cell carcinoma. Ulcerative, nodular, or scarlike neoplasm of the skin, especially facial skin.

Benign. Nonmalignant, nonrecurrent, slow-growing tumors that are not (by their location and histopathology) usually a threat to life.

"Blasts." Referring to immature leukocytes.

Blood-brain barrier. Neurophysiologic mechanism preventing access of certain blood substances to brain tissue (see further discussion in Chapter 4).

Breast-cyst fluid proteins (BCFP). Antigens which may be associated with breast carcinoma.

Burkitt's lymphoma. A malignant tumor in children causing gross swelling of the jaw.

Cancer. A group of malignant diseases characterized by abnormal cell growth.

Carcinoembryonic antigen (CEA). Antigens that may be associated with gastric malignancies.

Carcinogen. A substance that stimulates the formation of malignancies.

Carcinolysis. Destruction of cancer cells.

Carcinoma. A malignant tumor of epithelial tissues.

Cardiac tamponade. A condition characterized by an accumulation of excess fluid in the pericardium, often associated with lung cancer.

Cellular immunity. A form of immunologic activity involving sensitized lymphocytes, or T-cells, which are produced in the thymus and stored in lymphoid tissue. After stimulation of an antigen, the sensitized lymphocytes are released into the blood to either destroy the antigen or prepare the antigen for destruction by macrophages.

Chalone. A glycoprotein that is thought to inhibit growth and proliferation of normal cells.

Chemodectoma, glomus jugulare tumors. Referring to tumors (composed of nests of epithelioid cells and nerve fibers in a highly vascular stroma) of the chemoreceptors located in the carotid body, aortic body, vagus nerve, glomus tympanicum, auricular and tympanic nerves, and the jugular bulb in the region of the jugular vein. Patients with these tumors are usually female in the fourth or fifth decade of life who present with deafness, tinnitus, vertigo, otorrhea, bleeding, otalgia, facial palsy, ear canal mass, and deficits of the IXth and XIIth cranial nerves. They may present with dysphagia and a pulsatile pharyngeal mass.

Chondroma. Benign neoplasm of cartilaginous tissue.

Chondrosarcoma. Malignant tumor of the cartilage cells.

Chordoma. Tumors arising from remnants of the embryonic notochord (the structure giving rise to the spinal cord during fetal development).

Choriocarcinoma. Malignant tumor of the uterus.

Craniopharyngioma. A benign, congenital tumor that is cystic in nature, which appears in the midline, suprasellar region with involvement of the third ventricle, optic nerve, and pituitary gland.

Cystadenocarcinoma. Malignant, cystic growth of the glandular epithelium, especially the ovaries, salivary glands, breast, and thyroid.

Cystadenoma. Benign, cystic growth of the glandular epithelium.

Debulking. The surgical removal of the majority, but not all, of a tumor.

Dermoid cyst, cystic teratoma. A congenital tumor appearing commonly in the midline, suprasellar area and considered a benign tumor.

Diffuse malignancies. Widespread or systemic cancers, such as leukemia, multiple myeloma, and forms of lymphoma.

Distant metastases. Cancer spread outside of the regional lymphatics.

Duke's criteria. A method for staging large bowel cancers.

Encapsulated. Enclosed in a sheath.

Ependymoma. Common childhood tumor appearing in the membranous lining of the posterior fossa and the cerebral ventricles. This tumor tends to be slow-growing and may be benign or malignant.

Epidermoid carcinoma. Carcinoma of the skin and mucosa.

Erythroplakia. Velvety red patches. Erythroplakia, leukoplakia, and ulcerative lesions may be gross indicators of squamous cell carcinoma of the mucous membranes.

Ewing's sarcoma. Bone cancer involving the long bones or pelvis.

Fibrosarcoma. Cancerous tumor of the collagen-producing fibroblasts.

Functioning tumor. Referring to a neoplasm, usually of an endocrine gland, capable of synthesizing and releasing hormones into the blood.

Fungating. Growing rapidly in a fungus-like manner.

Ganglioneuroblastoma. Malignant ganglioneuroma.

Ganglioneuroma. Benign tumor of the ganglionic cells and neuroblasts.

Gastrinoma, Wollinger-Ellison syndrome. A syndrome characterized by hypersecretion of gastric acid due to a gastrin-producing tumor.

Glatosyl transferase isoenzyme II (GTI-II). An antigen thought to be a tumor marker for malignancies of the stomach, colon, and pancreas.

Glioblastoma multiforme. A highly invasive, destructive form of malignant tumor involving the glia (supportive cells) of the neurons; *malignant astrocytoma.*

Glioma. A family of tumors of the supportive cells of the brain (glia).

Glucagonoma. Alpha cell tumors of the pancreas.

Growth factor. In tumor growth, referring to the ratio of proliferating to nonproliferating malignant cells.

Hairy cell leukemia. A form of lymphoid malignancy characterized by significant anemia, pancytopenia, and hairlike cytoplasmic projections in the blood and bone marrow.

Heavy chain disease. A plasmacytic-lymphocytic neoplasm causing infiltration of tissues by malignant cells, especially into the small intestine and peripheral lymphoid tissues.

Hemangiosarcoma. Cancerous tumor of the blood vessels.

Hodgkin's disease. Lymphoma occurring in young adults characterized by a painless, progressive enlargement of lymph nodes, spleen, and general lymphoid tissues.

Hospice. A concept of care for terminally ill persons in which the notion of *intensive caring* replaces *intensive care.* In hospice care, the family is considered the primary caregiver, and medical treatment is directed toward optimizing the quality of life, alleviating pain, and reducing helplessness.

Human chorionic gonadotropin (HCG). A placental antigen known to be a tumor marker for choriocarcinoma and possibly a marker for testicular cancer.

Human T-cell leukemia-lymphoma virus (HTLV). Virus known to cause cancer in humans.

Hygroma. A sac, cyst, or bursa containing fluid.

Hyperkeratosis. Abnormal, horny, irregular growth that can be the result of noncancerous diseases or a premalignant condition.

Hypernephroma. Malignant tumor of the kidney.

Hyperplasia. Excessive growth of normal cells.

Induction therapy. Intensive chemotherapy directed at putting a malignancy into remission.

Infiltrative. Cancerous tumor growing or extending into normal tissue.

In situ. Not invading adjacent tissues.

Insulinoma. Beta cell tumors of the pancreas.

Interstitial. Between a space.

Invasive. Spreading.

Kaposi's sarcoma. Malignant neoplasm characterized by soft, bluish nodules of the skin with hemorrhages and lymphadenopathy.

Karnowsky scale. The Karnowsky scale, or Karnowsky Scale Placement, is a scaled method for describing the condition and functional performance abilities of patients with cancer.

Leiomyoma. Benign neoplasm of smooth muscle.

Leiomyosarcoma. Malignant tumor of the smooth muscle.

Lesion. An injured or altered area of tissue.

Leukemias. Cancers of the blood-forming bodies causing excessive formation of leukocytes.

Leukoplakia. Well-defined, white patches on mucous membranes which may be due to a fungus infection, lichen planus, or other oral disease, or may be early carcinoma.

Lipoma. Benign neoplasm of the adipose (fat) tissues.

Liposarcoma. Cancerous tumor of the adipose (fat) tissues.

Low-grade tumors. Referring to the histopathologic grades of tumor cells in which cells are well-differentiated or at less advanced stages (Grade 1, Grade 2).

Lumpectomy. The surgical removal of a tumor mass and a small amount of surrounding tissue.

Lymphangioma. Benign tumor of the lymph vessels.

Lymphangiosarcoma. Malignant tumor of the lymph vessels.

Malignant. Bad; tumors that spread to other areas and may ultimately be life-threatening if untreated.

Medullary. Term referring to soft tissues, the medulla, or bone marrow.

Medulloblastoma. Cancerous tumor arising in the fourth ventricle and base of the cerebellum. This malignant tumor of the posterior fossa is usually fast-growing and more commonly occurs in children.

Melanoma. Malignant tumor usually arising from a black mole.

Meningioma. Benign tumor arising from the arachnoid covering of the brain. These tumors tend to be slow-growing and are usually encapsulated.

Metastasis. Process of cancer spreading to secondary sites.

Moribund. Near death.

Mucositis. Mucosal inflammation associated with radiation therapy.

Myeloma, multiple myeloma. Malignant tumor arising from the bone marrow.

Natural killer (NK) immunity. A form of immunologic activity not mediated by B- or T-cells, but probably a type of lymphocyte stimulated by viral injections. (Also see Chapter 6.)

Necrosis. Dead tissue.

Neoplasm. Abnormal new growth of tissue cells.

Nerve block. Injection of neurolytic agents to achieve anesthesia.

Neurectomy. Neurosurgical sectioning of the peripheral nerve to produce anesthesia.

Neurilemoma. Benign, encapsulated neoplasm arising from a peripheral nerve.

Neuroblastoma. A highly malignant tumor of the neuroblasts in the adrenal gland, sympathetic nerve chains, jaw, lip, and viscera; usually found in children.

Neurofibroma. Benign tumors of the peripheral nerve sheaths.

Neurofibrosarcoma. A malignant tumor of the peripheral nerve sheaths.

Nevus. Pigmented mole or malformation of the skin.

Non-Hodgkin's lymphoma. Referring to a heterogeneous group of lymphoid malignancies, several of which are possibly related to viral or immunodeficiency causes. Non-Hodgkin's Lymphomas occur uncommonly in children, and the average age of onset for non-Hodgkin's lymphoma in adults is later than that of Hodgkin's disease (after young adulthood). Non-Hodgkin's lymphoma in children usually involves the mediastinum and abdomen and the disease tends to be more diffuse and has more bone marrow spread than is typical for adults.

Oatcell carcinoma. Very malignant, undifferentiated *small cell tumor* of the lung.

Ogliodendroglioma. An uncommon brain tumor with a slow growth rate arising from the ogliodendrocytes.

Oncogenic. Causing the formation of a tumor.

Opsonin. Antibody.

Optic gliomas. Referring to tumors arising from the optic nerve or optic chiasm.

Osteoid osteoma. Benign tumor arising from fibrous bone tissue.

Osteosarcoma. Malignant tumor arising from fibrous bone tissue.

Paget's disease. An inflammatory disease sometimes seen at the onset of the development of bone cancer. Paget's disease is characterized by local areas of bone destruction with development of porous bone and deformities. Beethoven may have had this disease.

Pain trajectory. The direction or pattern of pain.

Palliative. Alleviating symptoms without curing the disease.

Pancreotic oncofetal antigen (POA). A fetal protein felt to be a marker for pancreatic cancer.

Pap smear. *Papanicolaou* (named for the originator of the test) *Smear Test*; a method for early detection of uterine and cervical cancer which involves swabbing cells from uterine and cervical mucosa for microscopic examination.

Pineal tumor. Rare brain tumors occurring mainly in males during adolescence through early adulthood. Pineal tumors are usually *germ cell* tumors categorized as *germinal, parenchymal,* or *glial*, depending on the cell type of origin. This tumor is difficult to approach surgically; thus radiotherapy and shunt procedures to relieve intracranial pressure are used.

Pituitary adenoma. Tumors involving the pituitary gland, occurring more often in young or middle-aged adults.

Polyp. Nonspecific reference to tissue growth, usually on mucous membranes. *Sessile* polyps are fixed and attached with a broad base. *Pedunculated polyps* are attached with a narrow stalk and are mobile.

Primary tumor. Original tumor.

Proliferation. Rapid growth.

Prostatic acid phosphatase (PAP). An enzyme marker for prostate cancer.

Prostatic-specific antigen (PSA). A tumor marker for prostate cancer.

Reed-Sternberg cells. A type of malignant cell associated with Hodgkin's disease.

Remission. State in which no signs or symptoms of a disease are apparent.

"Rescue" technique. Term often applied to radiation therapy or chemotherapy when surgery has failed to eradicate a malignant tumor.

Retinoblastoma. A relatively rare, highly malignant tumor of the retina, more often found in children than adults.

Rhabdomyoma. Benign tumor arising from skeletal (striated) muscle tissue.

Rhabdosarcoma. Malignant tumor of the striated muscle tissue.

Rhizotomy. Neurosurgery on the nerve root to provide anesthesia.

Sarcoma. Highly malignant tumor composed of connective tissue, such as muscle, fat, bone, and blood vessels.

Scirrhus. Term used to designate a hard tumor.

Secondary tumor. Tumor that has metastasized from a primary site.

Seminoma. Malignant testicular neoplasm.

Squamous cell carcinoma. Malignant neoplasm of the squamous epithelial cells of the skin, mucosal linings, salivary glands, larynx, lungs, bladder, and elsewhere.

Squamous papilloma. Benign neoplasm arising from squamous epithelia, characterized by a flat pavement-like appearance.

Staging. A method for classifying malignancies with reference to the size and location of the primary lesion, nodal involvement, and metastases.

Stomatitis. Inflammation of the mucosa of the mouth.

Substance P. A neuropeptide involved in the transmission of painful, noxious stimuli.

Sympathectomy. Neurosurgery performed on the peripheral sympathetic ganglion chain.

Tennessee antigen (TennGen). A glycoprotein tumor marker felt to be associated with colonrectal cancer.

Teratoma. A tumor containing types of embryonic tissues that are not normally found at the site of the neoplasm (vestiges of hair, teeth, bone, etc).

Thanatology. The study of death and the dying process.

Thymoma. Tumor of the thymus gland.

Tractotomy. Neurosurgery, performed through occipital craniotomy in which the spinothalamic tract is cut at the level of the mesencephalon.

Trismus. Difficulty or pain with mouth opening; may follow radiation therapy to the mouth and oral cavity.

Tumor burden. Referring to the ratio of tumor cells to normal cells in a patient's body.

Tumor doubling time (TDT). An estimation procedure used to determine the preclinical stages of certain cancers, such as breast cancer.

Tumoricidal. Destructive to tumors.

Tumor marker. Biologic activities that indicate progression or regression of tumors.

Undifferentiated, dedifferentiated, differentiated. Histopathologic description of the cellular state when there is an alteration of the specialization of cells due to neoplastic growth. In tumor grading, pathologists usually describe cellular states from tissue biopsies as *well-differentiated*, or **Grade 1** (indicating that the normal morphologic characteristics of malignant cells are maintained); *moderately differentiated*, or **Grade 2** (indicating that some morphologic changes have taken place); *poorly differentiated*, or **Grade 3** (indicating a near total lack of normal cell differentiation); and *undifferentiated*, or **Grade 4** (indicating that features of normal cell specialization from the tissues of origin cannot be determined).

Verrucous carcinoma. The clinical manifestation of slowly progressive, warty growths that are histopathologically well-differentiated (low-grade) squamous cell carcinoma.

Vesicant. A drug that causes extreme irritation if there is extravasation (spread outside of the blood vessel) into surrounding tissues.

Wilms' tumor. Cancerous tumor of the kidney found mainly in children.

Wound seeding. Referring to the inadvertent spread of cancer from biopsy methods or tumor dissemination during surgery or other invasive procedures that might dislodge tumor cells into the blood or lymphatic circulation.

Xerostomia. Dry mouth.

Zinc glycinate marker (ZGM). An antigen thought to be associated with gastrointestinal malignancies.

II. ABBREVIATIONS

ACS. American Cancer Society

ACTH. Adrenocorticotropic hormone

Adeno CA. Adenocarcinoma

ADH. Antidiuretic hormone

AFP. Alpha fetoprotein

AJCC. American Joint Committee on Cancer

ALL. Acute lymphocytic leukemia

AML. Acute myelogenous leukemia

ANLL. Acute nonlymphytic leukemia

Astro. Astrocyte (star-shaped cell)

BhCG. Beta human chronic gonadotropin

Bx. Biopsy

CA. Cancer, carcinoma

chemo. Chemotherapy

CI. Continuous infusion

CIS. Carcinoma *in situ*

CML. Chronic myelogenous leukemia

CR. Complete remission

CS. Clinical stage

DNA. Deoxyribonucleic acid

5-FU. 5-fluorouracil

G. Grade

HD. Hodgkin's disease

HTLV. Human T-cell leukemia-lymphoma virus

IL-2. Interleukin-2

IUAC. International Union Against Cancer

LAK. Lymphokine-activated killer (cells)

MEN. Multiple endocrine neoplasia

Mets. Metastases

MUO. Metastasis of unknown origin

N. Node

NED. No evidence of disease

NGF. Nerve growth factor

NSD. Nominal single dose

PS. Pathologic state

RNA. Ribonucleic acid

SCCA. Squamous cell carcinoma

SI, SII, SIII, and so on. Stage one, two, three (etc.)

SIADH. Syndrome of inappropriate antidiuretic hormone secretion

TAA. Tumor associated antigens

Tis. Tumor *in situ*

TNF. Tumor necrosis factor

TNJ. Tongue, neck, jaw

TNM. Tumor, node, metastases

T0. No evidence of primary tumor

TX. Primary tumor cannot be assessed

III. CLASSIFICATION AND STAGING OF CANCER

The American Joint Committee on Cancer (AJCC) and the international Union Against Cancer (IUAC) have jointly developed a system for classifying and staging cancers which is internationally endorsed and applied in the field of Oncology. These classifications and stages are specific to particular region sites and malignancy types. For example, there is no staging system for some cancers, such as cancer of the pinna, external auditory canal, middle ear, and inner ear; and lymph node classifications do not apply to staging of brain tumors.

Certain types (solid tumors and lymphomas) and sites of cancer are staged based on **TNM,** or **tumor, node,** and **metastasis** status categories. Various qualifiers are applied to refine the TNM categories further. These include lowercase letter qualifiers applied to the TNM staging numbers. For example, clinical diagnostic staging of patients who have had biopsies but no treatment may be designated as *cTNM*. Post operative staging may be designated as *pTNM*. Staging at the time of retreatment for recurrent cancer may be designated as *rTNM*, and staging at the time of autopsy may be designated as *aTNM*. Pathologic classification of regional nodes, done from resected tissue samples, is indicated as *pN*; and additional qualifiers (pNa, pNb, pNbi, pNbii, etc.) will be used to denote the size of the nodal metastases. The TNM classification scores are made to determine the stages of cancer for a given tumor type and site, as this is critical to a determination of the prognosis and treatment choices. Lesion size is usually discussed as the most critical factor; however, for some sites, categorization and staging of the primary tumor depend on the extent of involvement of particular structures rather than the size of the lesion per se. The following section describes staging methods with head and neck cancer. Consult the *Manual for Staging Cancer* (3rd edition) for further elaboration and criteria for staging other sites.

A. Lymph Node Classification

N0. No regional lymph node metastasis.

N1. Metastasis in a single ipsilateral lymph node, 3 cm or less in dimension.

N2a. Metastasis in a single ipsilateral lymph node, more than 3 cm but not more than 6 cm in greatest dimension.

N2b. Metastases in multiple ipsilateral lymph nodes, none more than 6 cm in greatest dimension.

N2c. Metastases in bilateral or contralateral lymph nodes, none more than 6 cm in greatest dimension.

N3. Metastasis in a lymph node, more than 6 cm in greatest dimension.

B. Distant Metastases

M0. No known distant metastasis.

M1. Distant metastasis present.

C. Lymphoma (Hodgkin's and NonHodgkin's) Classification

Stage I. Limited to one area.

Stage II. Involvement of two or more areas on the same side of the diaphragm.

Stage III. Involvement of two or more areas on both sides of the diaphragm.

D. Primary Laryngeal Tumors

1. Supraglottal

TX. Primary tumor cannot be assessed.

Tis. Carcinoma *in situ.*

T0. No evidence of tumor.

T1. Normal cord movement, tumor limited to supraglottal larynx.

T2. Tumor involving adjacent supraglottic sites without glottic fixation.

T3. Tumor limited to larynx with fixation and/or extension to the precricoid area, medial wall of the pyriform sinus, or pre-epiglottic space.

T4. Massive tumor extending beyond the larynx to involve the oropharynx, soft tissues of the neck, or destruction of the thyroid cartilage.

2. Glottal

TX. Primary tumor cannot be assessed.

Tis. Carcinoma *in situ.*

T0. No evidence of tumor.

T1. Tumor confined to the vocal fold with mobility preserved at the anterior and posterior commissures.

T2. Supraglottic and/or subglottic extension of tumor, with normal or impaired cord mobility.

T3. Tumor confined to the larynx with fixation of the cords.

T4. Massive tumor with thyroid cartilage destruction and/or extension beyond the laryngeal confines.

3. Subglottal

TX. Primary tumor cannot be assessed.

Tis. Carcinoma *in situ.*

T0. No evidence of tumor.

T1. Tumor confined to subglottic region.

T2. Tumor extending to the vocal folds with normal or impaired movement.

T3. Tumor confined to the larynx with vocal fold fixation.

T4. Massive tumor with cartilage destruction, extension beyond the laryngeal confines, or both.

E. Primary Oropharyngeal Tumors

TX. Primary tumor cannot be assessed.

Tis. Carcinoma *in situ.*

T0. No evidence of tumor.

T1. Tumor 2 cm or less in greatest dimension.

T2. Tumor more than 2 cm but not more than 4 cm in greatest dimension.

T3. Tumor more than 4 cm in greatest dimension.

T4. Massive tumor invading adjacent structures (cortical bone, extrinsic tongue muscles, maxillary sinus, skin).

F. Staging

Tis. Carcinoma *in situ.*

Stage I. Tl, N0, M0.

Stage II. T2, N0, M0.

Stage III. T3, N0, M0; Tl, T2 or T3, N1, M0.

Stage IV. T4, N0 or N1, M0; any T, N2 or N3, M0; any T, any N, M1.

IV. STAGING BRAIN TUMORS

A. Primary Tumors

TX. Primary tumor cannot be assessed.

T0. No evidence of primary tumor.

1. Supratentorial Tumors

T1. Tumor is 5 cm or less in greatest dimension and limited to one side.

T2. Tumor is more than 5 cm in greatest dimension and limited to one side.

T3. Tumor invades or encroaches on the ventricular system.

T4. Tumor crosses the midline and invades the opposite side or invades infratentorially.

2. Infratentorial Tumors

T1. Tumor 3 cm or less in greatest dimension.

T2. Tumor more than 3 cm in greatest dimension and limited to one side.

T3. Tumor invades or encroaches on ventricular system.

T4. Tumor crosses the midline, invades the opposite side, or invades supratentorially.

B. Distant Metastases

MX. Presence of distant metastasis cannot be assessed.

M0. No evidence of distant metastasis.

M1. Distant metastasis is present.

C. Histopathologic Grade

Roman numerals are also used (e.g. G I).

GX. Grade cannot be assessed.

G1. Well-differentiated.

G2. Moderately well-differentiated.

G3. Poorly differentiated.

G4. Undifferentiated.

D. Staging

Stage IA. Gl, Tl, M0.

Stage IB. Gl, T2, M0; Gl, T2, M0.

Stage IIA. G2, Tl, M0.

Stage IIB. G2, Tl, M0; G2, T3, M0.

Stage IIIA. G3, Tl, M0.

Stage IIIB. G3, T2, M0; G3, T3, M0.

Stage IV. Gl, 2, 3, T4, M0; G4, any T, M0; any G, any T, M1.

V. CHEMOTHERAPY AND OTHER ANTINEOPLASTIC THERAPIES

A. Chemotherapy

Chemotherapy uses chemical agents and drugs to combat disease in anticancer therapies. At this time, there are approximately 40 drugs that have been approved as anticancer agents in the United States. These agents are selected to direct **antineoplastic effects** on certain malignant cells, but there will necessarily be toxic effects on normal cells as well. The normal tissues that are most susceptible to the toxic effects of antineoplastic agents are those that reproduce rapidly, such as hair follicles, cells lining the gastrointestinal tract and cells in the bone marrow, which is why people lose hair, feel ill, and are susceptible to infection while undergoing chemotherapy.

Cell-cycle dependent chemotherapy refers to antineoplastic drugs that have an effect on cells only at a particular stage of reproduction. **Cell-cycle independent** chemotherapy refers to antineoplastic drugs that exert anticancer effects at any stage of cellular reproduction. Chemotherapy is the treatment of choice in disseminated malignancies, such as leukemia. The advent of antineoplastic agents has dramatically changed cancer survival rates for a number of malignancy types.

Chemotherapy is used in conjunction with other therapies and as a palliative therapy for certain localized tumors that cannot be adequately treated with surgery or radiation therapy. **Combined-modality therapy**, or **adjuvant** therapy, refers to the use of chemotherapy following the completion of local therapy (surgery or radiation therapy). **Combination chemotherapy** refers to the simultaneous or sequenced use of two or more drugs to treat a particular cancer.

Forms of chemotherapy include *antimetabolites, hormone and hormone antagonists, alkylating agents, vinca ankaloids,* and *antibiotics*.

Antimetabolites. Referring to substances that interfere with the metabolic processes for manufacturing protein in the cells. Antimetabolite drugs include 5-fluorouracil (5-FU); methotrexate (MTX); 6-mercaptopurine; cytosine arabinoside (Cytarabine, Ara-C, Cytosar); and 6-thioguanine (6-TG).

Hormone and hormone antagonists. Referring to the use of endocrine manipulation as a therapy for neoplastic disease by influencing RNA-to-protein synthesis. Androgens are used to treat breast cancer. Estrogen is used to treat prostate and breast cancers. Adrenocortical hormones are used to treat leukemia, and progestines are used to treat endometrial, renal, breast, and prostatic cancers. Antiestrogens, such as tomoxifen citrate (Novadex), are used for metastatic breast carcinoma.

Alkylating agents. Referring to compounds that have the ability to produce breaks in DNA as well as cross-linking the strands to interfere with reduplication of DNA and transcription of RNA effectively. Such agents are a class of cell-cycle nonspecific antineoplastic drugs. Alkylating agents, such as cis-platinum (Platinol), nitrogen mustard, chlorambucil (Leukeran), busulfan (Myeleran), thio-TEPA (Triethylene Thiophosphoramide), melphalan, and cyclophosphamide (Cytoxan) are used in the treatment of leukemia, lymphomas, and other disseminated malignancies. Semustine (methyl-CCNU) is an oral alkylating agent that crosses the blood-brain barrier and may be used to treat brain tumors.

Vinca alkaloid antineoplastic drugs. Referring to anticancer drugs made from substances in the periwinkle plant that inhibit the formation of protein structures necessary for DNA activity and interfere with cell division. These agents may be used in the treatment of Hodgkin's disease, neuroblastoma, Wilms' tumor, sarcomas, and acute lymphoblastic leukemia. Vinca alkaloid agents include vincristine (Oncovin), vinblastine (Velban), and vindesine.

Antibiotics. Certain antibiotics stimulate natural processes that interfere with DNA and RNA synthesis. These drugs include streptozotocin, mitomycin-C (Mutamycin), mithramycin (Mithracin), bleomucin (Blenoxane), dactinomycin (Actinomycin-D), doxorubicin (Adriamycin), and daunorubicin (Daunomycin).

B. Immunotherapy

Immunotherapy uses certain antigens to stimulate the host's immune response and resistance to specific cancers. Immunotherapy is usually described as **active specific** (the use of agents to produce a specific host-immune response), **nonspecific** (the use of agents to produce a generalized immune reaction), and **passive** (the use of agents from an immunocompetent donor to elicit an immune response in the recipient).

C. Biologic Response Modifiers

Genetically engineered immunotherapeutic drugs are used to treat certain types of cancer. Interleukin-2 (IL2) stimulates an immune system to produce lymphokine-activated killer (LAK) cells. Recombinant interferon is felt to strengthen the immune system and has been used efficaciously with hairy cell leukemia. These drugs are known to produce behavioral and cognitive changes, delusion, and hallucinations.

D. Hyperthermia

A treatment termed "selective tumor heating," or hyperthermia, uses ultrasound, microwaves, radio frequency waves, induction coils, and magnet loops for direct **tumoricidal** therapy. Regional hyperthermia is sometimes used to treat cancers in the extremities by perfusion with prewarmed blood. Whole body hyperthermia (raising the body temperature to 108° F) is felt to enhance the effect of other therapies. Hyperthermia is nearly always combined with another cancer therapy, usually chemotherapy.

E. Photodynamic Therapy

The systemic administration of hematoporphyrin dye followed by red laser light exposure to specific sites has been used for treatment of certain cancers, such as recurrent breast cancer and certain skin cancers.

F. Bone Marrow Transplants

Bone marrow transplantation is an effective treatment for certain types of malignancies. Bone marrow transplants allow other therapies to be escalated to more effective levels and can, thus, increase sensitivity to other therapies. The three major categories of bone marrow transplantation are **syngeneic transplants** (between genetically identical twins), **allogenic transplants** (from a non-twin donor), and **autologous transplants** (from the patient's own harvested bone marrow). The efficacy of bone marrow transplants has been established in treating acute myelogenous leukemia, acute lymphoblastic leukemia, chronic myelogenous leukemia, lymphoma, Hodgkin's disease, and neuroblastoma. Bone marrow transplants may also have some benefit for oat cell carcinoma, breast carcinoma, Ewing's sarcoma, and glioblastoma multiforme.

VI. NOTES

_____

_____

_____

_____

_____

_____

_____

_____

NOTES *(continued)*

_____

_____

_____

_____

_____

_____

_____

_____

_____

_____

VII. REFERENCES

Beahrs, O. H., Henson, D. E., Hutter, R. V. P., & Myers, M. H. (Eds.). (1988). *Manual for staging of cancer* (3rd ed.). Philadelphia: J. B. Lippincott.

Friedman, M. (Ed.). (1986). Nonsquamous tumors of the head and neck: I. *The Otolaryngologic Clinics of North America* (Vol. 19). Philadelphia: W. B. Saunders.

Gomella, L. G. (Ed.). (1993). *Clinician's pocket reference*. (7th ed.). Norwalk, CT: Appleton & Lange.

McIntire, S. N., & Cioppa, A. L. (Eds.). (1984). *Cancer nursing*. New York: John Wiley & Sons.

Rice, D. H., & Spiro, R. H. (1989). *Current concepts in head and neck cancer.* New York: The American Cancer Society.

Shapshay, S. M., & Ossoff, R. H. (Eds.). (1985). Squamous cell cancer of the head and neck. *The Otolaryngologic Clinics of North America* (Vol. 18). Philadelphia: W. B. Saunders.

Snyder, C. C. (1986). *Oncology nursing*. Boston: Little, Brown.

CHAPTER

12

Surgeries and
Other Procedures

Surgeries involving the oral, pharyngeal, and laryngeal structures are likely to result in changes in speech or swallowing which require attention from a speech-language pathologist. Neurologic, cardiothoracic, and vascular surgeries are frequent features in the histories of patients with neurogenic speech, language, and swallowing disorders. This chapter reviews terminology and abbreviations that may be encountered as a part of the patient's surgical history or in summary reports of an operation procedure ("op. reports"). This chapter also provides brief descriptions of some of the more common surgeries as well as other procedures usually performed by surgeons. Collaborative therapies for cancer surgeries are described in Chapter 11, and terminology related to rehabilitation is found in Appendix B.

I. TERMINOLOGY USED IN SURGICAL PROCEDURES

Abscess. Localized area of pus.

Abdominal pad. Drainage dressing used over large abdominal suture sites.

Abdominal tray. Instruments and supplies for abdominal surgeries.

Absorbable suture. Temporary suture (surgical "thread") that is absorbed in the body.

Administration set. Devices and materials used to deliver or dispense fluids (e.g., intravenous fluid administration set).

Amputation. Removal of a limb or body appendage.

Anastomosis. Joining two tubular or hollow organs; for example, coronary artery bypass grafts involve anastomoses of heart vessels.

Anesthesia. Complete or partial loss of feeling and/or consciousness resulting from administration of an anesthetic agent or from disease or injury.

Approach. Referring to the method used and the route taken to reach a body structure in surgery.

Approximate. Bringing tissues together by suturing or other means.

Atraumatic. In surgery, techniques causing little tissue trauma.

Bed specs. Graduated plastic or metal containers for measuring urine output.

Bifurcated. Y-shaped.

Biopsy needle. Hollow needle used to extract tissue samples.

Bistoury. A slender surgical knife, used most frequently to open an abscess.

Bladder irrigation. Washing of the urinary bladder with a solution.

Bleeder. Severed blood vessel.

Blood administration set. Tubing and devices used to dispense whole blood to the patient.

Blood gas tray. Equipment used to measure oxygen and carbon dioxide levels in the blood.

Blunt dissection. Use of a sponge or blunt instrument to separate tissues.

Body restraint. Belts, bands, or vests used to immobilize a patient.

Bougienage dilation. Stretching and expanding a tubular structure with bougies (flexible tubes of increasing sizes), done often in cases of esophageal stricture.

Brown and Sharp (B & S) sizing. System for sizing stainless steel suture.

Brushing. Removing debris from a hollow organ or tube by means of a brush and basket.

Burr. A round instrument used for cutting holes into bone.

Butterfly bandaids. Adhesive bandages cut in a butterfly shape.

Butterfly infusion set. Scalp vein set with intravenous catheter and tubing used for intravenous fluid administration with children and infants.

Cadaver. Referring to a dead body or the tissues and organs harvested from a dead body.

Cannula. Inner lining within a hollow tube, such as a tracheostomy tube; tube used to aid in insertion of a drain or to inject medication.

Catgut. Suture material made from the intestines of sheep; it is eventually absorbed into the body.

Catheterization. Introduction of a flexible tube to inject fluids into or drain fluids from the body.

Cautery. Destroying tissue by heat, electricity, or caustic chemicals.

Cavitron. A motorized scalpel that cuts through delicate flesh, but leaves blood vessels and ductal tissues intact; used in brain and liver surgeries.

Chest stripper. Instrument used to remove tissues from ribs.

Chest trocar, thoracic trocar. Large handled, sharp instrument with a triangular tip.

Chux. Absorbent underpads used with incontinent patients.

Cisternal puncture. Spinal puncture of the cervical vertebrae.

Clip remover. Instrument used to remove surgical staples from wounds.

Closure. The suturing of a wound.

Clyster. An enema.

Compound F tray. Instruments and supplies used to remove fluid from a joint.

Connecting tube. Plastic or rubber devices used to connect drainage tubes, catheters, pumps, and air supplies.

Conscious sedation. A minimally depressed level of consciousness in which the patient retains the ability to respond to physical and/or verbal stimulation and maintains protective (swallow, cough) reflexes.

Cryosurgery. Surgery using methods to destroy tissue by extreme cold.

Currette. A spoon-like instrument used to scrape away diseased tissues and growths.

Cutdown. Surgery to expose a vein.

Cutdown tray. Instruments and supplies used to perform a venous cutdown.

Cystectomy. Removal of a cyst.

Debridement. Removal of dead and/or diseased tissue.

Deep sedation. A controlled state of depressed consciousness or unconsciousness in which there may be a partial or complete loss of protective reflexes and purposeful response to physical and/or verbal stimulation and from which the patient is not easily aroused.

Dehiscence. Splitting or opening wound.

Desiccation. Drying out (of tissues).

Detritus. Dead epithelial tissue, such as that sloughed from the surface of the skin.

Dilator. Instrument used to expand a hollow organ.

Dissection. Separating tissues.

Divinyl ether. An inhaled anesthetic agent.

Drainage bag. Plastic bag with tubing connectors used to collect urine from indwelling catheters.

Dressing. External covering or bandage for a wound.

Electrocoagulation. The use of electrical current to produce coagulation and wound closure.

Emerson suction pump. Three bottle suction apparatus used for withdrawing fluid from the chest.

Emesis basin. Kidney-shaped container for collecting vomitus or other secretions.

Epistaxis tray. Instruments and supplies to control nasal hemorrhages.

Ethyl chloride. A local anesthesia that freezes the tissues it contacts.

Evacuation. Removal of drainage from a natural passage.

Eviscerate. In surgery, splitting open a surgical wound and removing, or spilling out, its contents. Evisceration also refers to the opening of the abdomen to remove or pull out the intestines.

Excision. Removal of a piece of tissue.

Exploration. Surgical opening to examine internal organs.

Fenestrated. Having openings.

Finger cot. Small rubber or plastic shield used to protect a finger or a wound from soil or infection.

Flatus bag. Plastic tubing attached to a bag inserted to remove gas from the colon.

Fluffs. Pressure dressings for post-operative wound coverings with certain surgeries, such as hemorrhoidectomies and thyroidectomies.

Fowler's position. Position in which the patient is sitting in a reclined posture with head raised by about 20 inches to aid in draining fluids from the peritoneum or as a preferred positioning for endotracheal suctioning.

Fracture. Breaking a bone. A *compound fracture* refers to a fracture that penetrates adjacent soft tissue; *open fractures* penetrate the skin; *greenstick fractures* are partial breaks in bone; *comminuted fractures* refer to bone splintered into many fragments; *impacted fractures* refer to bones that have penetrated other bone; *spiral fractures* are bones twisted apart in a spiral pattern; *transverse fractures* have fracture lines perpendicular to the length of the bone; and *pathologic fractures* are bone breaks caused by disease rather than injury.

French catheter scale. A scaled method of measurement in which "1" equals ⅓ mm diameter and each incremental size increase is increased by ⅓ mm (e.g., #2 French equals ⅔ mm diameter, #3 French equals 1 mm, etc.).

Friable. Tissue that is easily torn.

Frozen section. Process by which a piece of tissue is frozen for microscopic examination; tissue analysis is often done during the surgery to provide a diagnosis before closure.

Furacin pads. Gauze dressings soaked in antibacterial ointment.

Gastric connecting tubing. Flexible tubing used to connect nasogastric tubing with a suction machine.

Gelfilm. Trademarked name for a gelatin film used to stop local bleeding.

Gelfoam. Trademarked name for a product used to stop bleeding.

General anesthesia. A controlled state of unconsciousness accompanied by a loss of protective reflexes and purposeful response to physical or verbal stimulation.

Graduate. Container with graduated markings used for liquid measurements.

Graft. Transplanting tissue from a donor or from one part of the body to another.

Hagedorn needle. A surgical needle with a cutting edge, used to sew up skin and as a finger-pricking needle used to draw blood.

Halo brace. Halo ring with brace suprastructure used to immobilize the neck of a patient with a high spinal cord injury.

Head halter. Device made of foam rubber and cotton used to secure head positioning for cervical traction.

Hemostat. A device or agent that stops the flow of blood.

Hot pack. Moist, hot dressing.

Huck towels. Specially woven towels used to dry hands after a surgical scrub or for surgical draping and to absorb fluids during surgery.

Hypodermic. Below the skin.

Incision. A cut into soft tissue with a sharp instrument.

Infusion. Introduction of fluid into a vein.

Intracatheter. Narrow tubing inserted into a vein for infusion of fluids, injection, or venous pressure monitoring.

Iodoform. Iodine compound used as an antiseptic.

Irrigation. Cleansing of a body cavity, surface, or wound with a stream of fluid solution or water.

Jackson tracheostomy tubes. Variable-sized silver, stainless steel, or silver-plated tracheostomy tubes.

Javid shunt. Trademarked name for a type of plastic tubing used to bypass, temporarily, the carotid artery during carotid endarterectomy.

Kelly forceps. Forceps with scissor-like handles used as hemostats to stop blood flow.

Kerlix bandage. A soft, woven rolled bandage.

Lancet. A surgical knife used for puncturing.

Laparotomy. Opening used for freeing adhesions and/or exploring the abdomen.

Leg bag. Drainage bag for urinary catheter that is attached to the leg with two rubber straps.

Lidocaine. A local anesthesic agent.

Ligate. To tie something together.

Ligation clips. Special metal clips placed around a structure to ligate vessels, nerves, or ducts.

Local anesthesia. A limited loss of sensation.

Logan bow. External metal loop used to close skin and reduce tension on deep muscles and fascia.

Loupes. Magnifying lenses used by the surgeon during microsurgery; may be fitted to glasses.

Lumen. The channel or opening into a tubular or other hollow structure.

Lumpectomy. Removal of a tumor or other mass.

Malecot catheter. Wing-tipped catheter used for fluid drainage from the body cavities.

Mask. Facial covering.

Microtome. A laboratory device used to slice thin sections of tissue for examination under a microscope.

Nasal cannula. Plastic tubing with a nose piece used to administer oxygen through the nose.

Nasal speculum. Instrument used to expand or dilate the nares.

Necrotic. Dead tissue.

Nidus. Point where a pathologic lesion has developed.

Nitrous oxide. The anesthetic gas used for light anesthesia, known as "laughing gas."

Operative monitoring. During surgeries, there is continuous monitoring of heart rate, respiratory rate, and blood pressure as well as visual monitoring of the patient's color every 5 minutes.

Osteoclasis. The deliberate rebreaking of a bone to more accurately set alignment.

Osteophyte. Bony outgrowth.

Osteotome. A surgical bone chisel.

Paracentesis. Puncture and drainage of a body cavity.

Penrose drain. A rubber tube with a gauze center inserted into a wound to drain fluids; *cigarette drain.*

Pentothal. An intravenous anesthetic agent.

Percutaneous needle biopsy. A procedure usually done under fluoroscopy in which a biopsy needle is inserted through a small incision, and cells are aspirated for analysis.

Phantom limb pain. Sensation sometimes following amputations in which pain from the missing limb is felt as if the limb were still there.

Pipette. A calibrated, open-ended glass tube used to measure or transfer small volumes of fluids.

Pledget. Small compress of gauze, such as a "2 × 2" or "4 × 4" gauze square.

Politzer's bag. A device used to inflate the middle ear.

Prosthesis. An artificial body part.

Radiosurgery. Using radium in surgical treatment.

Ratchets. Interlocking clasps that hold the finger rings of an instrument together (such as the clasps found on a hemostat).

Resection. Cutting off; removal of all or part of an organ or structure.

Robinson catheter. A round-tipped, double-ported plastic or rubber tube used for wound drainage or aspirating fluids.

Rongeur. A pliers-like instrument with sharp edges.

Scalp vein needle. An intravenous catheter used to administer fluids to infants.

Scalpel blade. A thin, disposable blade that attaches to a scapel handle.

Section. Cutting through a structure.

Serrated. Referring to a notched or saw-toothed margin.

Sheepskin. Fleece pad used to reduce risks for pressure sores in immobile patients.

Skin bond cement. Adhesive paste used to attach prostheses or stomal bags to the skin.

Snare. An instrument fitted with a wire loop used to snare and sever a tumor or polyp.

Sponge. Gauze pad.

Staples. Fine stainless steel surgical wires formed into a "B" shape when inserted through the skin; used to approximate surfaces.

Stents and keels. Silastic or Teflon devices used to fix tissues into place to prevent closures. Stents may be used to keep fistulae open, when desirable; and keels may be used to prevent re-formation of webs after glottic webs have been sectioned or excised.

Stereotaxis. The use of a three-dimensional apparatus to precisely locate structures.

Sterile tape. Paper tapes that are adhesive on one side; used to approximate edges of skin wounds.

Stilet, stylet. Sharp instrument used to probe or to guide catheters during insertion.

Stryker frame. Positioning frame; trademarked name for an apparatus used to move and position patients.

Suppuration. Pus formation in infected tissue.

Suture. To sew up a wound, also the thread or wire used to sew up a wound.

Swab. Small pledget, or gauze pad.

Tamponade. Stopping blood flow by pressure.

T.B.C. syringe. Referring to a tuberculin calibrated syringe.

T-drain. Small tubing used especially for bile drainage following gall bladder surgery.

Telfa. Trademarked name for absorbent, nonadherent dressings used on burns and superficial wounds.

Tenaculum. A tongs-like instrument used to hold a body part during surgery.

Tissue forceps. Fine-tipped, tweezer-like instrument used to grasp tissue.

Tracheostomy ties. Twill tape used to secure tracheostomy tubes.

Triage. System used to classify emergencies by the severity of the injury or illness.

II. ABBREVIATIONS

AB. Abortion

A.B. Ace bandage

AE, BE. Above the elbow, below the elbow

AKA, BKA. Above the knee amputation; below the knee amputation

A & O, A & T. Alert and oriented, awake and talking

ASD. Atrial septal defect

ASU, DSC. Ambulatory Surgery Unit, Day Surgery Center

AVF. Ateriovenous fistula

AVM. Arteriovenous malformation

AVR. Aortic valve replacement

AXR. Abdominal X ray

BLE, BUE. Both lower extremities, both upper extremities

Bleph. Blepharoplasty

BND. Bilateral neck dissection

BOT. Base of tongue

BT. Bladder tumor

BTL. Bilateral tubal ligation

BTS. Brain tumor suspect

BVL. Bilateral vas ligation

Bx. Biopsy

C1, C2, and so on. Cervical (spinal nerve) 1, 2, etc.

CAB. Coronary artery bypass

CABG × 2, 3, 4, 5, 6. Coronary artery bypass graft times (involving) 2, 3, 4, 5, or 6 vessels

Cath. Catheter

CDH. Congenital dislocation of the hip

CEA. Carotid endarterectomy

CHI. Closed head injury

CIS. Carcinoma *in situ*

cm. Centimeter

CMB. Carbolic methylene blue

C & P. Cystoscopy and panendoscopy

CPB. Cardiopulmonary bypass

CT. Connective tissue

CU. Cystourethrocele

CVL. Central venous line

DD. Dry dressing

D & C. Dilation and curettage

D & E. Dilation and evacuation

DISH. Diffuse idiopathic skeletal hypertrophy

DMFT. Decayed, missing, and filled teeth

DNS. Deviated nasal septum

DSD. Dry sterile dressing

E.N.T., E.E.N.T. Ear, nose, and throat; eye, ear, nose, and throat

ET. Endotracheal tube

FB. Foreign body

FD. Fully dilated

FOM. Floor of mouth

FP. Floor procedure

fr. French (measurement scale for catheters)

FTSG. Full thickness skin graft

FX. Fracture

GB. Gall bladder

G-tube. Gastrostomy tube

G-View. Gastraview (x-ray study)

HNP. Herniated nucleus proposus (spinal disk)

HNV. Has not voided

HOB. Head of bed

I & D. Incision and drainage

Irrig. Irrigate

J.P. Jackson-Pratt (type of drainage tube)

L.A. Local anesthesia

Lap. Laparotomy

Lx. Larynx

MT. Multiple trauma

MVA. Motor vehicle accident

MVP. Mitral valve prolapse

NAI. No acute infiltration

neg. Negative

NKA. No known allergies

N/T, N-T. Nasotracheal

N & T. Nose and throat

NWB. Nonweight bearing

OC. Oral cavity

OG, SGT. Operative gastrostomy, surgically placed gastrostomy tube

OP. Oropharynx

Ortho. Orthopedics

Panendo. Panendoscopy

Path. Pathology

P.B. Piggyback

PDA. Patent ductus arteriosus

PEG, PEJ. Percutaneous endoscopic gastrostomy, percutaneous endoscopic jejunostomy

Perf. Perforation

PMVA. Pedestrian (in a) motor vehicle accident

PORP. Partial ossicular replacement prosthesis

PSD. Post surgical day

PTCA. Percutaneous transluminal coronary angioplasty/angiogram

PTFE. Polytetrafluoroethylene (Teflon)

RND. Radical neck dissection

SAH. Subarachnoid hemorrhage

SBD. Straight bag drain

SBO. Small bowel obstruction

SCCA. Squamous cell carcinoma

SDH. Subdural hemorrhage

S Hx. Surgical history

SICU. Surgical Intensive Care Unit

SOD. Surgical officer of the day

S/P. Status post

Sq. Squamous

SR. Suture removal, staple removal

STSG. Split thickness skin graft

TBI. Traumatic brain injury

TCC. Transitional cell tumor

T.E. Transesophageal

TEF. Tracheoesophageal fistula

TEP. Tracheoesophageal puncture

THA. Total hip arthroplasty

THR. Total hip replacement

TKA. Total knee arthroplasty

TKR. Total knee replacement

TM. Tympanic membrane

TMJ. Temporomandibular joint

TNJ. Tongue, neck, jaw

TNM. Tumor, node, metastasis

TOAA. To all affected areas

Top. Topical

TORP. Total ossicular replacement prosthesis

TPC. Total proctocolectomy

Trach. Tracheostomy, tracheotomy

TRB. Transrectal biopsy

TSR. Total shoulder replacement

TUR. Transurethral resection

TURB. Transurethral resection of the bladder

TURP. Transurethral resection of the prostate

WD. Wet dressing

Z-plasty. Z-shaped incision (in plastic surgery)

III. COMMON SURGERIES AND PROCEDURES

A. Head and Neck Surgeries and Procedures

Also see Section H.

Adenectomy. Removal of a gland.

Adenotonsillectomy. Removal of the pharyngeal lymphatic tissue (adenoids) and the lymphatic tissue of the fauces (palatine and lingual tonsils).

Arytenoidectomy. Removal of an arytenoid.

Arytenoid-epiglottic flap. Procedure to close off the entrance to the larynx by folding the epiglottis posteriorly and suturing it to the arytenoid cartilage to prevent aspiration.

Arytenoid rotation. Repositioning of the arytenoid, usually following traumatic dislocation.

Atticotomy. Surgical opening into the attic of the middle ear.

Botulinum toxin injection. Needle injection of botulism, a neurotoxin into muscles with electromyographic guidance; usually done for treatment of certain facial, neck and laryngeal dystonia.

Cheiloplasty. Plastic surgical repair of the lip.

Cheilostomatoplasty. Plastic surgical repair of the lip and mouth, as in cleft lip repairs.

Cochlear implantation. A surgical technique in which a hole is drilled into the mastoid bone (specific approach is called a *facial recess approach*) into the middle ear space to get access to the round window. Electrodes are then threaded into the round window opening to provide direct stimulation of the cochlea from a receiver which has been secured into the temporal (mastoid) bone.

Cordectomy. Removal of a vocal fold.

Cricopharyngeal myotomy. Surgical dissection of the cricopharyngeous muscle to cause a relaxation of the upper esophageal sphincter in an effort to discourage recurrence of a Zenker's diverticulum, to treat chronic aspiration and vocal fold paralysis, and to improve alaryngeal voice with the tracheo-esophageal fistula voice prostheses.

Dilatation of the larynx. Stretching the laryngeal structures with instruments.

Epiglottectomy. Removal of the epiglottis.

Frenulum clipping. Surgically cutting a shortened frenulum to relieve "tongue tie."

Full mouth extraction. Removal of all of the patient's teeth.

Gastric transposition (pull-up) operation. Method for reconstructing the gullet usually after esophageal cancer surgery, by creating an end-to-end anastomosis of the hypopharynx and stomach.

Gingivectomy. The surgical removal of part of the gums.

Glossectomy, hemi or partial glossectomy. Removal of all or part of the tongue.

Hemilaryngectomy. Removal of one half of the structures of the larynx in the vertical plane; **vertical laryngectomy** is synonymous.

Hemimandibulectomy. Removal of up to half of the mandible.

Laryngectomy. Removal of the larynx, hyoid bone, and strap muscles along with creating a permanent tracheostomy and closing any communication between the trachea and the oropharynx.

Laryngofissure. Surgical incision to create a "wide window" with medial opening into the thyroid cartilage, usually done to remove a cancerous tumor.

Laryngostomy. Opening into the larynx.

Mandibulectomy. Removal of all or most of the mandible.

Near-total laryngectomy. An operation designed to ablate (remove) all of a laryngeal tumor but not all of the larynx. Most techniques leave a mucosal bridge over the uninvolved arytenoid, and the recurrent laryngeal nerve on the unaffected side of the larynx is spared. A primitive tracheopharyngeal sphincter with the laryngeal "leftovers" and a mucosal flap from the pharynx are techniques used to allow for a prosthesis-free method of speech and to prevent aspiration.

Nerve-muscle pedicle graft to the larynx. A technique for reinnervating a paralyzed larynx using the ansa hypoglossal nerve and the omohyoid muscle as a nerve-muscle pedicle.

Palatoplasty. Surgical repair of the palate, as in cleft palate surgeries.

Parotidectomy. Resection of the parotid gland.

Partial laryngectomy. Subtotal removal of the larynx.

Periapical tissue biopsy. Biopsy of tissue from the roots of the teeth to examine for a malignant process.

Pharyngectomy. Removal of pharyngeal tissue.

Phonosurgeries. Surgeries done for the purpose of improving phonation; include *thyroplasties; recurrent nerve resection; laser therapy* for plica ventricularis; and injection of bulking substances into the vocal folds (Teflon injection, lipoprotein [fat] injections, collagen injections).

Septectomy. Surgical correction of a deviated nasal septum.

Stoma revisions, Z-plasties of the stoma. Plastic surgical technique to reduce stoma scar tissue stenosis by releasing the circular tension on the stoma.

Stomatoplasty, stoma plasty. Plastic surgical repair of the mouth, or stoma.

Supraglottic laryngectomy. Removal of the endolaryngeal structures from the tip of the epiglottis down to the upper laryngeal structures without sacrificing the remaining larynx; **subtotal horizontal laryngectomy** is synonymous.

Thyroidectomy, partial thyroidectomy, hemi-thyroidectomy, parathyroidectomy, partial parathyroidectomy. Excision of all or part of the thyroid gland or parathyroid gland.

Thyroplasties, laryngeal framework surgeries. Referring to surgeries which involve creating a window in the ala of the thyroid between the inner and outer perichondrium on the side of a weakened vocal fold and implanting a Silastic wedge to medialize the fold for improved phonation.

Tracheoesophageal puncture (TEP) voice restoration. Creation of a fistula from the tracheal wall of the tracheostoma after laryngectomy into the esophagus for the purpose of fitting a tracheoesophageal puncture prosthesis for alaryngeal speech. This surgery may be performed as a part of the **primary procedure** (at the time of the laryngectomy) or may be a **secondary procedure**, performed sometime following the total laryngectomy.

Tracheostomy. Opening into the trachea. (See Figure 12–1).

Tracheotomy. Incision into the trachea.

Uvulopalatopharyngoplasty (UP). Either a laser-assisted (LAUP) or cold steel procedure to remove wedges of the uvular tissue bilaterally to improve or eliminate snoring.

Vocal fold fusion. Surgical technique closing the glottis to prevent severe aspiration. Patients require a tracheostomy following this surgery and an alaryngeal method for speech.

Voice restoration techniques. Surgeries designed to provide a phonation alternative following removal of all or most of the larynx. These surgeries may involve anatomical reconstructions without the use of mechanical aids or other prostheses or reconstructions performed to accommodate either implanted or removable prostheses. Reconstructive surgeries include construction of a *neoglottis* (such as the Staffieri technique), creating a *mucoarytenoid shunt* of the airway into the esophagus, creating a *pharyngo-esophageal mucosal flap,* creating a *reed-fistula* from the trachea to the hypopharynx, and creating a *tracheo-esophageal fistula* to insert a valved prosthesis (see tracheo-esophageal puncture voice restoration).

B. Neurosurgeries and Procedures

Aneurysm repair. Surgical clipping or ligation of an artery to correct an aneurysm (ballooning out of a weakened vessel wall). In some cases, vascular bypass may be performed to prevent ischemia distal to the affected vessel.

Brain resections. Removal of brain tissue to treat intractable epilepsy or to remove all or a portion of brain tumors.

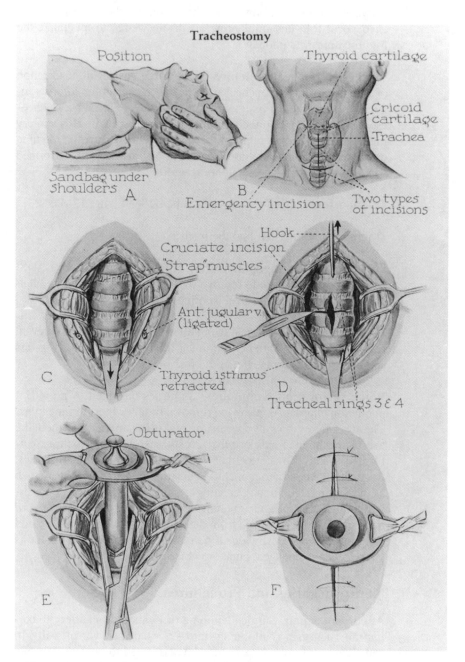

Figure 12–1. Tracheostomy (From Thorek, P. *Atlas of Surgical Techniques*. Philadelphia: J. B. Lippencott, Co., 1970; used with permission).

Cerebral artery bypass, enarterectomy, and anastomosis. Microvascular surgeries on the cerebral arteries to treat cerebrovascular disease.

Cervical fusion. Excision of one or more herniated cervical intervertebral disc(s) and placement of bone grafts to cause fusion of the discs.

Commissurotomy. Sectioning the anterior commissure or some part of the corpus callosum of the brain.

Cordotomy. Sectioning of the lateral pathways of the spinal cord to alleviate pain.

Cranioplasty. Replacement of an area of cranial bone with an autograft, metal prosthesis, or methylmethacrylate plate.

Craniotomy. Creating an opening into the skull to expose the brain or its coverings.

Evacuation of a hematoma (hemorrhage). Aspiration and drainage of a blood mass located in or causing pressure on the brain.

Laminectomy. Creating an opening into the lamina of the spinal cord, usually to repair a herniated disc.

Lobectomy. Resection of a large portion of the brain.

Neurorrhaphy. Peripheral nerve repair with anastomosis of a severed nerve.

Rhizotomy. Sectioning a nerve root. *Neurectomy* refers to removing a nerve segment.

Shunts. Diverting cerebrospinal fluid away from the ventricles to another location to correct or prevent hydrocephalus, such as with *ventriculo-atrial shunts* (in which a thin catheter with a valve to prevent reflux is tunneled under the scalp from a ventricle to an exit site through the common facial vein and reinserted percutaneously through the internal jugular vein to the superior vena cava) or *ventriculo-peritoneal shunts* (in which the shunt tube is placed into the peritoneal cavity for drainage).

Sympathectomy. Sectioning of a sympathetic nerve.

Thalamotomy. Removal of a part of the thalamus.

C. Cardiothoracic and Pulmonary (Chest) Surgeries and Procedures

Atrial septal defect correction. Surgical closure of a congenital anomaly which had allowed blood from the left atrium to flow across into the right atrium.

Balloon catheterization. Placement of a catheter having a distal, inflatable (helium-filled) balloon into a blood vessel or heart chamber.

Cardiac catheterization. Passage of a long, thin catheter, specially designed for passage through the blood vessels, into the heart chambers for examination and to take special samples of blood, blood pressure, and cardiac output measures.

Cardiopulmonary bypass. Temporary diversion of the blood from the heart and lungs to be able to perform surgery on the heart or major vessels.

Closure of a patent ductus arteriosus. Surgical closure of an unnatural communication between the pulmonary artery and the thoracic aorta.

Coronary artery bypass grafts. Surgery to improve blood flow to the heart which involves taking an autogenous vein graft (vein from elsewhere in the patient's body), such as the saphenous vein from the lower leg, and anastomosing one end of the grafted vein to the ascending aorta and the other end to one or more of the arteries supplying the heart.

Correction of a coarctation of the thoracic aorta. Surgical correction of a congenital stenosis of the thoracic aorta.

Insertion of chest tubes. Surgical insertion of drainage tubes into the pleural cavity to remove blood or air that has accumulated after a thoracotomy.

Lobectomy. Removal of a lobe of the lung.

Lung biopsy. Excision of a small piece of lung tissue for microscopic analysis to establish a diagnosis of lung disease.

Pacemaker insertion. Suturing electrodes (with external batteries) to the heart to correct bradycardia, heart block, or arrhythmias.

Percutaneous transluminal coronary angioplasty (PTCA). The use of catheterization guided by x-ray imaging to examine and repair coronary artery disease.

Pneumonectomy. Removal of a lung.

Resection of an aneurysm of the ascending aorta. Surgical removal of an aneurysm section in the ascending aorta which typically has caused the aorta valve to become incompetent.

Resection of an aneurysm of the descending thoracic aorta. Surgical removal of an aneurysm section from the descending aorta.

Sternotomy. Cutting through the sternum to gain access to the heart.

Thoracotomy. Surgical opening into the thoracic region.

Valve replacements. Surgical implantation of prosthetic valves in place of irreversibly damaged, stenosed heart valves (*aortic valve, mitral valve,* and *tricuspid valve*).

D. Orthopedic Surgeries and Procedures

Amputation. Surgical removal of a limb, most often necessitated by severe peripheral vascular insufficiency or malignancy.

Arthroplasty. Reconstructive surgery to a joint.

Arthroscopy. Direct visualization of a joint through a fiberoptic instrument.

Hand tendon surgeries. Surgical treatment of diseases affecting the hand tendons, such as tendon release surgery for *Dupuytren's contracture* (disease causing finger contractures) or surgery to release pressure on the median nerve of the wrist found with *carpal tunnel syndrome.*

Joint replacement surgeries. Surgical implantation of prosthetic joints (e.g., hip, knee, and shoulder joint replacement prostheses); Total Hip Arthroplasty (THA), Total Knee Arthroplasty (TKA).

E. Vascular and Lymph System Surgeries

Abdominal aortic aneurysm and aortic femoral bypass. The surgical removal of an abdominal aortic aneurysm and insertion of a bifurcated vessel prosthesis.

Carotid endarterectomy. Surgical removal of atherosclerotic plaque from an obstructed carotid artery.

Femoral-popliteal bypass. Surgical implantation of an artificial or autogenous (from elsewhere in the parent's body) vessel graft into the femoral and popliteal arteries.

Lymphadenectomy. Excision of lymph nodes.

Lymphadenotomy. Incision and drainage of a lymph gland.

Portacaval shunt. The surgical anastomosis of a portal vein of the liver to the vena cava to alleviate portal hypertension.

Portal shunt. Surgical method used to treat variceal hemorrhaging by diverting the blood of a hypertensive portal liver system into a normal systemic venous system.

Vein stripping. Surgical removal of the saphenous veins to alleviate severe varicose veins in the legs.

F. Gastrointestinal and Other Abdominal Surgeries and Procedures

Adrenalectomy. Removal of all or part of the adrenal gland(s).

Antrectomy. Removal of the gastrin-producing pyloric gland of the stomach.

Appendectomy. Removal of the appendix.

Brunschwig's operation. Removal of all of the pelvic organs in order to stop massive spread of cancer.

Celiotomy. Any surgery that opens the abdomen.

Cholecystectomy. Removal of the gall bladder.

Cholecystogastronomy. Surgically joining of the gall bladder to the stomach.

Choledocholithotomy. Removal of stones from the common bile duct leading from the gall bladder.

Colectomy. Removal of a section of the colon.

Colostomy. Surgical creation of an abdominal output (Stoma) from the colon, usually following a colectomy.

Diverticulectomy. Surgical correction of an outpouching, or diverticulum, of the esophagus (or intestines).

Esophageal myotomy. Surgical dissection of a portion of esophageal muscle.

Esophagectomy. Removal of all or part of the esophagus.

Esophagojejunostomy. Surgical joining of the esophagus and jejunum.

Fundic patch. Surgical repair of a ruptured esophagus or an acid-peptic stricture at the distal esophageal-stomach juncture.

Fundoplication. Surgical procedure to relieve gastroesophageal reflux and improve gastroesophageal competence.

Gastric resection. Removal of the majority of the stomach and joining the resected stomach to the duodenum (Billroth I procedure) or to the jejunum (Billroth II procedure).

Gastrostomy tube placement. Creation of an opening into the stomach for insertion of a permanent or temporary tube. *Operative gastrostomy* (OG) refers to procedures done under general anesthesia, usually by a general surgeon (see Figure 12–2). Gastrostomies performed by percutaneous methods, *percutaneous endoscopic gastrostomies* (PEGs), are usually done under local anesthesia by surgeons or a gastroenterologist. Complications associated with gastrostomies include wound infections, gastric wall hematoma, gastrocolic fistula, and benign pneumoperitoneum (air entering the lining of the body cavity).

Hemorrhoidectomy. Removal of hemorrhoids.

Hepatic lobectomy. Removal of a lobe of the liver.

Hiatus (hiatal) hernia repair. Surgical procedures to correct a defect which permitted the esophagus to pass through the diaphragm.

Ileostomy. Creating an opening into the ileum.

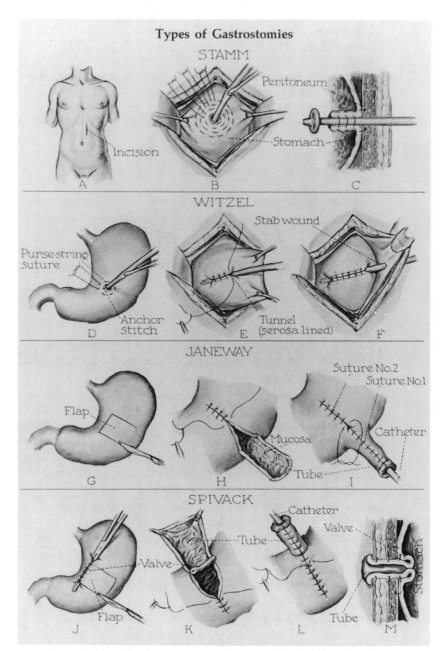

Figure 12–2. Gastrostomy (From Thorek, P. *Atlas of Surgical Techniques.* Philadelphia: J. B. Lippincott, Co., 1970; used with permission)

Imperforate anus repair. Surgical creation of an anal opening when one has failed to develop.

Inguinal hernia repair. Surgical correction of a tear or defect in the abdominal wall in the groin area of a male which had allowed abdominal contents to protrude.

Jejunostomy. Creating an opening into the jejunum.

Jejunostomy tube placement. Procedure for placing an enteral feeding tube into the jejunum. A percutaneous endoscopic jejunostomy placement is similar to a PEG (see above), except that a dual-lumen tube is used. The distal tip of the feeding tube is directed into the duodenum endoscopically, with the proximal port left to decompress the stomach.

Pancreatectomy. Removal of part or all of the pancreas. The *Whipple procedure*, or pancreaticojejunostomy, refers to a large surgical resection of the pancreas as well as the duodenum, part of the stomach, and bile duct.

Percutaneous endoscopic gastrostomy (PEG). See Gastrostomy.

Pharyngostomy and esophagostomy tube placement. Procedures performed under general or local anesthesia to place an enteral feeding tube in the pharynx or esophagus.

Proctoplasty. Removal and reconstruction of the rectum.

Resection of esophageal stricture. Removal of a narrowed portion of the esophagus followed by a colonic bypass anastomosis.

Sialadenectomy. Removal of a salivary gland.

Sialolithotomy. Removal of a salivary stone.

Thymectomy. Removal of all or part of the thymus gland(s).

Vagotomy. Denervation of the vagal nerve branch to the stomach to eliminate excessive stimulation of acid production to treat chronic gastric or duodenal ulcers.

G. Urogenital Surgeries and Procedures

Adenectomy. Removal of the glands of the uterus, tubes, and ovaries.

Circumcision. Removal of a part of the prepuce to expose the glans penis.

Cystectomy. Removal of part or all of the bladder.

Cystoplasty. Surgical repair of the bladder.

Hysterectomy. Removal of the uterus.

Nephrectomy. Excision of one or both kidneys.

Nephrotomy. Incision into a kidney.

Orchiectomy. Removal of the testes.

Orchioplasty. Surgical repair of the testes.

Pyeloplasty. Surgical repair of the renal pelvis.

Renal transplantation. Removal of irreversibly diseased kidneys and replacement with a donor kidney from a tissue-matched living donor or cadaver organ donor.

Transurethral resection of the bladder (TURB). Endoscopic resection of the bladder to remove nonelastic tissues causing poor bladder control.

Transurethral resection of the prostate (TURP). Endoscopic resection of some portion of a hypertrophic prostate gland (in males).

Tubal ligation. Sectioning and ligating the uteral tubes.

Ureteral resection. Excision of a ureteral lesion.

Ureterectomy. Removal of the ureter.

Vasectomy. Removal and ligation of the vas deferens.

H. Plastic, Aesthetic, Reconstructive, and Other Eye, Ear, and Nose Surgeries and Procedures

Blepharoplasty. Surgical repair of the eyelid, usually to remove redundant tissue.

Blephrectomy. Excision of an eyelid.

Cataract surgery. Removal of an opaque lens.

Corneal surgery. Surgical repair of cornea defects *Cornea transplant* surgery involves replacing a full thickness cornea with a donor graft.

Dacryocystectomy. Removal of a lacrimal gland.

Ectropion repair. Plastic surgical repair of a sagging lower eyelid.

Enucleation. Removal of an eye.

Evisceration of the eye. Removal of the contents of an eye.

Functional endoscopic sinus surgery (FESS). Surgery using endoscopic instruments to correct nasal sinus abnormalities.

Labyrinthectomy. Destruction of the labyrinth of the inner ear to treat intractable vertigo.

Mammoplasty. Plastic surgery to breast, usually to improve the appearance.

Mastoidectomy. Removal of diseased mastoid tissue.

Myringoplasty. Surgical repair of the tympanic membrane with a graft.

Myringotomy. Opening into the tympanic membrane, usually as a result of surgery.

Otoplasty. Surgical repair of a deformed pinna.

Ptosis correction. Plastic surgical correction of a drooping eyelid, often caused by weakness of the levator palpebrae muscle.

Reduction mammoplasty. Plastic surgery to reduce the size of the breasts.

Rhinoplasty. Reconstruction of the nose.

Rhytidectomy. Plastic surgery to remove wrinkles.

Stapedectomy. Removal of the stapes, usually followed by prosthetic repairs (TORP, PORP).

Tarsorrhaphy. Surgical closure of an eyelid.

IV. SURGICAL INSTRUMENTS

A variety of instruments are used in head and neck surgery, neurosurgery, cardiothoracic and pulmonary, orthopedic, vascular and lymph systems, gastrointestinal and abdominal, urogenital, and plastic reconstructive surgeries. Figure 12–3 illustrates a few of the more common types of surgical instruments.

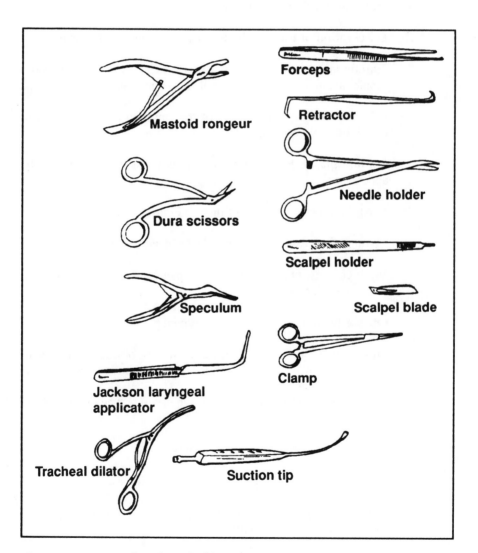

Figure 12–3. Examples of surgical instruments

V. NOTES

VI. REFERENCES

Bailey, B. J., & Biller, H. F. (1985). *Surgery of the larynx.* Philadelphia: W. B. Saunders.

Casper, J. K., & Colton, R. H. (1993). *Clinical manual for laryngectomy and head/neck cancer rehabilitation.* San Diego: Singular Publishing Group.

Friedman, M. (Ed.). (1986). Nonsquamous tumors of the head and neck: I. *The Otolaryngologic Clinics of North America* (Vol. 19). Philadelphia: W. B. Saunders.

Fuller, J. R. (1981). *Surgical technology: Principles and practices.* Philadelphia: W. B. Saunders.

Keith, R. L., & Darley, F. L. (Eds.). (1986). *Laryngectomee rehabilitation* (2nd ed.). San Diego, CA: College-Hill Press.

Lucente, F. E., & Sobol, S. M. (1983). *Essentials of otolaryngology.* New York: Raven Press.

Schedd, D. P., & Weinberg, B. (Eds.). (1980). *Surgical and prosthetic approaches to speech rehabilitation.* Boston: G. K. Hall.

Shapshay, S. M., & Ossoff, R. H. (Eds.). (1985). Squamous cell cancer of the head and neck. *The Otolaryngologic Clinics of North America* (Vol. 18). Philadelphia: W. B. Saunders.

Thorek, P. (1970). *Atlas of surgical techniques.* Philadelphia: J. B. Lippincott.

Wind, G. G., & Rich, N. M. (1987). *Principles of surgical technique* (2nd ed.). Silver Spring, MD: Urban & Swartzenberg.

APPENDIX

A

Anatomical Figures

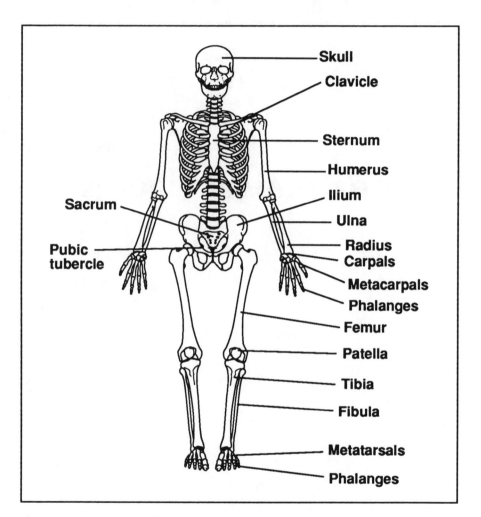

Figure A-1. Human skeleton: Anterior view

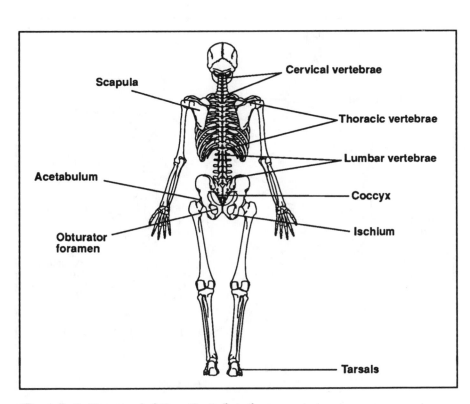

Figure A–2. Human skeleton: Posterior view

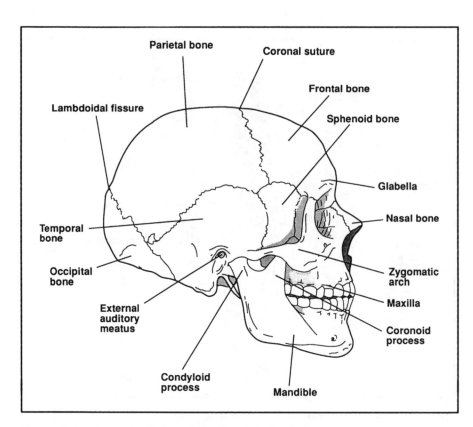

Figure A-3. Bony structures of the head: Lateral view

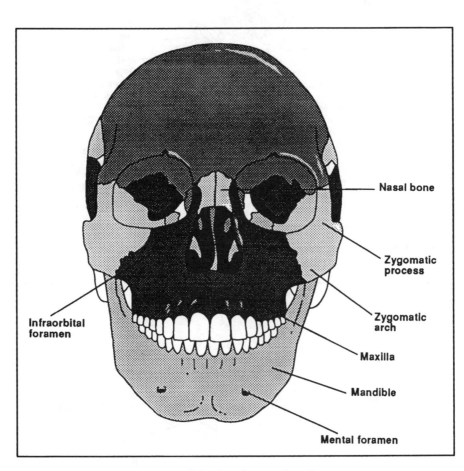

Figure A-4. Bony structures of the head: Anterior view

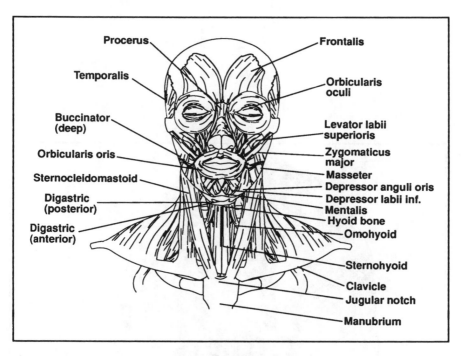

Figure A-5. Head and neck muscles and structures

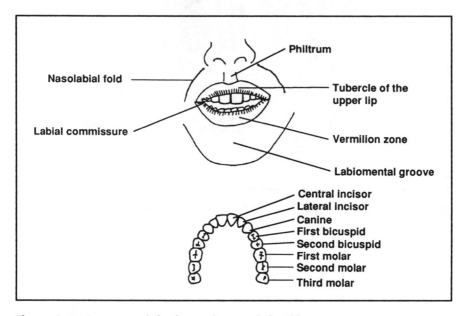

Figure A-6. Anatomy of the lower face and dentition

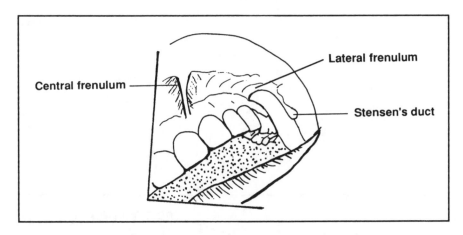

Figure A-7. Anatomy of the upper buccal space

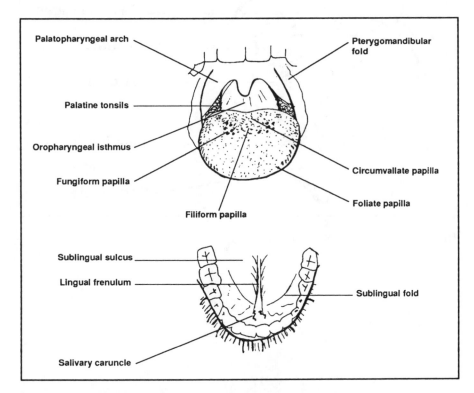

Figure A-8. Anatomy of the oral cavity, tongue, and floor of the mouth

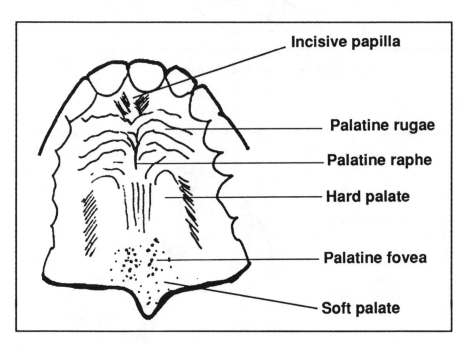

Figure A-9. Anatomy of the palate

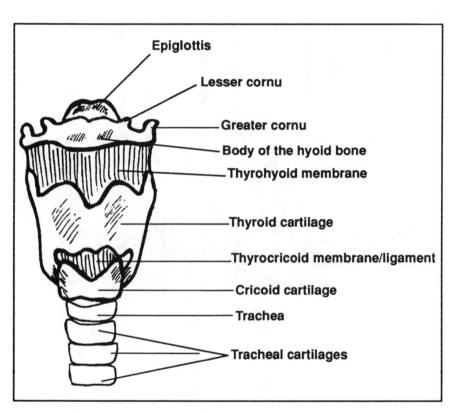

Epiglottis

Lesser cornu

Greater cornu

Body of the hyoid bone

Thyrohyoid membrane

Thyroid cartilage

Thyrocricoid membrane/ligament

Cricoid cartilage

Trachea

Tracheal cartilages

Figure A-10. External laryngeal anatomy

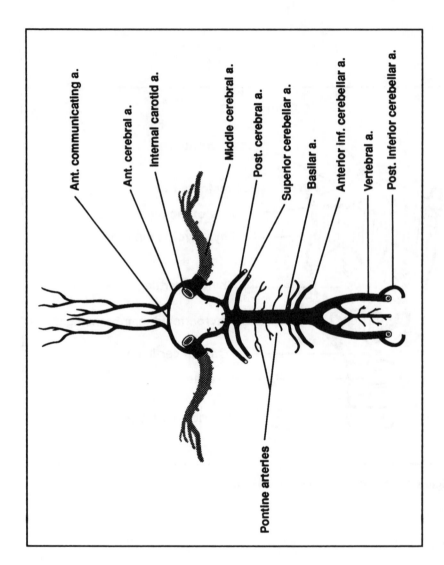

Ant. communicating a.

Ant. cerebral a.

Internal carotid a.

Middle cerebral a.

Post. cerebral a.

Superior cerebellar a.

Basilar a.

Anterior Inf. cerebellar a.

Vertebral a.

Post. Inferior cerebellar a.

Pontine arteries

Figure A–11. Circle of Willis

APPENDIX

B

Terminology and Abbreviations Used in Rehabilitation Medicine

Additional terminology related to rehabilitation medicine is found in Chapters 3, 4, 7, 9, and 12.

I. TERMINOLOGY

Abducted gait. Swinging the leg through a step in an abducted position.

Active. Motion performed with voluntary muscle action.

Active-assisted. Movements using voluntary muscles with gravity effects removed by assistance from another person, device, or from an unaffected limb.

Acupressure. The application of pressure to acupuncture sites.

Adaptive equipment. Devices that support or compensate for an impaired function.

Ambulation. Walking.

Amputation. Removal, usually by surgery, of a body extremity or protrusion.

Amputee chair. Wheelchair with rear wheels set back to compensate for a change in the user's center of gravity.

Ankylosing spondylitis. A group of nonspecific, chronic inflammatory spondyloarthropathies which include Reiter's syndrome, psoriatic arthritis, and other spondyloarthropathies. Patients with ankylosing spondylitis complain of stiff necks and back pain and have radiographic evidence of large cartilaginous and small synovial joints of the axial skeleton.

Anti-tips. A right-angled extension to the tipping lever on a wheelchair which prevents backward tipping of the chair.

Cardiac rehabilitation. Multi-staged (Phase I, II, III, and IV) cardiac fitness programs usually prescribed for post MI or bypass surgery patients.

Cervical orthoses. Various types of cervical braces or collars used for the purpose of treating pain and instability after cervical injury or dysfunction. Types of cervical orthoses include *Halo vests, head-cervical thoracic orthoses* (HCTOs), *sternal-occipital-mandibular immobilizers* (SOMIs), and *skull cervical thoracic lumbar-pelvic orthoses* (SCTLOs).

Complex lymphedema massage therapy. Treatment for edematous swelling (usually after mastectomy or other surgery) using massage and pneumatic pumps.

Conditioning. Referring to exercises or activities that improve fitness.

Cryokinetics. Referring to cold pack (iced) massage.

Decubitus ulcers. Pressure sores caused by a combination of several factors including pressure on a body part, shearing (rubbing) forces, malnutrition, edema, sensory loss, weakness, sepsis, maceration, and inactivity.

Degenerative joint disease (DJD). A noninflammatory disease of the joints characterized by the degeneration of articular hyaline cartilage and secondary hypertrophy of a subchondral and marginal bone.

Diathermy. Therapeutic deep-heating modality of treatment using high-frequency electromagnetic radiation.

Effleurage. Superficial or deep massaging motions.

Facilitation. Stimulation to increase muscle tone.

Foot drop. Foot posturing lacking dorsiflexion.

Footplate. Metal support for the foot attached to a wheelchair.

Footrest. Part on a wheelchair which supports only the feet, without calf support.

Forward stabilizers. An attachment to the front of a wheelchair which prevents forward tipping.

Friction. Deep circular massaging motions.

Functional ratings. Functional status for mobility, activities of daily living, speech, transportation, and so forth are often rated with the following qualifiers: *independent* (no assistance from others is required), *with supervision* (stating how much and in what manner), *with assistance* (stating what manner), and *dependent*.

One copyrighted system for formal ratings of functional status that is commonly used in inpatient rehabilitation programs is the **Functional Independence Measure** (FIM). This assessment methodology was developed by the State University of New York's Department of Rehabilitation Medicine as a method for rating functional outcomes in rehabilitation and contributing that information to a "Uniform Data Set for Medical Rehabilitation." Eighteen functional status variables are rated by seven qualifiers from "complete independence" (7) to "total assistance" (1) (Research Foundation, SUNY, 1990). An adjunctive system suggested for head injured patients, which adds ratings for parameters related to cognitive, behavioral, communication, and community functioning, is the Functional Assessment Measure (FAM) (Hall, 1993).

Genu recurvatum. Hyperextension of the knee on the weight-bearing, or stance, leg.

Gluteus maximus gait. Backward lurching of the trunk producing lordosis and shortened step.

Grip strength. Measurement in weight (pounds or kilograms) of the patient's grasp strength; grip strength is measured by a **goniometer**.

Hubbard tank. Tank with a mechanical lift and whirlpool used as a form of hydrotherapy to treat open wounds (such as burns), pressure sores, rheumatoid arthritis, tendon surgery and joint replacement surgeries, and fractures.

Inhibition. Stimulation to reduce muscle tone.

Jobst stocking. Type of compression stocking worn to reduce leg edema.

Local cooling. Cold packs or immersion therapy to reduce spasticity.

Lower extremity orthoses. Brace or splint supports to parts of the lower extremity, including *above the knee orthoses* (AKOs), *ankle-foot orthoses* (AFOs), *knee-ankle-foot orthoses* (KAFOs), and *hip-KAFOs.*

Mobilization. Referring to the use of passive movements to regain fluidity and range of movement between joint parts.

Neurogenic bladder or bowel. Inhibition of the reflex for urinary or fecal voiding due to a disturbance in neurologic control of the bladder or bowel. The forms of neurogenic bladder and bowel disorders include *uninhibited neurogenic, sensory paralytic, motor paralytic, reflex neurogenic,* and *autonomous neurogenic.*

One-arm drive. Wheelchair with both hand rails on the same side of a chair with each controlling a different wheel; used with patients who have only one functional upper extremity.

Orthoses. Braces or splints; devices which support dysfunctional body parts.

Paraffin bath. Tub of very warm (melted) paraffin used for emersion of the hands for relief of painful joints and to improve joint mobility.

Passive. Referring to movements assisted by another person or with assistance from the functional extremity.

Percussion. Repeated tapping motions.

Petrissage. Compression or kneading massage motions.

Phantom pain. A sensation of pain coming from a missing part following an amputation.

Plinth. Padded table, or platform, upon which the patient performs therapeutic exercises.

Pneumatic lymphedema device. Pump "sleeves" or "stockings" which apply pressure on extremities that are lymphedematous.

Prone cart. Self-propelled stretcher.

Prosthesis. An artificial body part.

P.U.L.S.E.S. Acronym for a profile for evaluating independence in self-care and mobility where **P** refers to physical condition; **U** refers to upper limb functions (such as dressing, grooming, etc.); **L** refers to lower extremity functions (walking, transferring, etc.); **S** refers to sensory components (speech, hearing, and vision); **E** refers to excretory functions; and **S** refers to support from the caregivers (intellectual, emotional, financial).

Short opponens orthosis. Hand-wrist brace which maintains the thumb in opposition with the index and middle finger.

Sjögren's syndrome. A syndrome found in postmenapausal women thought to be a form of a collagen disease, characterized by rheumatoid arthritis, xerostomia, and keratoconjunctivitis sicca.

Spinal orthoses. Spinal support braces, including *trochanteric belts, sacroiliac orthoses* (SIOs), *thoracic-lumbro-sacral orthoses* (TLSOs), and *lumbosacral orthoses* (LSOs).

Stance phase, Trendelenburg sign. Abnormal angle or drop of the pelvis contralateral to affected limb, noted by observing the gluteral fold. When standing on the affected limb, the gluteral fold of the unaffected side will fall instead of rise when the unaffected leg swings forward through a step. A positive Trendelenburg sign will be seen in poliomyelitis, fractures of the femoral neck, and congenital dislocations.

Syme's amputation. Removal of the foot, sparing the heel.

Tapotement. Clapping-type percussion motions made with a cupped hand.

Transportation. Moving from one place to another.

Vibratory. Referring to the use of a vibratory mechanical device in massage or to promote bronchial drainage.

II. ABBREVIATIONS

Abd. Abduction

Add. Adduction

ADL. Activities of daily living

AFO. Ankle foot orthosis

AKO. Above the knee orthosis

AROM. Assisted range of motion

B & B. Bowel and bladder

BFO. Balanced-frame orthosis

BoS. Base of support

CoG. Center of gravity

CTS. Carpal tunnel syndrome

F. Fair

FES. Functional electrical stimulation

F.I.M. Functional Index Measure

G. Good

KD . Knee disarticulation

LE. Lower extremity

Left hemi. Left hemiparesis/plegia

MHB. Maximal hospital benefits

N. Normal

NDT. Neurodevelopmental Therapy

P. Poor

PNF. Proprioceptive neuromuscular facilitation

PREs. Progressive resistive exercises

PROM. Passive range of motion

PULSES. Physical, upper extremity, lower extremity, sensory, excretory, support

Right hemi. Right hemiparesis/plegia

ROM. Range of motion

ROM (p). Range of motion (passive)

St. c. Standard cane

T. Trace

TENS. Transcutaneous electrical nerve stimulation

UE. Upper extremity

WFL. Within functional limits

WNL. Within normal limits

WO. Wrist orthosis

APPENDIX

C

Selected Normal Laboratory Values and Ranges

The values in this appendix are adapted from Gomella (1989, 1993), Kenner (1992), Rothstein, Roy, and Wolf (1991), and Thomas (1985).

I. NORMAL VALUES

Ranges for "normal" laboratory **values will vary slightly between laboratories;** and for some values, expected **levels for normal will differ between men and women and children and adults.** Other factors also affect acceptable ranges for normal values, including diet, nutrition and hydration status, medications, activity level, and medical status. Some of the ranges for normal values likely to appear in medical records of adults are listed below. Most of these values are referenced in units from the *Systeme International d'Unites (SI)*. The SI units for reporting laboratory values are generally preferred. Most medical dictionaries contain a complete list of laboratory norms with equivalent units for both *conventional* and *SI* values, and laboratory parameters and reference groups that are not included in this list.

II. NORMAL ADULT LAB VALUES

A. Blood Counts and Chemistry

Albumin (Alb). 3.0–5.0 g/dL

Alkaline phosphatase (Ark. Pho). 50–136 U/L

Amylase. 44–128 U/L

Bicarbonate (HCO_3). 24–30 mmol/L

Calcium (Ca). 8.5–10.5 mg/dL

Chloride (Cl). 100–106 mmol/L

Creatine Phosphokinase (CPK). 3–350 U/L

Creatinine. 0.6–1.5 mg/dL

Glucose. 70–110 mg/dL (fasting)

Iron (Fe). 35–142 µg/dL

LDH. 300–650 U/L

Lipase. 40–210 U/L

Lipids. *Cholesterol* < 200 mg/dL; *HDL* 35–50 mg/dL; *LDL* < 159 mg/dL; *Triglycerides* 35–200 mg/dL

Phosphate (PO_4). 2–4 mg/dL

Potassium (K). 3.4–5.3 mmol/L

Prealbumin (PAB). 17–42 mg/dL (well-nourished)

Protein (total). 6.0–8.4 g/dL

Magnesium (Mg). 1.4–2.4 mg/dL

Sodium (Na). 135–145 mmol/L

Transaminase (AST, SGOT). 0–50 U/L

Urea nitrogen (BUN). 5–25 mg/dL

B. Blood Gases

HCO$_3$. –23 to –25 mmol/L

Oxygen saturation (arterial) (O$_2$ sat.). 96–100%

Partial pressure of arterial carbon dioxide (PaCO$_2$). 35–45 mm Hg

Partial pressure of arterial oxygen (PaO$_2$). 75-100 mm Hg when breathing room air (dependent upon age)

pH. 7.35–7.45

C. Urinalysis

Bacteria. None; negative

Calcium (Ca). 100–250 mg/24 hrs

Chloride (Cl). 110–250 mmol/24 hrs

Creatinine. 15–25 mg/kg of body weight/24 hrs

Creatinine clearance. 140–180 liters/24 hrs

Glucose. None; negative

Potassium (K). 40–80 mmol/24 hrs

Protein. Less than 150 mg/24 hrs

Sodium (Na). 130-200 mmol/24 hrs

D. Hematologic Values

Differential cells. Segmenteds 41–71%; eosinophils 1–3%; basophils 0–1%; lymphocytes 24–44%; monocytes 3–7%; and stab neutrophils 5–10%

Erythrocytes (RBC). 4.2-5.9 million/mm^3

Mean corpuscular hemoglobin (MCH) 27–32 pg

Mean corpuscular volume (MCV) 80–94 μm^3

Mean corpuscular hemoglobin concentration (MCHC) 33–37 g/dL

Erythrocyte sedimentation rate. Male: 1–13 mm/h; Females: 1–20 mm/h

Hematocrit (HCT). 45–52% (males); 37–48% (females)

Hemoglobin (HgB). 13–19 g/dL (males); 12–16 g/dL (females)

Leukocytes (WBC). 4,300–10,800/mm^3

Platelets. 150,000–350,000/mm^3

E. Cerebrospinal Fluid Analysis

Bacteria. None; negative

Cell count. 0–5 mononuclear cells (lymphs)

Glucose. 45–100 mg/dL

Pressure (initial). 70–180 mm of water

Protein. 15–45 mg/dL

III. NORMAL LAB VALUES FOR NEONATES

A. Blood Chemistry

Bicarbonate (HCO$_3$). 18–23 mmol/L

Calcium (Ca). 7–10 mg/dL

Carbon dioxide (CO$_2$). 15–25 mmol/L

Chloride (Cl). 90–114 mmol/L

Glucose. 40–80 mg/dL

Potassium (K). 4–6 mmol/L

Protein. 4–7 g/dL

Sodium (Na). 135–148 mmol/L

B. Hematologic Values

Differential cells. Segmenteds 9,400/mm^3 (52%); eosinophils 400/mm^3 (2.2%); basophils 100/mm^3 (.6%); lymphocytes 5,500/mm^3 (31%); monocytes 1,500/mm^3 (5.8%); and stab neutrophils 1,600/mm^3 (9%)

Hematocrit (HCT). 51–56%

Hemoglobin (HgB). 16.5 g/dL (cord blood)

Platelets. 1,500,000 to 4,000,000/mm^3

White cells total. 18,000/mm^3

GENERAL TEXT
AND APPENDIX
REFERENCES

Andreoli, T. A., Carpenter, C. J., Plum, F., & Smith, L. H. (1990). *Cecil essentials of medicine* (2nd ed.). Philadelphia: W. B. Saunders.

Boggs, R. L., & Wooldridge-King, M. (1993). *AACN procedure manual for critical care* (3rd ed.). Philadelphia: W. B. Saunders.

Chabner, D. -E. (1991). *The language of medicine* (4th Ed.). Philadelphia: W. B. Saunders.

D'Angelo, H. H., & Welsh, N. P. (1988). *The signs and symptoms handbook.* Springhouse, PA: Springhouse Corp.

DeGowin, E. L., & DeGowin, R. L. (1987). *Bedside diagnostic examination* (4th ed.). New York: Macmillan.

Detmer, W. M., McPhee, S. J., Nicoll, D., & Chou, T. M. (1992). *Pocket guide to diagnostic tests.* Norwalk, CT: Appleton-Lange.

Dorland's illustrated medical dictionary (27th ed.). (1988). Philadelphia: W. B. Saunders.

Firkin, B. G., & Whitworth, J. A. (1987). *Dictionary of medical eponyms.* Trenton, NJ: The Parthenon Publishing Group.

Frenay, S. A. C. (1977). *Understanding medical terminology.* St. Louis, MO: The Catholic Hospital Association.

Garb, S., Krakauer, E., & Justice, C. (1987). *Abbreviations and acronyms in medicine and nursing.* New York: Springer.

Geigy Pharmaceuticals. (1977). *The medical and health sciences word book.* Boston: Houghton-Mifflin.

Gomella, L. G. (Ed.). (1989). *Clinician's pocket handbook* (6th ed.). East Norwalk, CT: Appleton & Lange.

Gomella, L. G. (Ed.). (1993). *Clinician's pocket reference* (7th ed.). Norwalk, CT: Appleton & Lange.

Gomez, G. E., Hord, E. V., & Gettrust, K. V. (1988). *Fundamentals of clinical nursing skills.* New York: John Wiley.

Hall, K. M., Hamilton, B., Gordan, W. B., & Zafler, M. D. (1993). Characteristics and comparisons of functional assessment indices: Disability Rating Scale, Functional Independence Measure, and Functional Assessment Measure. *Journal of Head Trauma Rehabilitation, 8*(12), 60–74.

Hyde, L. (1988). *McGraw-Hill essential dictionary of health care.* New York: McGraw-Hill.

Kelly, W. J. (Ed.). (1992). *Clinical skillbuilders: Better documentation.* Springhouse, PA: Springhouse Publishers.

Kenner, C. A. (1992). *Nurse's clinical guide: Neonatal care.* Springhouse, PA: Springhouse Corp.

Melanakos, K. (1990). *Saunders pocket reference for nurses.* Philadelphia: W. B. Saunders.

Melloni, B. J., & Eisner, G. M. (1985). *Melloni's illustrated medical dictionary* (2nd ed.). Baltimore: Williams & Wilkins.

Nicolosi, L., Harryman, E., & Kresheck, J. (1983). *Terminology of communication disorders* (2nd ed.). Baltimore: Williams & Wilkins.

Research Foundation, SUNY. (1991). *Functional Independence Measure.* Buffalo, NY: Uniform Data Management Service, SUNY.

Rice, J. (1990). *Medical terminology* (2nd ed.). East Norwalk, CT: Appleton & Lange.

Rothstein, J. M., Roy, S. H., & Wolf, S. L. (1991). *The rehabilitation specialist's handbook.* Philadelphia: F. A. Davis.

Saxton, D., Nugent, P. M., & Pelikan, P. K. (1987). *Mosby's comprehensive review of nursing* (12th ed.). St. Louis, MO: C. V. Mosby.

Thomas, C. L. (Ed.). (1985). *Taber's cyclopedic medical dictionary* (15th ed.). Philadelphia: F. A. Davis.

INDEX